Master the Boards
USMLE®

Step 3

Sixth Edition

Other USMLE Titles by Conrad Fischer

Master the Boards USMLE® Step 2 CK

Other USMLE Titles from Kaplan Medical

USMLE Step 3 Lecture Notes

Dr. Pestana's Surgery Notes

Master the Boards
USMLE®

Step 3

Sixth Edition

Conrad Fischer, MD

© 2020 by Conrad Fischer, MD
Images courtesy of Conrad Fischer, MD, unless otherwise noted

Published by Kaplan Publishing, a division of Kaplan, Inc.
750 Third Avenue
New York, NY 10017

10 9 8 7 6 5 4 3 2 1

ISBN: 978-1-5062-5445-6

Kaplan Publishing books are available at special quantity discounts to use for sales promotions, employee premiums, or educational purposes. For more information or to purchase books, please call the Simon & Schuster special sales department at 866-506-1949.

For Test Changes or Late-Breaking Developments

kaptest.com/publishing

The material in this book is up-to-date at the time of publication. However, the Federation of State Medical Boards (FSMB) and the National Board of Medical Examiners (NBME) may have instituted changes in the test after this book was published. Be sure to carefully read the materials you receive when you register for the test. If there are any important late-breaking developments—or any changes or corrections to the Kaplan test preparation materials in this book—we will post that information online at *kaptest.com/publishing*.

Table of Contents

**Additional resources available at
kaptest.com/usmlebookresources**

About the Authors

Conrad Fischer, MD, is vice chairman of Medicine and director of the Internal Medicine residency program at Brookdale University Hospital and Medical Center and professor of medicine at Touro College of Medicine in New York City. He teaches USMLE Steps 1, 2, and 3, Internal Medicine Board Review and Attending Recertification, and USMLE Step 1 Physiology.

Niket Sonpal, MD, FACP (Surgery, Pediatrics, and Psychiatry sections) is associate program director of the internal medicine residency at Brookdale Hospital Medical Center in Brooklyn and assistant professor at Touro College of Medicine in New York City. He is a fellow of the American College of Physicians and co-author of the best-selling books *Master the Boards: USMLE Step 2 CK* and *Master the Boards: USMLE Step 3*. Dr. Sonpal teaches all three steps of USMLE, COMLEX, and American Board of Internal Medicine review.

Victoria Hastings, DO, MPH, MS (Obstetrics and Gynecology sections) is a resident physician in obstetrics and gynecology at New York Presbyterian Brooklyn Methodist Hospital. She received her master of public health degree in biostatistics and epidemiology from Saint Louis University and her doctorate in osteopathic medicine with a master of science from NYIT College of Medicine. She is section editor of the obstetrics and gynecology chapters in *Master the Boards: USMLE® Step 2 CK* and *Master the Boards: USMLE Step 3*. She teaches obstetrics, gynecology, and biostatistics for USMLE Steps 1, 2, and 3.

Previous contributions by Elizabeth August, MD, and Sonia Reichert, MD.

Peer Reviewers/Section Editors

Pharmacology: Ed El Sayed

Cardiology: Yury Malyshev, Gautham Uppadya

Infectious Disease: Richard Cofsky

Endocrinology: Chris Paras

Pulmonology: Sonu Sahni

Rheumatology: Marium Khan

Hematology: Hamza Minhas

Gastroenterology: Niket Sonpal

Neurology: Volodymyr Vulkanov

Nephrology: Samuel Spitalewitz

Oncology: Hamza Minhas

Preventive Medicine: Herman Lebovitch

Surgery: Ravi Kothuru

Psychiatry: Jason Hershberger

Acknowledgments

This book represents the consolidation of 25 years in the classroom teaching Step 3. You can be fully confident that you have—in one volume—**everything** you need to do well on Step 3.

The authors wish to recognize the excellent support of David Rose, MD, Chair of Medicine at Brookdale, and the administrative and emotional support of Ms. Juliette Akal.

Conrad Fischer wishes to dedicate this book to Edmund Bourke, MD as my "Fearless Leader," teacher, and protector these many years. You represent the best compilation of a "Gentleman Scholar," lifelong student, and teacher. A wise counselor and loyal friend. You are a "man for all seasons" whose kindness spills over onto all who are in contact with you. "Oh, for a muse of fire!"

Niket Sonpal wishes to acknowledge his mother and father, without whose support and sacrifice I would not be where I am today.

Victoria Hastings wishes to acknowledge her husband, who lifts me up and pushes me to achieve great things.

Introduction

About the Step 3 Exam

The USMLE© Step 3 exam is the last in a series of 3 USMLE examinations that all physicians applying for a license to practice medicine in the United States are required to pass. After successfully completing the 3 steps of the USMLE, a physician is eligible to practice medicine in an independent, unsupervised setting (some period of U.S. postgraduate training is also required).

This test is not merely a more advanced and detailed version of the Step 2 CK or CS exams. Understanding this concept is key to this challenging exam. Step 3 tests whether a physician not only can assimilate data and diagnose clinical conditions but also has acquired the ability to make clinical decisions about patient management in a way that ensures appropriate management in an unsupervised setting. In addition, Step 3 will test your understanding of basic science correlations.

How can the Step 3 test all first-year interns if they are working in such varied subspecialty settings? The same concepts that medicine house-officers learn about managing a diabetic with heart failure can be equally applied to the postsurgical patient with heart failure.

How Is Step 3 Different?

Unlike the Step 2 exams, which emphasize diagnosis of medical conditions, Step 3 evaluates your ability to evaluate the severity of a patient's condition and discern the most appropriate clinical management based on the presenting scenario. This assessment of your *clinical judgment* distinguishes Step 3 from Step 2. In Step 3, you are required to think beyond the diagnosis (which is often implicit in the question itself) and make decisions in management. The cases presented will include options that may all appear appropriate; however, for the presented situation, there is only ever one correct answer. Your interpretation of laboratory data, imaging, and elements of the presenting history and physical examination will assist you in selecting the correct management.

Clinical Encounter Frames

Multiple-choice and case-simulation questions are presented in one of three *clinical encounter frames:* initial care, continuing care, and urgent care. The encounter frame determines the amount of history, as well as clinical and laboratory test results, that are available to you. More importantly, the encounter frame influences how you'll proceed with management. For example, a long-standing patient with a history of repeated hospitalizations for asthma who presents with shortness of breath would be approached differently than if she were presenting for the first time to a clinic complaining of periodic dyspnea or if she presented to the emergency department with an acute asthma attack. The majority of test items (50 to 60 percent) in Step 3 involve the management of continuing-care patients. In the continuing-care setting, you are tested on your ability to recognize new problems in an existing condition, assess severity, establish prognosis, monitor therapy, and perform long-term management.

Clinical Settings

There are 3 clinical settings in Step 3: office/health center, inpatient facility, and the emergency department. As with the encounter frame, knowing the clinical setting influences your management decisions. As will be discussed in the "Examination Structure" section, test questions will be arranged in blocks based on one of the three clinical settings.

Physician Tasks

For any given clinical encounter frame in a clinical setting, you'll be challenged with a finite number of skills. The 6 physician tasks that are tested on the Step 3 exam are representative of what all physicians practicing unsupervised medical management are expected to know.

Task	Tests your ability to...
Obtaining a history and performing a physical examination	• identify key facets of the history or physical exam and relate them to the presenting problem or condition. • predict the most likely additional physical finding or examination technique that would result in the finding.
Using laboratory and diagnostic studies	• select the appropriate *routine* or *initial* lab or diagnostic test either to ensure effective therapy or to establish diagnosis. • predict the most likely lab or diagnostic test result.
Formulating the most likely diagnosis	• determine the diagnosis and use it to manage the patient.
Evaluating the severity of the patient's problems	• assess the severity of a patient's condition and identify indications for consultations or further diagnostic workup. • recognize factors in history, physical exam, or lab studies that affect prognosis or determine a change in therapy.
Managing the patient	• manage a patient in the following 4 areas: 1. Health maintenance (i.e., implementing preventative measures by identifying risk factors) 2. Clinical intervention (i.e., knowing appropriate postsurgical/ postprocedural management and follow-up measures) 3. Clinical therapeutics (i.e., properly utilizing pharmacotherapeutic options) 4. Legal/ethical and health care system issues, including patient autonomy, physician-patient relationships, and managed-care protocols
Applying scientific concepts	• identify processes responsible for an underlying condition and interpret results of clinical or epidemiologic experiments

Step 3 Examination Structure

The USMLE Step 3 is a 2-day computerized examination. The first day and a half tests your knowledge with a total of 412 traditional multiple-choice questions, which are arranged in blocks organized by one of the 3 clinical settings. Within a block, you may answer the items in any order, review responses, and change answers. However, after exiting a block, you can no longer review questions or change answers within that block. A link to view standard lab values, as well as access a calculator, is available at any time within the block of questions.

Day 1 includes 232 multiple-choice items divided into six 60-minute blocks of 38–39 items. A total of 60 minutes is allowed for completing each block of questions. The first day of testing is approximately 7 hours. There are 45 minutes of break time and an optional 5-minute tutorial complete the 8-hour day. Extra break time can be gained by completing question blocks or the tutorial before the allocated time.

Day 2 includes 180 items divided into 6 blocks of 30 questions. There are approximately 9 hours in the test session on the second day. You will have 45 minutes to complete each of these blocks. The time allotted for these blocks is 3 hours. The second day also includes 13 clinical case simulations (CCS), preceded by a 5-minute tutorial. CCS cases vary from 10 to 20 minutes in duration. As with the first day, a minimum of 45 minutes of break time is allocated for the day.

The multiple-choice questions contribute 75 percent of your score on Step 3. They are the largest component of your exam. Don't get so caught up worrying about CCS that you forget about the rest of the exam!

Traditional multiple-choice questions may either be single-item questions, multiple-item sets, or cases. The examination will also be given on 2 test days; however, examinees will be able to schedule the 2 test days on nonconsecutive days.

Day 1: Step 3 Foundations of Independent Practice (FIP). Day 1 will focus on assessment of knowledge of foundational medicine and science essential for effective health care. This test day will be entirely devoted to multiple-choice questions and will include some of the newer item formats, such as those based on scientific abstracts, pharmaceutical advertisements, and basic science correlates.

Day 2: Step 3 Advanced Clinical Medicine (ACM). Day 2 will focus on assessment of applying comprehensive knowledge of health and disease in the context of patient management. This test day will include multiple-choice questions and computer-based case simulations (CCS).

Single Items

These questions are the traditional, multiple-choice format that you encountered in Step 1 and Step 2 CK. These items include a patient vignette followed by four or five response options. Other options may be partially correct, but there is only *one best* answer.

Multiple Item Sets

A single patient-centered vignette may be associated with 2 or 3 consecutive questions that are linked to the initial patient vignette but test different points. Questions are designed to be answered independently of each other. You are required to select the one best answer for each question. As with single items, any of the options may be partially correct, but there is only *one best* answer.

Cases

A single-patient or family-centered vignette may ask 2 or 3 questions, each related to the initial opening vignette. The difference in these case sets is that additional information is added as the case unfolds. *Always* answer the questions in the order presented. You may find your response to earlier questions is altered by the additional information in subsequent questions; however, resist the urge to change your prior answers. If you do skip questions, be sure to answer earlier questions with only the information presented to that point in the case. Each question is intended to be answered independently.

Guide to the CCS

The Primum computer-based case simulations (CCS) is a testing format that allows you to provide care for a simulated patient. You decide which information to obtain and how to treat and monitor the patient's progress. The computer records each step you take in caring for the patient and scores your overall performance.

In the CCS software, you will be required to choose additional elements of the presented history, as well as select the components of the physical examination you wish to perform. You have the flexibility to order any laboratory study, procedure, request, and consultants, and you can begin medications and other therapies. Any of the thousands of possible entries that you type on the "order sheet" are processed and verified by the "clerk," and there is no limit to the number of entries into the order sheet. However, each order has a corresponding "virtual time" in which the test result may be available or procedure can be performed. Advancing the virtual time allows you to obtain results and submit the requested procedures. As virtual time passes, the patient's condition changes based on the underlying problem and the sequence and priority of your interventions. You are responsible for managing the results of tests and interventions and making subsequent management decisions based on the first sequence of tests you ordered. While you cannot go back in virtual time, you can change your orders to reflect your updated management plan. In addition, you have the option to move patients between the office, home, emergency department, intensive care unit, and hospital ward. An important aspect of correctly managing CCS patients is recognizing the most appropriate sequence of management and the most appropriate location where that patient should be treated.

The challenge of the CCS is twofold:

1. You need to manage the case itself. The management steps are case-dependent and based on acceptable standards of care. It is assumed that you will have reviewed the management of the most common presenting complaints during your year of internship and/or during your Step 3 review.
2. You will manage a patient by initiating the most appropriate course of action, such as ordering tests or transferring the patient to another setting. The computer will not cue you on what to do—*you* must decide independently what you need to do and the sequence in which it should be done.

Each case can be divided into 3 parts: the case introduction, vital signs, and initial history (first 1 to 2 minutes); the management of the case (10 to 12 minutes maximum, often less); and the conclusion of the case (last 5 minutes).

Case Introduction Screen

The first screen is called the case introduction and provides a one- or two-sentence description of the patient's chief complaint, the patient's location at presentation, and time of day. After reading this screen, click the **OK** button.

Vital Signs Screen

These initial vital signs are the most important indicator of whether this condition is acute-emergent or chronic-stable. Review for any abnormalities before hitting the **OK** button.

Initial History Screen

The initial history screen gives you a comprehensive description of the history of present illness, medical history, family history, social history, and review of systems. Read this section carefully, as key diagnostic information is given here. After reading the history of present illness, you should be able to establish a short differential diagnostic list. Make note of any key features in the past medical, family, and social history and review of systems that support or refute your differential diagnosis. At the end of the initial history, click the **OK** button; this will mark the end of the prompted section of the case.

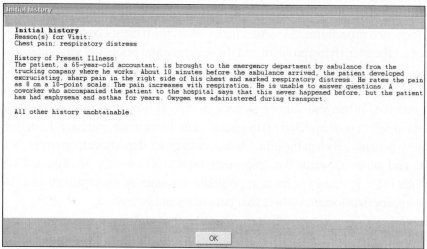

(courtesy **http://usmle.org**)

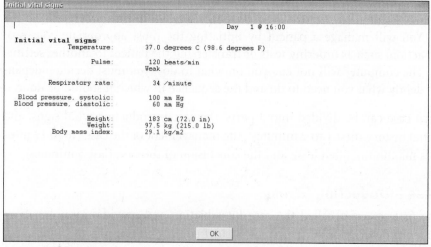

(courtesy **http://usmle.org**)

Case Management

This section of the case is driven by your actions rather than prompts from the software. There are 4 buttons at the top of the screen, which you will use to manage the case. You will be able to access any of these buttons until the last 5 minutes, at which point you are automatically brought to the final stage.

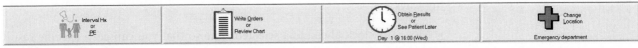

(courtesy **http://usmle.org**)

The **History/Physical** button allows you to order a follow-up history, as well as either a comprehensive or system-focused physical exam.

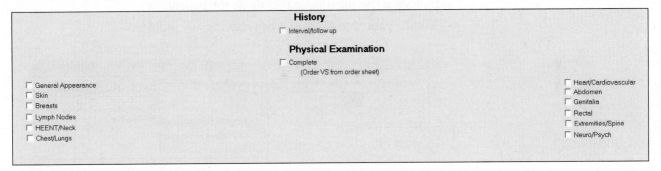

(courtesy **http://usmle.org**)

The **Write Orders/Review Chart** button brings up a number of other chart options, including an order sheet, progress notes, vital signs, lab reports, imaging studies, other tests, and a treatment record.

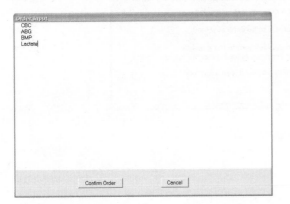
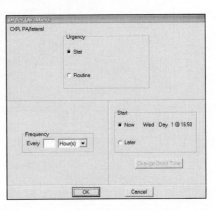

(courtesy **http://usmle.org**)

The **clock button** allows you to manipulate the **case time clock (virtual time).** This is a completely separate from the real-time clock, found at the bottom right part of the screen throughout the case. In real test time, you have up to a maximum of 10 to 25 minutes to manage the case from beginning to end. But to get results or schedule a time to reevaluate the patient, you'll need to move the **case time clock** ahead. You may move the clock ahead in any of the following ways:

- Move the clock ahead to a selected time so that you can get a specific result back.
- Move the clock automatically to when the first result comes back. Remember that you will still need to manage the case in the interim period before the next available result may come back.
- Indicate a specific time to reevaluate the patient.
- Ask the patient to call you if he is having any problems.

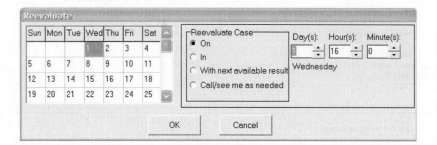

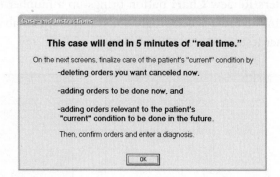

At the end of the case, you must enter your diagnosis on the screen provided. When you click **OK,** the case closes, and you move on to the next case.

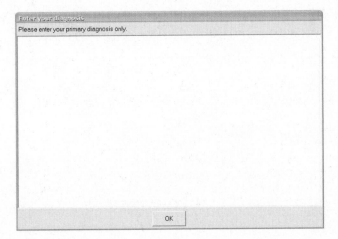

Score Reporting

The minimum passing score for Step 3 is 196. This corresponds to answering 60–70% of the items correctly.

The USMLE does not report performance as a percentile; rather, you will be given a 3-digit score. On the reverse side of the score report will be a graph of your performance, indicating your relative strengths and weaknesses. You are the only one who will see this graph, ie, it is not sent to any institutions or licensing bodies.

Registration for Step 3

For registration and more information, contact:

FSMB

Department of Examination Services
Website: *fsmb.org*
Telephone: (817) 868-4041
Fax: (817) 868-4098
Email: usmle@fsmb.org

Or contact your state **medical licensing authority;** see the USMLE website at *http://usmle.org.*

PART 1

Internal Medicine

Neurology 1

Stroke and TIA

A 67-year-old man with a history of hypertension and diabetes comes to the ED with a sudden onset of weakness in the right arm and leg over the last hour. On exam he is unable to lift the bottom half of the right side of his face. What is the best initial step?

a. Head CT with contrast
b. Head CT without contrast
c. Aspirin
d. Thrombolytics
e. MRI

Answer: **B.** Before giving thrombolytics or any anticoagulation, you need to rule out hemorrhagic stroke, which is a contraindication to thrombolytics. You cannot even give aspirin without doing a head CT first. Thrombolytics are indicated within the first 3 hours of the onset of the symptoms of a stroke. Remember, 20% of strokes are hemorrhagic. You do not need contrast to visualize blood; contrast is used to detect cancer or infection, such as an abscess.

Stroke and transient ischemic attack (TIA) present with the sudden onset of weakness on one side of the body. Weakness of half of the face and aphasia are common as well. Partial or total loss of vision may be present, which may be transient. The cause is decreased or altered cerebral blood flow.

Stroke is distinguished from TIA **based on time**.

- With **stroke**, symptoms last ≥24 hours. There will be permanent residual neurologic deficits, caused by ischemia (80% of cases) or hemorrhage (20%).
  - Stroke spares the upper third of the face, from the eyes up.
  - Ischemic stroke can result from emboli or a thrombosis; emboli present with more sudden symptoms.
- With **TIA**, symptoms last <24 hours and resolve completely. The only symptom may be transient loss of vision in one eye (amaurosis fugax) (the first branch of the internal carotid artery is the ophthalmic artery).
  - TIA is always caused by emboli or thrombosis and never caused by hemorrhage (hemorrhage does not resolve in 24 hours).
  - TIA does not spare the upper third of the face.

Cryptogenic stroke means there is no known etiology. It can be labeled "cryptogenic" only after 1–3 months of EKG monitoring has been done.

- Carotids normal (<70% stenosis)
- Echo normal (no clots or vegetation)
- EKG and telemetry: no A-fib
- Holter: no A-fib
- 30 day and up to 90-day monitoring with Holter or implantable loop recorder: no A-fib

With stroke, the younger the patient, the more likely the cause is a vasculitis or hypercoagulable state.

Arterial lesions are a subtype of stroke and TIA. On the Step 3 exam, you will likely be asked to identify or localize a lesion based on characteristic symptoms.

Cerebral Artery	Symptoms
Anterior cerebral artery	• Profound lower extremity weakness (contralateral in the case of unilateral arterial occlusion) • Mild upper extremity weakness (contralateral in the case of unilateral arterial occlusion) • Personality changes or psychiatric disturbance • Urinary incontinence
Middle cerebral artery	• Profound upper extremity weakness (contralateral in the case of unilateral arterial occlusion) • Aphasia • Apraxia/neglect • The eyes deviate toward the side of the lesion. • Contralateral homonymous hemianopsia, with macular sparing
Posterior cerebral artery	• Prosopagnosia (inability to recognize faces)
Vertebrobasilar artery	• Vertigo • Nausea and vomiting • May be described as a "drop attack," loss of consciousness • Vertical nystagmus • Dysarthria and dystonia • Sensory changes in face and scalp • Ataxia • Bilateral findings
Posterior inferior cerebellar artery	• Ipsilateral face • Contralateral body • Vertigo and Horner syndrome
Lacunar infarct	• Absence of cortical deficits • Ataxia • Parkinsonian signs • Sensory deficits • Hemiparesis (most notable in the face) • Possible bulbar signs
Ophthalmic artery	• Amaurosis fugax

Diagnostic testing for both stroke and TIA is as follows.

- Head CT without contrast (**best initial diagnostic test**)
  - Extremely sensitive for blood
  - Within first several days, all nonhemorrhagic stroke should be associated with a normal head CT
  - Needs 3–5 days to achieve >95% sensitivity in the detection of nonhemorrhagic stroke

Add statins to all nonhemorrhagic strokes.

- MRI achieves 99% sensitivity for a nonhemorrhagic stroke within 24 hours but is not often done because CT is more widely available, less expensive, and more sensitive for blood
- MRA (**most accurately images the brain for stroke**) can be positive within 60 minutes of stroke

Treatment is as follows:

- **Within 3–4.5 hours of onset** of stroke symptoms
  - **Thrombolytics** if stroke is not severe (NIH stroke scale >25) and patient meets all of the following conditions: age <80; not a diabetic with a previous stroke; does not use anticoagulation
  - Absolute **contraindications** to thrombolytic therapy
    - History of hemorrhagic stroke
    - Presence of intracranial neoplasm/mass or a bleeding disorder
    - Active bleeding or surgery within 6 weeks; cerebral trauma or brain surgery within 6 months; or non-hemorrhagic stroke within 1 year
    - CPR within 3 weeks that was traumatic (e.g., chest compressions)
    - Suspicion of aortic dissection
- **After 4.5 hours of onset** of stroke symptoms
  - Remove clot with a catheter (useful up to 24 hours after stroke, unlike angioplasty; angioplasty would rupture the vessel, whereas a catheter pulls the clot out like a corkscrew)
  - **Aspirin (best initial therapy)** for those coming too late for thrombolytics; also indicated after the use of thrombolytics
  - Antiplatelet medication: aspirin or clopidogrel (or aspirin + dipyridamole) is acceptable medication to prevent a subsequent stroke, but aspirin first is the standard of care
  - If patient develops a stroke on aspirin, switch to clopidogrel
  - If patient is already on aspirin when a new stroke or TIA occurs, add dipyridamole or switch to clopidogrel
  - For all nonhemorrhagic stroke, add a statin

Don't forget to control hypertension, diabetes, and hyperlipidemia in a patient who has had a stroke. Hypertensive urgency is a relative contraindication to thrombolytic therapy.

Heparin has no clear evidence of benefit for stroke, and ticlopidine is always a wrong answer (no advantage over clopidogrel and has more adverse effects [TTP, neutropenia]).

Do not use prasugrel for TIA/stroke.

tPA between 3–4.5 hours:
- Age <80
- NIH stroke scale <25
- Not diabetic with previous stroke
- Not on anticoagulation

Always do a head CT without contrast before anticoagulating to rule out a hemorrhagic stroke.

For the exam, know that catheter retrieval provides a definite benefit up to 24 hours after stroke onset. It decreases both focal neurological findings and mortality, and the benefit persists for years after the stroke.

- Thrombolytic use 3–4.5 hours after the onset of stroke symptoms is useful in select patients.
- Fewer than 20% of patients with a stroke come in time to get thrombolytics (<3 hours).
- The goal of the thrombolytic is to achieve resolution of symptoms; if symptoms have already resolved, there is no reason to give thrombolytics.

With cerebral vein thrombosis, a type of stroke, clotting in cerebral veins presents with headache developing over several days (can mimic subarachnoid hemorrhage). Many patients present with the same weakness and speech difficulty seen in stroke. LP is normal.

Magnetic resonance venography (MRV) is the **most accurate test**. Treat with LMW heparin followed by warfarin for a few months.

Further management includes:

- Stroke: after the head CT and administration of thrombolytics or aspirin, move the clock forward on CCS. On subsequent screens, the most important issue is to determine the origin of the stroke.
- TIA: management is same as stroke, except that thrombolytics are not indicated.
  - Paradoxical emboli through a patent foramen ovale need closure with a catheter device.
  - Use dual antiplatelet therapy (DAPT) with aspirin and clopidogrel for the first several weeks.

The following are indicated in all patients with stroke or TIA:

- Echocardiogram: anticoagulation for clots, possible surgery for valve vegetations
- Carotid Doppler/duplex: endarterectomy for stenosis >70%, but not if it is 100%
  - Do only if patient is symptomatic
  - Stenosis of the carotids, even when the passage is narrowed 70–99%, is not an indication for endarterectomy if patient is asymptomatic
- EKG and a Holter monitor if EKG is normal: warfarin, dabigatran, or rivaroxaban for A-fib
- In young patients age <50 with no past medical history (diabetes, hypertension), do sedimentation rate; VDRL or RPR; ANA; double-stranded DNA; protein C, protein S; factor V Leiden mutation; antiphospholipid syndromes

Condition	Goal
Hypertension	<140/90 mm Hg in a diabetic
Diabetes	Same tight glycemic control as general population
Hyperlipidemia	LDL <70 mg/dL add statins for all nonhemorrhagic strokes

When is **closure of patent foramen ovale (PFO)** the next step in management?

- When patient has an embolic-appearing cryptogenic ischemic stroke, and right-to-left shunt detected by bubble study

PFO closure is conducted in conjunction with antiplatelet therapy and is done with a percutaneous device.

Use MRI/MRA for the brainstem.

Anterior stroke and middle cerebral artery stroke are managed the same way.

24–48 hour Holter is not enough to exclude A-fib.

KAPLAN MEDICAL

Seizures

In seizure disorders, only the management of status epilepticus is clear. Status epilepticus therapy is as follows:

- Benzodiazepines, such lorazepam
- If seizure persists after moving the clock forward 10–20 minutes, add fosphenytoin
- If seizure persists after moving the clock forward another 10–20 minutes, add phenobarbital
- If seizure persists after moving the clock forward another 10–20 minutes, add general anesthesia (e.g., pentobarbital, thiopental, midazolam, propofol)

Diagnostic tests include:

- Sodium, calcium, glucose, oxygen, creatinine, and magnesium level
- Head CT (urgently); if negative, consider MRI later
- Urine toxicology screen
- Liver and renal function
- Electroencephalogram (EEG) only if the other tests do not reveal the etiology

Neurology consult should be ordered for all seizure patients. On the exam, you will be asked your reason for the consult in 10 words or less.

> Liver failure and renal failure can cause seizures, but potassium disorders cannot.

CCS Tip: On CCS, consultants never say anything. CCS is testing your knowledge of when you are expected to need help.

Treatment is as follows:

- **Single seizure**: chronic antiepileptic drug therapy is generally not indicated, with some exceptions: strong family history of seizures; abnormal EEG; status epilepticus that required benzodiazepines to stop the seizure; or non-correctable precipitating cause, e.g., brain tumor
- **Chronic seizures**: no single agent is the best initial therapy
  - **First-line**: levetiracetam, valproic acid, carbamazepine, phenytoin (all equal in efficacy); lamotrigine is also effective but is associated with severe skin reactions, e.g., Stevens-Johnson (HLA B*1502 testing can predict Stevens-Johnson)
    - In pregnancy, most dangerous is valproic acid while safest is levetiracetam/lamotrigine
    - OCPs/estrogen increase metabolism of lamotrigine to ineffective level
  - **Second-line**: gabapentin, phenobarbital, lacosamide, zonisamide
- Ethosuximide: best for absence or petit mal seizures
- Carbamazepine for hyponatremia

Parkinson Disease

Parkinson disease (PD) is predominantly a gait disorder. Symptoms include trembling/shaking with a slow, abnormal "festinating" gait. Orthostasis is often seen.

Physical findings include:

- "Cogwheel" rigidity; everything is slow, bradykinesia
- Resting tremor (resolves when patient moves or reaches for something)
- Hypomimia (a masklike, underreactive face)
- Micrographia (small writing)
- Orthostasis
- Intact cognition and memory

There are no specific diagnostic tests to confirm PD.

Treatment is as follows:

- **Mild disease**
  - Anticholinergic, e.g., benztropine or trihexyphenidyl if age <60
  - Amantadine if age >60 (has fewer side effects than anticholinergics so better for older patients)
- **Severe disease** (unable to perform activities of daily living, i.e., cooking, shopping)
  - Levodopa/carbidopa: greater efficacy but "on-off" phenomena with uneven long-term effects and more adverse effects
  - Dopamine-agonists (pramipexole, ropinirole, cabergoline, rotigotine [given by patch], apomorphine): fewer side effects but less efficacy

If these medications cannot control the patient's symptoms, then use:

- COMT inhibitors (tolcapone, entacapone) to block the metabolism of dopamine and extend the effect of dopamine-based medications (by themselves, they are not effective)
- MAO inhibitors (selegiline, rasagiline, safinamide)
- Deep brain stimulation when medical therapy does not control symptoms
- Dopamine-receptor agonist (apomorphine)
- 5HT inhibitor (pimavanserin) to minimize psychotic symptoms (note that this antipsychotic medication does not worsen PD because its mechanism is not dopamine-inhibition)

Shy-Drager syndrome is PD characterized by orthostatic hypotension. Add fludrocortisone or midodrine. Fludrocortisone is pure mineralocorticoid (aldosterone) and midodrine is an oral alpha 1 agonist raising blood pressure.

Progressive supranuclear palsy can be misdiagnosed for PD; the patient can't look up or down (vertical gaze palsy).

A man with severe parkinsonism is admitted for hip fracture. On admission, the medicine reconciliation form is not recorded, and his multiple Parkinson medications are not continued in the hospital. Which of the following can happen?

a. Seizure or stroke
b. Arrhythmia/MI
c. Fever/rhabdomyolysis
d. Diarrhea or malabsorption

Answer: **C.** It is an idiosyncrasy of parkinsonism and its medical therapy that the sudden withdrawal of medications can result in rhabdomyolysis. The reason for this is not known.

Essential Tremor

Essential tremor is a tremor that occurs both at rest and with action (or "intention"). This is a tremor not associated with another illness.

There is no specific diagnostic test.

Treatment is beta blockers, specifically propranolol.

In a CCS case, move the clock forward 1–2 weeks for a repeat meeting, choose "interval history," and repeat the neurological exam.

- If tremor is still there, add primidone (antiepileptic medication)
- If tremor still persists, switch to topiramate or gabapentin
- If multiple medical therapies fail and severe tremor interferes with functioning (i.e., computer use), choose thalamotomy
  - Unilateral thalamotomy is standard, not experimental.
  - Magnetic resonance–focused ultrasound to ablate the thalamus with local heat will help improve the tremor.

Type of Tremor	Resting Tremor	Tremor with Intention (Action) Only	Tremor Both at Rest and with Intention
Diagnosis	Parkinson disease	Cerebellar disorders	Essential tremor
Treatment	Amantadine	Treat etiology	Propranolol

Multiple Sclerosis

Multiple sclerosis (MS) presents with abnormalities in any part of the CNS; these improve only to have another defect develop several months to years later.

- Optic neuritis (most common)
- Motor and sensory problems
- Defects of the bladder (e.g., an atonic bladder)
- Fatigue, depression
- Hyperreflexia, spasticity

Diagnostic testing includes:

- MRI (**best initial** and **most accurate diagnostic test**)
  - Allergic reactions to gadolinium (contrast agent used with MRI) are less frequent than they are with iodinated contrast material used with CT scan.
  - Those with renal insufficiency may have a systemic overreaction with increased collagen deposition in soft tissues ("nephrogenic systemic fibrosis"); hardened fibrotic nodules develop on the skin and (in severe cases) the heart, lung, and liver. There is no specific treatment.
- CSF (lumbar tap): shows presence of oligoclonal bands only if MRI is non-diagnostic
- CT scan of the head: not needed, less sensitive than MRI
- Visual and auditory evoked potential studies: never used

Treatment is as follows:

Anti-CD20 drugs decrease the progression of MS.

- Steroids (**best initial therapy for acute exacerbation**)
- Vitamin D and calcium for all cases
- Disease-modifying therapy:
  - Beta interferon, glatiramer, mitoxantrone, natalizumab (but causes PML), daclizumab, fingolimod, or dimethyl fumarate
  - Ocrelizumab (anti-CD20 drug that is disease-modifying)
  - Alemtuzumab (anti-CD52 drug that inhibits lymphocytes and deters progression)
- Amantadine for fatigue

Oral therapy for MS is dimethyl fumarate, fingolimod, and teriflunomide.

- Dalfampridine to increase walking speed
- Baclofen or tizanidine for spasticity

Dementia

With dementia syndromes, all patients have memory loss.

All patients with memory loss must receive:

- Head CT
- B12 level
- Thyroid function testing (T4/TSH)
- RPR or VDRL

Alzheimer Disease (AD)

AD presents with slowly progressive memory loss exclusively in older patients (age >65). There are no focal deficits such as motor or sensory problems, but patients do develop apathy and, after several years, imprecise speech.

Exercise slows the progression of dementia.

AD is a diagnosis of exclusion. The **best diagnostic test** is head CT scan showing diffuse, symmetrical atrophy.

Treatment is anticholinesterase medications (donepezil, rivastigmine, and galantamine). Memantine provides only modest benefit. Combinations are not effective.

- Preventing falls in the elderly is essential, as a fall in that population is far more deadly than a myocardial infarction.
- Strength training and exercise are the only proven way to prevent falls. Nearly any form of exercise helps: walking, yoga, tai chi, dancing, and weight training.
- Screening for visual problems and removing tripping hazards in the home should be done as well.

Frontotemporal Dementia (Pick Disease)

Personality and behavior become abnormal first. Memory is lost afterward. Movement disorder is not present.

Head CT or MRI shows focal atrophy of the frontal and temporal lobes.

Treatment is the same as for AD, but the response will be less.

Creutzfeldt-Jakob Disease (CJD)

CJD is caused by prions, transmissible protein particles. It manifests as rapidly progressive dementia and the presence of myoclonus. Patients are younger than those with AD.

Diagnostic testing is as follows:

- EEG (abnormal)
- Brain biopsy (**most accurate diagnostic test**)
- In a CCS case, perform MRI as well, although there is nothing on MRI to suggest CJD.
- CSF: the presence of the 14-3-3 protein spares the need for brain biopsy

There is no treatment for CJD.

"Lewy Body" Dementia

Lewy body dementia is PD plus dementia. It is associated with very vivid, detailed hallucinations.

Treat both the AD and the PD. Remember, PD is primarily a gait disorder.

Normal Pressure Hydrocephalus

This condition generally presents in older males, but it can affect women as well.

Symptoms can be remembered as WWW: wet, weird, wobbly.

- Wet: urinary incontinence
- Weird: dementia
- Wobbly: wide-based gait/ataxia

Diagnostic testing includes CT of the head. Lumbar puncture (LP) will show normal pressure, and this should be done on CCS.

Treatment is placement of a shunt.

Huntington Disease (HD)/Chorea

HD presents in a young patient (age 30s), far below the age for AD. On the exam you will likely be asked about family history. Symptoms are the following:

- Dementia
- Psychiatric disturbance with personality changes
- Chorea/movement disorder

Diagnose with specific genetic testing. Inheritance is autosomal dominant.

Treatment is antipsychotics for symptomatic control.

Which of the following treats movement disorders, such as tardive dyskinesia and HD?

- **Deutetrabenazine**, **tetrabenazine**, and **valbenazine**, which alter levels of monoamines (e.g., dopamine, serotonin, norepinephrine)

Headache

Migraine

Of migraines, 60% are unilateral, and 40% are bilateral. Triggers include cheese, caffeine, menstruation, and OCPs.

The following symptoms may precede the headache:

- Aura of bright flashing lights
- Scotomata
- Abnormal smells

Diagnostic testing is head CT or MRI when the headache has any of the following characteristics:

- Sudden and/or severe
- Onset after age 40
- Associated with focal neurological findings

Treatment is as follows:

- Sumatriptan or ergotamine (**best initial therapy**, i.e., abortive)
  - All triptans are interchangeable for aborting acute migraine; others include almotriptan, eletriptan, naratriptan, zolmitriptan
  - When a contraindication is involved (e.g., coronary disease, pregnancy), give NSAIDs or antiemetics that work through dopamine inhibition (e.g., chlorpromazine, metoclopramide, or prochlorperazine)
- If status migrainosus or cannot give triptans/ergotamine
  - Dopamine antagonists: prochlorperazine, metoclopramide, chlorpromazine
  - Use with diphenhydramine to prevent dystonic reaction
  - All can prolong QT
- Transcranial magnetic stimulation may be needed for acute migraine if other treatments do not work
- Prophylactic therapy (requires several weeks to take effect):
  - When ≥4 headaches per month, give prophylactic therapy with beta blockers (propranolol)
  - Alternate prophylactic medications are CCBs, tricyclic antidepressants, or SSRIs

> Dopamine antagonist antiemetics treat status migrainosus not responsive to triptans.

Which migraine drug makes Parkinson disease worse?

a. Prochlorperazine
b. Metoclopramide
c. Chlorpromazine
d. All of the above

Answer: **D.** All worsen Parkinson disease symptoms because all are antidopaminergic.

Basic Science Correlate

Mechanism of Triptans

Migraine is thought to be vasoconstriction followed by vasodilation, then pain. Triptans constrict vessels; they function by reconstricting the cerebral vessels, but they constrict vessels in the heart as well and can provoke cardiac ischemia. That is why they are dangerous in hypertension, pregnancy, and coronary disease.

Cluster Headache

Cluster headache is exclusively unilateral with redness and tearing of the eye and rhinorrhea. Men > women 10:1.

Treatment is as follows:

- Triptans or 100% oxygen (**best initial abortive therapy**)
  - Triptans: generally used, easy to give at home
  - Sumatriptan, used in same way as with migraine headache
  - Steroids
- CCBs such as verapamil (**best initial prophylactic therapy**)
  - Cluster headache occurs multiple times in a short period and then resolves
  - "Cluster" is often over by the time prophylactic therapy has taken effect
  - Verapamil does prevent cluster headache

Headache Type	Migraine	Cluster
Gender	More common in women	More common in men
Presentation	• Unilateral or bilateral • Aura	• Only unilateral • Tearing and redness of eye; rhinorrhea • No aura
Abortive therapy	• Sumatriptan	• Sumatriptan • Special: 100% oxygen
Prophylactic therapy	• Propranolol	• Verapamil

Temporal Arteritis

Temporal arteritis presents with jaw claudication and tenderness of the temporal area.

Diagnostic testing includes erythrocyte sedimentation rate (ESR) and temporal artery biopsy (**most accurate diagnostic test**).

Give steroids first and fast if these are available. A delay may result in permanent vision loss.

Pseudotumor Cerebri

Pseudotumor = headache plus:

- Sixth nerve palsy
- Visual field loss
- Transiently obscure vision
- Pulsatile tinnitus

Look for an obese young woman with headache and double vision. On exam there is papilledema but normal CT/MRI. Vitamin A use is suggestive.

Lumbar puncture with opening pressure measurement (**most accurate diagnostic test**) will show a markedly elevated pressure.

Treatment is weight loss and acetazolamide. If those fail, consider surgery for VP shunt and optic nerve sheath fenestration.

Intracranial Hypotension

- From CSF leak after LP
- Look for orthostatic headache
- MRI abnormal (80% of cases); confirm with low CSF pressure, <60 mm Hg

Treatment is blood patch to close off the leak.

Central Nervous System Infections

When a CNS infection is suspected, perform a head CT before a lumbar puncture (LP) in the following circumstances:

- History of CNS disease
- Focal neurologic deficit
- Presence of papilledema
- Seizures
- Altered consciousness
- Significant delay in the ability to perform an LP

If these findings are present, get blood cultures and start empiric antibiotic therapy before ordering the head CT.

Bacterial Meningitis

A 45-year-old man comes to the ED with fever, headache, photophobia, and a stiff neck. What is the next best step in management?

a. LP
b. Head CT scan
c. Ceftriaxone and vancomycin
d. Penicillin
e. Move to ICU

Answer: **A.** When you suspect bacterial meningitis, administer antibiotics quickly. Further, do blood cultures stat simultaneously with an LP, or immediately prior. Penicillin can never be used as empiric therapy for meningitis; it is not sufficiently broad in coverage to be effective empiric therapy. In this case, perform the LP.

> Vaccination for group B meningococcus is given at age 10–25.

The **most accurate diagnostic test** is a culture, but you cannot wait for the results of culture before starting therapy. Preliminary analysis of the cerebrospinal fluid (CSF) is useful.

- Gram stain is only 50–60% sensitive for bacterial meningitis, so a negative stain excludes nothing. On the other hand, a positive Gram stain is extremely useful and specific.
  - Gram-positive diplococci: Pneumococcus
  - Gram-negative diplococci: *Neisseria*
  - Gram-negative pleomorphic, coccobacillary organisms: *Haemophilus*
  - Gram-positive bacilli: *Listeria*

> The Gram stain has poor sensitivity but good specificity for bacterial meningitis.

> CSF cell count is the most important criterion to determine the need to treat a patient. Thousands of polys (neutrophils) indicate bacterial meningitis until proven otherwise.

- Elevated CSF protein is of marginal diagnostic benefit, as it is nonspecific (any form of CNS infection can elevate the CSF protein); a normal CSF protein level essentially excludes bacterial meningitis
- Glucose <60% of serum level is consistent with bacterial meningitis
- CSF cell count (**best initial diagnostic test**)
  - Not as specific as a culture, but available much sooner
  - Cell count with a differential is much more specific than an elevated CSF protein
  - If thousands of neutrophils are present in CSF, start IV ceftriaxone, vancomycin, and steroids; steroids have been associated with a decrease in mortality in bacterial meningitis

Cryptococcus

This infection is slower than bacterial meningitis and may not give severe meningeal signs, such as neck stiffness, photophobia, and high fever, all at the same time. Look for an HIV-positive patient with <100 CD4 cells.

- India ink positive in 60–80%
- Cryptococcal antigen (**most accurate diagnostic test**)

Treatment is amphotericin and 5-flucytosine (5FC), followed by oral fluconazole.

- If CD4 count does not rise, continue fluconazole indefinitely.
- If CD4 count rises >100, fluconazole can be stopped.

Lyme Disease

Look for a patient who has recently returned from a camping or hiking trip. Tick exposure is remembered only by 20% of patients.

Symptoms include joint pain, 7th cranial nerve palsy, and a rash with central clearing (target lesion). Note that 7th CN is not CNS.

There are no characteristic CSF findings to confirm a diagnosis of CNS Lyme.

Specific serologic or Western blot testing on the CSF is the **most accurate diagnostic test**.

Treatment is IV ceftriaxone or penicillin.

Rocky Mountain Spotted Fever

Look for a camper or hiker with a rash that starts on the wrists and ankles and moves centripetally toward the center. Fever, headache, and malaise precede the rash. Tick bite is remembered only by 60% of patients.

Diagnose with specific serology. Doxycycline is the most effective therapy.

TB Meningitis

It is very difficult to be precise about diagnosing TB meningitis. Look for an immigrant with a history of lung TB. The presentation is very slow over weeks to months:

- Very high CSF protein level
- Positive acid fast (mycobacterial) stain of CSF (≤10% of cases); for acid-fast culture, you need 3 high-volume taps that are centrifuged

If the case describes fever, headache, and neck stiffness over hours, it is not TB.

Culture is the **most accurate diagnostic test** in TB of CSF but it will take weeks. PCR is the **most accurate test you can get quickly**.

Treatment is rifampin, isoniazid, pyrazinamide, and ethambutol (RIPE) as you would give for pulmonary TB, but add steroids and extend the length of therapy longer.

- Ethambutol has poor CNS penetration
- If a fluoroquinolone is an answer choice, choose it instead of ethambutol

Viral Meningitis

Viral meningitis is oftentimes a diagnosis of exclusion. There is a lymphocytic pleocytosis in the CSF.

There is no specific treatment.

An elderly man comes to the ED with fever, headache, a stiff neck, and photophobia. He is HIV-positive with <50 CD4 cells and a history of pneumocystis pneumonia. Head CT is normal. CSF shows 2,500 white cells that are all neutrophils; Gram stain is normal. What is the best initial therapy?

a. Ceftriaxone and metronidazole
b. Cefoxitin and mefloquine
c. Ceftriaxone, ampicillin, and vancomycin
d. Fluconazole
e. Amphotericin

Answer: **C.** *Listeria monocytogenes* is a cause of meningitis that is not adequately treated by any form of cephalosporin. Ampicillin is added to the usual regimen of ceftriaxone and vancomycin to cover *Listeria*. This cannot be fungal meningitis, because the CSF is characterized exclusively by a high number of neutrophils; neutrophils are not consistent with fungal meningitis.

A 17-year-old man comes to the ED with fever, headache, stiff neck, and photophobia. He has a petechial rash. CSF shows 2,499 neutrophils. Ceftriaxone and vancomycin are started. What is the next step in management?

a. Test for HIV
b. Wait for results of culture
c. Add ampicillin
d. Droplet isolation
e. Droplet isolation and prescribe rifampin for close contacts

Answer: **E.** When an adolescent presents with a petechial rash and increased neutrophils on CSF, it is suggestive of *Neisseria meningitidis*. These patients should be placed on droplet isolation, and close contacts should receive prophylaxis.

Listeria

Look for elderly, neonatal, and HIV-positive patients and those who have no spleen, are on steroids, or are immunocompromised with leukemia or lymphoma.

There will be elevated neutrophils in the CSF.

Add ampicillin to treatment.

Neisseria meningitidis

Look for patients who are adolescent, in the military, or asplenic or who have terminal complement deficiency.

Treatment is as follows:

- Patient: droplet isolation for 24 hours
- Close contacts (household members/those who kiss and share cups/utensils): prophylaxis with rifampin, ciprofloxacin, or ceftriaxone
- Routine contacts (school/work): no prophylaxis needed

> The nurse or medical student taking care of a patient with *Neisseria* does not need prophylaxis. Those with kissing and other saliva-type contact do need prophylaxis.

Amoebic Meningitis

Naegleria fowleri and *Acanthamoeba* are free-living, thermophilic (warm water) amoebae that can infect swimmers in fresh water. The amoebae swim up the nose and through the cribriform plate into the brain.

Look for anosmia in the question stem.

- Without treatment, 95% of cases are fatal: emergency care required
- Wet mount of CSF shows mobile amoebae
- Treatment is miltefosine and maybe amphotericin; steroids may help

Encephalitis

Almost all encephalitis in the United States is caused by herpes simplex. The patient does not have to recall a herpes infection in the past for the condition to be herpes encephalitis. Varicella is a treatable form of encephalitis.

> Fever + Confusion = Encephalitis

Look for a patient with fever and altered mental status over a few hours. If the patient also has photophobia and a stiff neck, you will not be able to diagnose encephalitis.

Testing includes:

- Head CT scan (**best initial diagnostic test**)
- PCR of the CSF for HSV and VZV (**most accurate diagnostic test**)

"Brain biopsy" is the most common wrong answer on questions about encephalitis diagnosis. A brain biopsy is not necessary. Do a PCR instead.

Treatment is acyclovir for both HSV and VZV. With acyclovir-resistant patients, use foscarnet.

Basic Science Correlate

Mechanism of Acyclovir

Acyclovir, valacyclovir, famciclovir, and ganciclovir all have the same mechanism: to inhibit DNA polymerase. All need to be activated by thymidine kinase, except foscarnet. This is why ganciclovir cannot be used to treat acyclovir-resistant herpes and why foscarnet (with a different mechanism) is used instead.

Autoimmune (NMDA) Encephalitis

- Fever, headache, confusion, normal head CT like any encephalitis
- Psychiatric symptoms and dystonias
- Ovarian teratomas in history
- Diagnose with specific antibodies in CSF
- Treatment is IVIG, steroids, and removal of the teratoma

Brain Abscess

A brain abscess presents with fever, headache, and focal neurological deficits. CT scan reveals a "ring" (or contrast-enhancing) lesion. Contrast ("ring") enhancement basically means infection or cancer.

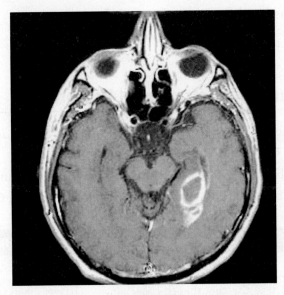

Brain Abscess

Consider HIV status in the context of a brain abscess as follows:

- HIV-negative: brain biopsy (**next best step**); ceftriaxone and metronidazole while awaiting culture results
- HIV-positive: treat for toxoplasmosis with pyrimethamine and sulfadiazine (2 weeks) and repeat head CT

Progressive Multifocal Leukoencephalopathy

These brain lesions in HIV-positive patients are not associated with ring enhancement or mass effect.

There is no specific treatment. Treat HIV and raise the CD4. When HIV is improved, the lesions will disappear.

Neurocysticercosis

Look for a patient from Mexico with a seizure.

Head CT shows multiple 1 cm cystic lesions. Over time, the lesions calcify. Confirm diagnosis with serology.

Treatment is albendazole and praziquantel when the lesions are still active and uncalcified (but not when there is only calcification; in those cases, use anti-epileptic drugs). Steroids are used to prevent a reaction to dying parasites.

Posterior Reversible Encephalopathy Syndrome

This is an autoregulatory failure leading to cerebral ischemia. Look for headaches, altered consciousness, visual disturbance, and seizures in a setting of hypertensive crisis, preeclampsia, or cytotoxic medications such as cyclosporine.

MRI shows vasogenic edema in posterior lobes.

Most patients recover in 2 weeks.

Head Trauma and Intracranial Hemorrhage

With head trauma, do not use skull x-ray. If the head trauma is severe, diagnosis requires a CT scan of the head without contrast.

- If there has been **loss of consciousness (LOC)**, diagnosis requires a CT scan.
- If there has been **altered mental status**, diagnosis requires a CT scan.

	Concussion	Contusion	Subdural Hematoma	Epidural Hematoma
Focal deficits	Never	Rarely	Yes or no	Yes or no
Head CT	Normal	Ecchymosis	Crescent-shaped collection	Lens-shaped collection

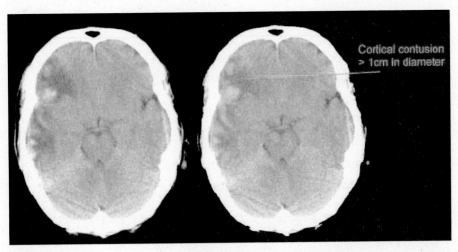

Cerebral Contusion

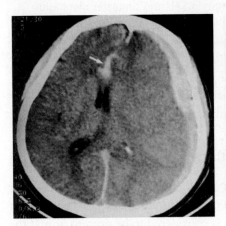

Subdural Hematoma   Epidural Hematoma

Treatment for head trauma is as follows:

- Concussion: none
- Contusion: admit as inpatient, but most cases require no treatment
- Subdural and epidural: large ones are drained; small ones are left alone to reabsorb on their own
- Large intracranial hemorrhage with mass effect
    - Decrease intracranial pressure with intubation/hyperventilation. Decrease pCO_2 to 28–32, which will constrict cerebral blood vessels.
    - Mannitol (osmotic diuretic) to decrease intracranial pressure
    - Surgical evacuation

Prophylaxis against stress ulcer (in the form of PPIs) is required for patients with any of the following conditions:

- Head trauma
- Burns
- Endotracheal intubation with mechanical ventilation

> Steroids do not help intracranial hemorrhage.

Subarachnoid Hemorrhage

Subarachnoid hemorrhage (SAH) is like the sudden onset of meningitis with LOC but without fever. Look for the following symptoms:

- Sudden, severe headache
- Stiff neck
- Photophobia
- LOC (50% of patients)
- Focal neurological deficits (30% of patients)

Basic Science Correlate

Mechanism of Blood Causing Symptoms in SAH

Blood is an irritant. It irritates the meninges in SAH and simulates meningitis. It stimulates the bowel and causes diarrhea with melena. Blood is cathartic.

Diagnostic testing is as follows:

- Head CT without contrast is 95% sensitive (**best initial test**): if that is conclusive for an SAH, no need for a lumbar puncture
- EKG: T-wave inversion
- Lumbar puncture (**most accurate test**): not needed if head CT shows blood

To determine whether increased white cells in CSF are caused by infection or are just from blood, look for the ratio: a normal number of white cells is 1 for every 500 red cells (1:500). An infection is considered to be present only if the number of white cells is greater than that.

> Normal white cell count = 1
> WBC:500 RBC

Treatment is as follows:

- Perform angiography to determine site of bleeding
- Embolize the site of the bleeding (superior to surgical clipping)
- If hydrocephalus develops, insert a ventriculoperitoneal shunt
- Prescribe nimodipine orally (CCB which prevents stroke)

When SAH occurs, an intense vasospasm can lead to a nonhemorrhagic stroke. You must embolize (or clip) the source of bleeding before it can rebleed. If it rebleeds, there is a 50% chance that the patient will die.

Spine Disorders

Spine disorders and their symptoms:

Lumbosacral Strain	Cord Compression	Epidural Abscess	Spinal Stenosis
Nontender	Tender	Tender and fever	Pain on walking downhill

Syringomyelia

Syringomyelia is a defective fluid cavity in the center of the cord. It is caused by trauma, tumor, or a congenital problem.

It presents with loss of sensation of pain and temperature in the upper extremities bilaterally in a cape-like distribution over the neck, shoulders, and down both arms.

Diagnostic testing is with an MRI. Treatment is surgical.

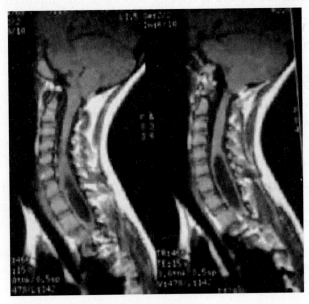

Syringomyelia

Cord Compression

Metastatic cancer presses on the cord, resulting in pain and tenderness of the spine. Lumbosacral strain does not give tenderness of the spine itself.

Scan with an MRI. The **most accurate test** is biopsy, if the diagnosis is not clear from the history.

Treatment depends on the cause. The most urgent step with cord compression is to reduce swelling with steroids.

- Spinal trauma can present with the same symptoms as cord compression: bilateral lower extremity weakness, hyperreflexia, and possible bowel/bladder dysfunction.
- There is no singular effective treatment for spinal trauma; steroids are not clearly the answer.

Spinal Epidural Abscess

A spinal epidural abscess presents with back pain with tenderness and fever.

Scan the spine with MRI. Give antibiotics against *Staphylococcus*, such as oxacillin or nafcillin. Large accumulations require surgical decompression.

Spinal Stenosis

This condition presents with leg pain on walking and can look like peripheral arterial disease. The pulses will be intact, and the pain is worse upon walking downhill, when the patient is leaning backward, but improved when walking uphill.

Diagnose with an MRI. Treat with surgical decompression.

Anterior Spinal Artery Infarction

All sensation is lost except position and vibratory sense, which travel down the posterior column. There is no specific treatment.

Brown-Sequard Syndrome

Brown-Sequard results from traumatic injury to the spine, such as a knife wound. The patient loses ipsilateral position, vibratory sense, contralateral pain, and temperature.

A 58-year-old woman with metastatic breast cancer comes in with back pain. The spine is tender. She has hyperreflexia of the legs. What is the most urgent step?

a. X-ray
b. CT
c. MRI
d. Biopsy
e. Steroids
f. Chemotherapy
g. Radiation

Answer: **E.** The most urgent step with cord compression is to relieve pressure on the cord with steroids. Imaging is done afterward if the diagnosis of cord compression is clear (as it is in this case with pain, tenderness, and signs of hyperreflexia in the legs).

Neuromuscular Disorders

Amyotrophic Lateral Sclerosis (ALS)

ALS is an idiopathic disorder of both upper and lower motor neurons.

- **Upper motor neuron signs**: hyperreflexia; upgoing toes on plantar reflex; spasticity; weakness
- **Lower motor neuron signs**: wasting; fasciculations; weakness

ALS is treated with riluzole, a unique agent that blocks the accumulation of glutamate. CO_2 retention from respiratory muscle weakness needs CPAP. Edaravone (an antioxidant) is also used in treatment.

> If an exam question asks which medication decreases progression of ALS, the answer is riluzole or edaravone. You will not be asked to choose between them.

Pseudobulbar Affect

This is a form of emotional lability or emotional incontinence characterized by intermittent episodes of inappropriate laughter or crying.

- 50% of patients with ALS have pseudobulbar affect
- Can also be caused by stroke and MS

Treatment is dextromethorphan combined with quinidine. SSRIs are effective in some patients.

Peripheral Neuropathies

Diabetes

Diabetes is the most common cause of peripheral neuropathy by far. A specific test, such as an electromyogram or nerve conduction study, is not necessary in most cases.

Treatment is gabapentin or pregabalin. Tricyclic antidepressants are less effective and have more adverse effects.

Carpal Tunnel Syndrome

Look for pain and weakness of the first 3 digits of the hand. Symptoms may worsen with repetitive use.

Initial management is a splint. In CSS, inject steroids when you move the clock forward if symptoms persist or worsen. If muscle atrophy, do surgical release.

Radial Nerve Palsy

Also known as "Saturday night palsy," this results from falling asleep or passing out with pressure on the arms underneath the body or outstretched, perhaps draped over the back of a chair. Radial nerve palsy results in a wrist drop.

Peroneal Nerve Palsy

This results from high boots pressing at the back of the knee. It results in foot drop and the inability to evert the foot. May see "high boots" in the case. Treatment is not needed; this condition will resolve on its own.

Trigeminal (5th Cranial Nerve) Neuralgia

Look for excruciating pain in the face with minor contact or touching of the tongue behind the teeth. Try carbamazepine. If not effective, try another medication such as an AED. If 2–3 sets of medications do not work, use ablation methods such as glycerol injection or laser. Carbamazepine has the highest risk of hyponatremia.

Bell Palsy (7th Cranial Nerve)

Bell palsy results in hemifacial paralysis of both the upper and lower halves of the face. There is also loss of taste on the anterior two-thirds of the tongue, hyperacusis, and the inability to close the eye at night. Hyperacusis results in the inability to control the stapedius muscle of the middle ear, which acts as a kind of "shock absorber" for sounds. Bell palsy is believed to result from a viral infection. Treatment is steroids. It is not clear that acyclovir helps.

Reflex Sympathetic Dystrophy

Reflex sympathetic dystrophy (or chronic regional pain syndrome) is seen in patients who have previous injury to the extremity. Light touch, as in a bed sheet touching the foot, results in extreme pain that is "burning" in quality. Bone abnormalities can be detected via bone scan. Treat with NSAIDs, gabapentin, and occasionally nerve block. Surgical sympathectomy may be necessary.

Restless Legs Syndrome

Restless legs syndrome (RLS) is associated with iron deficiency. It is often identified when the bed partner comes in complaining of pain and bruises in the legs. The patient experiences an uncomfortable feeling in the legs, which is relieved by movement. Treat with pramipexole or ropinirole. Iron replacement may help.

Guillain-Barré Syndrome

A man comes to the ED with weakness in his legs that has been getting markedly worse over the last few days. He has weakness and loss of deep tendon reflexes in the legs. He recalls an upper respiratory illness about 2–4 weeks ago which resolved. What is the most urgent step?

a. Steroids
b. IV immunoglobulins
c. Peak inspiratory pressure
d. Intubation
e. Lumbar puncture

Answer: **C.** Ascending weakness with loss of deep tendon reflexes is characteristic of Guillain-Barré. Peak inspiratory pressure diminishes as the diaphragm is weakened, and it predicts who will have respiratory failure before it happens. This is the most important factor in determining the need for therapy with IVIG or plasmapheresis. Steroids are not effective. Lumbar puncture will show elevated protein with no cells.

Miller Fisher syndrome is a variant of Guillain-Barré. There is descending weakness; ocular/oculomotor palsies; and antibodies against GQ1b.

Treatment is the same as for Guillain-Barré.

Myasthenia Gravis

Myasthenia gravis presents with weakness of the muscles of mastication, making it hard to finish meals. Blurry vision from diplopia results from the inability to focus the eyes on a single target. The case may classically report drooping of the eyelids as the day progresses.

- Anti-acetylcholine receptor antibodies (ACHR) (**best initial test**)
- Anti–muscle specific kinase antibodies are the answer if there is a falsely negative ACHR antibody test
- Clinical presentation and ACHR (**most accurate test**) are more sensitive and specific than an edrophonium or "Tensilon" stimulation test

Treatment is as follows:

- Pyridostigmine or neostigmine (**best initial treatment**); if no response, do thymectomy in patients age <60
  - Glycopyrrolate may reduce the side effects of pyridostigmine and neostigmine (drooling and diarrhea); it blocks adverse effects at the muscarinic receptors of the salivary gland without blocking the nicotinic receptors at the neuromuscular junction
  - Glycopyrrolate helps with COPD and decrease oral secretions during intubation
- If still no response, use prednisone; use azathioprine and cyclosporine to help keep patient off of long-term steroids
- For **acute myasthenic crisis**, assess for impending respiratory failure with peak inspiratory pressure and vital capacity. Use IV immune globulins or plasmapheresis as you would for Guillain Barre.
- Steroids

Basic Science Correlate

Mechanism of Azathioprine

Cyclosporine and azathioprine inhibit the immune system. They decrease the function of T-cells, which control cellular immunity such as organ transplant rejection. The drugs do not decrease T-cell numbers, just function.

Lambert-Eaton Myasthenic Syndrome (LEMS)

- Weakness improved by repetitive movement
- Hyporeflexia
- Test for anti-voltage gated calcium channel antibodies
- Lung cancer in 50%
- Treatment is amifampridine or dalfampridine

Cardiology 2

Ischemic Heart Disease

Coronary artery disease (CAD) is the most common cause of death in the United States by far and kills 10 times more women than breast cancer.

Risk factors include:

- Diabetes mellitus (most dangerous risk factor)
- Hypertension
- Tobacco use
- Hyperlipidemia
- Peripheral arterial disease (PAD)
- Obesity
- Inactivity
- Family history (family member must be young, i.e., females age <65, males age <55)

Stress is not a clear risk factor since it cannot be measured precisely.

Risk factors are useful for answering diagnostic questions in equivocal cases. They are useful in that modifying them can lower mortality.

- Symptoms include chest pain that does not change with body position or respiration
- Besides chest pain, other clues to ischemic disease as the cause of chest pain are dull pain; lasts 15–30 minutes; occurs on exertion; substernal location; and radiates to the jaw or left arm
- Not associated with chest wall tenderness

When any one of the following features is present, the patient has something *other* than CAD.

- Pleuritic pain (changes with respiration): pulmonary embolism; pneumonia; pleuritis; pericarditis; pneumothorax
- Positional pain (changes with body position): pericarditis
- Tenderness (pain on palpation): costochondritis

> The most common cause of chest pain that is not cardiac in etiology is a gastrointestinal (acid reflux) problem.

a. A patient comes to the ED with chest pain. The pain also occurs in the epigastric area and is associated with a sore throat, a bad metallic taste in the mouth, and a cough. What do you recommend?

b. An alcoholic patient comes to the ED with chest pain. There is nausea and vomiting and epigastric tenderness. What do you recommend?

c. A patient comes to the ED with chest pain. There is right-upper quadrant tenderness and mild fever. What do you recommend?

Answers:

a. Proton pump inhibitor

b. Check amylase and lipase levels

c. Abdominal sonogram for gallstones

There is nothing unique or pathognomonic about the physical findings of ischemic heart disease. Physical findings such as tenderness only tell you the patient does not have ischemic disease. There is no buzzword for physical examination of CAD that indicates, "Aha! This is coronary disease."

However, for CCS, it is critical to know what could be abnormal so you know which pieces of the physical to choose.

Piece of Physical Exam	Findings That Could Be Abnormal
Cardiovascular (CV)	S3 gallop: Dilated left ventricle S4 gallop: Left ventricular hypertrophy Jugulovenous distention Holosystolic murmur of mitral regurgitation
Chest	Rales suggestive of congestive heart failure
General exam	Distressed patient, short of breath, clutching chest
Extremities	Edema

Basic Science Correlate

Mechanism of S3 and S4 Gallop

- **S3 gallop** is rapid ventricular filling during diastole. As soon as the mitral valve opens, blood rushes into the ventricle, causing a splash sound transmitted as an S3.

- **S4 gallop** is the sound of atrial systole into a stiff or noncompliant left ventricle. It is heard just before S1 and occurs with any left ventricular hypertrophy. S4 is the bang of atrial systole.

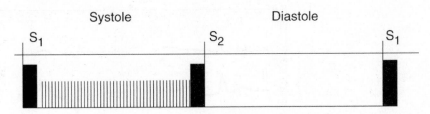

Holosystolic Murmur: Mitral Regurgitation

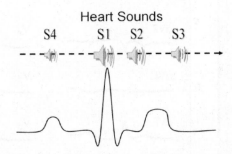

Heart Sounds

CCS Tip: Jugular veins on Step 3 CCS are in the CV exam, not the HEENT exam.

On Step 3, most cases of chest pain will have a clear diagnosis and will ask for the next step in management.

- **Best initial test** for ischemic-type pain: EKG (always)
- **Wrong "best initial test"**: troponin, CK-MB, stress test, echocardiogram, angiography
  - Do not eliminate the need for aspirin first
  - In a computerized CCS, however, answer all of these at the same time
- In a clear case of ischemic pain, if you are asked to choose between EKG and aspirin, nitrates, oxygen, and morphine, choose treatment first.
- CK-MB and troponin (**best tests to detect a reinfarction a few days after the initial infarction**): both CK-MB and troponin rise at 3–6 hours after the start of chest pain; they have nearly the same specificity. CK-MB stays elevated for only 1–2 days, while troponin stays elevated for 1–2 weeks.
- Myoglobin (rises first of all cardiac enzymes, as early as 1–4 hours after the start of chest pain)
- Stress test (when case is not acute and initial EKG/enzyme tests do not establish the diagnosis)

CCS Tip: When the question asks for the **most accurate test**, answer CK-MB or troponin.

CCS Tip: LDH isoenzymes or LDH level is always the wrong answer.

> Do not answer "consultation" for single best answer questions. However, "consultation" is okay to answer as a part of CCS management.
>
> In single best answer questions, a consultant should not be necessary when ordering an EKG, checking enzymes, and giving aspirin to a patient with acute coronary syndrome.

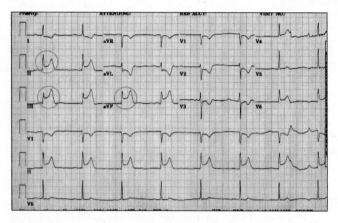

ST Elevation

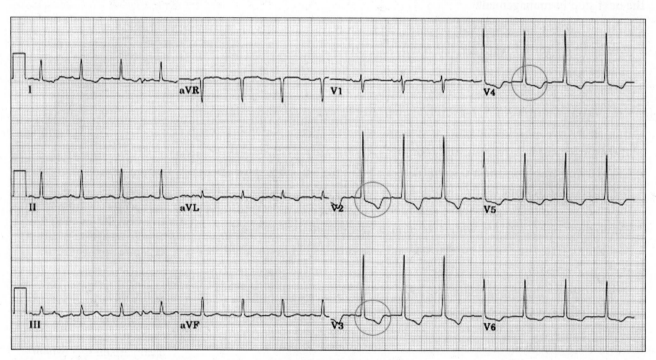

ST Depression

T-Wave Inversion

Basic Science Correlate

- Troponin **C** binds to calcium to activate actin:myosin interaction
- Troponin **T** binds to tropomyosin
- Troponin **I** blocks or inhibits actin:myosin interaction

A 56-year-old man comes to the office a few days after an episode of chest pain for which he went to the ED. This was his first episode of pain and he has no risk factors. In the ED, he had a normal EKG and normal CK-MB and was released the next day. Which of the following is most appropriate next step?

a. Repeat CK-MB
b. Statin
c. LDL level
d. Stress (exercise tolerance) test
e. Angiography

Answer: **D.** Stress test is needed when the case is equivocal or uncertain about the presence of CAD. Exercise tolerance, or "stress test" detects CAD when heart rate is raised and ST segment depression is detected. Do not do angiography unless the stress test is abnormal. This case is asking you to know that a stress test is a way to increase the sensitivity of detection of CAD beyond an EKG and enzymes.

> The Step 3 exam loves the phrase "further management."

When is **dipyridamole or adenosine thallium stress test or dobutamine echo** the answer?

- When patients cannot exercise to target heart rate >85% of maximum: COPD; amputation; deconditioning; weakness/previous stroke; lower extremity ulcer; dementia; obesity

When is **exercise thallium test or stress echocardiogram** the answer?

- When EKG is unreadable for ischemia: left bundle branch block; digoxin use; pacemaker in place; left ventricular hypertrophy; any baseline abnormality of ST segment of EKG

A 63-year-old woman comes in for evaluation of an abnormal stress test that shows an area of reversible ischemia. She has no risk factors for CAD. What is the best next step in management?

a. Troponin level
b. Angiography
c. Coronary bypass
d. Echocardiogram
e. Nuclear ventriculogram (MUGA scan)

Answer: **B.** Angiography is the next diagnostic test to evaluate an abnormal stress test that shows "reversible" ischemia. Reversible ischemia is the most dangerous thing a stress test can show. If the test shows "fixed" defects, i.e., defects unchanged between exercise and rest, those are scars from previous infarctions which require no angiography. Coronary bypass would be the next step only if the angiogram has already been done. Echocardiogram would be the **best initial test** to evaluate valve function or ventricular wall motion. MUGA scan would be the most accurate method to evaluate ejection fraction.

> Sestamibi nuclear stress testing is used in obese patients and those with large breasts because of its ability to penetrate tissue.

> **Basic Science Correlate**
>
> **Mechanism of Thallium**
>
> Nuclear isotopes are picked up by the Na/K ATPase of normal myocardium. If cardiac tissue is alive and perfused, it will pick up the nuclear isotope. To the myocardium, thallium looks like potassium.
>
> **Decreased uptake = Damage**

A patient admitted 5 days ago for a myocardial infarction has a new episode of chest pain. Which of the following is the most specific method for establishing the diagnosis of a new infarction?

a. CK-MB

b. Troponin

c. Echocardiogram

d. Stress testing

e. Angiography

Answer: **A.** CK-MB level should return to normal 2–3 days after a myocardial infarction. If a reinfarction has occurred, the level will elevate again 5 days later, while the troponin level will still be up from the original infarction. Troponin can be elevated for 2 weeks after an infarction. Angiography can detect obstructive, stenotic lesions but cannot detect myocardial necrosis. Stress test should never be performed if the patient is having current chest pain (and chest pain is a reason to stop a stress test). Echo will show decreased wall movement, but this could have been present from the previous cardiac injury.

Acute Coronary Syndrome (ACS)

ACS can be defined as follows:

- Causes acute chest pain
- Can be with exercise or at rest
- Can have ST segment elevation, depression, or even a normal EKG
- Not based on enzyme levels, angiography, or stress test results
- Based on a history of chest pain with features suggestive of ischemic disease

The Step 3 exam is very big on knowing which treatments will lower mortality.

Treatment is as follows:

- Aspirin (**best initial treatment**) administered orally, chewed, or absorbed under the tongue; has an instant effect on inhibiting platelets.
  - Aspirin alone reduces mortality by 25% for acute myocardial infarction
  - Aspirin alone reduces mortality by 50% for "unstable angina," which may become a non-ST segment elevation myocardial infarction
- Clopidogrel or ticagrelor for acute myocardial infarction

- Prasugrel if angioplasty is done
- Nitrates and morphine (have no effect on mortality)
- Oxygen if patient is hypoxic

> Clopidogrel, ticagrelor, or prasugrel is given to everyone getting angioplasty and a stent. These medications inhibit ADP activation of platelets.

Basic Science Correlate

Mechanism of P2Y$_{12}$ Antagonists

Clopidogrel, prasugrel, and ticagrelor block aggregation of platelets to each other by inhibiting ADP-induced activation of the P2Y$_{12}$ receptor. Clopidogrel and prasugrel are in the thienopyridine class.

ST Segment Elevation Myocardial Infarction (STEMI)

Angioplasty and **thrombolytics** both lower mortality in STEMI, but the timing of their administration is critical. Their benefit markedly diminishes with time.

- Angioplasty, a type of percutaneous coronary intervention (PCI), must be performed within 90 minutes of arrival at the ED for a STEMI; in stable angina it does not decrease mortality in more than medical therapy alone (aspirin, beta blockers, and statins).
  - Infarction is the single best evidence for mortality benefit with angioplasty.
  - Primary angioplasty is angioplasty during an acute episode of chest pain.
- If angioplasty cannot be performed within 90 minutes, give thrombolytics. Give thrombolytics within 30 minutes of arrival at the ED.
- One indication for thrombolytics is when chest pain <12 hours and there is ST segment elevation in ≥2 leads.
- Another indication is new LBBB.

> Re when to give angioplasty, the Step 3 exam question will state that "the patient is at a small rural hospital" or "the nearest catheterization facility is 90 minutes away." The question must be clear on this point.

Beta blockers lower mortality, but the timing of their administration is not critical.

- Beta blockers such as metoprolol can be given, but that is less urgent than aspirin, thrombolytics, or primary angioplasty.
- Angiotensin converting enzyme (ACE) inhibitor or angiotensin receptor blocker (ARB) should be given to all patients with an ACS, but mortality will be lowered only if there is left ventricular dysfunction or systolic dysfunction.
- Start every patient with CAD on HMG CoA reductase inhibitors.
- Treatment with HMG CoA reductase inhibitors is not based on a specific LDL level.

Statins such as atorvastatin should be given to all patients with an ACS—regardless of EKG result, troponin level, or CK-MB level.

Prasugrel is added only for angioplasty.

When is **urgent angioplasty or PCI** the answer?

- When the question asks, "What has the single greatest efficacy?" in lowering mortality in STEMI and a contraindication to the use of thrombolytics is included.

CCS Tip: CCS requires you to know the route of administration of medications.

Basic Science Correlate

Mechanism of Thrombolytics

Thrombolytics activate plasminogen into plasmin. Plasmin chops up fresh or newly formed fibrin strands into D-dimers.

That is why all clots elevate levels of D-dimers. After several hours, the fibrin clot has been stabilized (made more permanent) by factor XIII. Once stabilized by factor XIII, plasmin will not cleave fibrin.

Basic Science Correlate

Mechanism of Beta Blockers in Myocardial Infarction

The most common cause of death in both CHF and MI is a ventricular arrhythmia brought on by ischemia.

Beta blockers are both anti-arrhythmic and anti-ischemic. Slower heart rate means more time for coronary artery perfusion. Increased left ventricular filling time increases both stroke volume and cardiac output.

CCS Tip: CCS and Step 3 do not require you to know doses.

A 72-year-old man comes to the ED with chest pain for the last hour. Initial EKG shows ST segment elevation in leads V2–V4. Aspirin is given. Which of the following will most likely benefit this patient?

a. CK-MB
b. Stress test
c. Angioplasty
d. Metoprolol
e. Diltiazem
f. Atorvastatin
g. Digoxin
h. Amiodarone
i. Oxygen, morphine, and nitrates
j. Thrombolytics

$P2Y_{12}$ = ADP receptor antagonist

Answer: **C.** Angioplasty will lower the risk of mortality most, if it can be obtained within 90 minutes. Metoprolol lowers mortality but is not dependent on how soon you give it, as long as the patient receives it before going home.

Therapies Used in ACS		
Always Lower Mortality	**Lower Mortality in Certain Conditions**	**Do Not Lower Mortality**
• Aspirin • Thrombolytics • Primary angioplasty • Metoprolol • Statins • Clopidogrel, prasugrel, or ticagrelor	• ACE inhibitors if ejection fraction is low • ARBs if ejection fraction is low • Heparin if ST depression	• Oxygen • Morphine • Nitrates • CCBs • Lidocaine • Amiodarone

When is **prasugrel, clopidogrel,** or **ticagrelor** the answer?

- When there is aspirin allergy, the patient is to undergo angioplasty, or there is an acute infarction occurring
- Ticlopidine is associated with neutropenia
- With acute MI, add one of these drugs to aspirin

When is **verapamil** or **diltiazem** the answer?

- When patient has an intolerance to beta blockers, such as severe reactive airway disease (asthma); cocaine-induced chest pain, or coronary vasospasm/ Prinzmetal angina

When is **lidocaine** or **amiodarone** the answer for acute MI?

- When there is ventricular tachycardia (VT) or ventricular fibrillation
- Do not give prophylactically

When is a **pacemaker** the answer for acute MI?

- Third-degree AV block
- Mobitz II, second-degree AV block
- Bifascicular block
- New LBBB
- Symptomatic bradycardia

Complications of Myocardial Infarction (MI)

All the complications of MI lead to hypotension. The Step 3 exam will typically give you the diagnosis and ask for next steps in management.

- Clopidogrel or ticagrelor is used in the following scenarios:
  - Acute MI
  - Patient undergoes angioplasty and stenting
  - Aspirin allergy
- Prasugrel has greater efficacy than clopidogrel but it increases bleeding in those age >75 and weight <60 kg.
- Do not use with stroke because it increases CNC bleeding.

Diagnosis	Diagnostic Test	Treatment
Cardiogenic shock	Echo, Swan-Ganz (right heart) catheter	ACEI, urgent revascularization
Valve rupture	Echo	ACEI, nitroprusside, intra-aortic balloon pump as a bridge to surgery
Septal rupture	Echo, right heart catheter showing a step up in saturation from the right atrium to right ventricle	ACEI, nitroprusside, and urgent surgery
Myocardial wall rupture	Echo	Pericardiocentesis, urgent cardiac repair
Sinus bradycardia	EKG	Atropine, followed by pacemaker if there are still symptoms
Third-degree (complete) heart block	EKG, canon "a" waves	Atropine and a pacemaker even if symptoms resolve
Right ventricular infarction	EKG showing right ventricular leads	Fluid loading

---

Basic Science Correlate

Mechanism of Septal Rupture Systolic Murmur

Left ventricular pressure is greater than right ventricular pressure. This causes left-to-right shunt of oxygenated blood.

Oxygen saturation in the right ventricle is markedly increased compared with the right atrium.

All patients post-MI should go home on aspirin, clopidogrel (or prasugrel), a beta blocker, a statin, and an ACE inhibitor.

A patient's wife comes to take her husband home after an MI and asks how long they should wait before they have sex. What do you tell her?

a. No waiting necessary
b. 2–6 weeks
c. After echocardiography
d. Wait for a normal angiography

Answer: **B.** Some waiting is necessary to have sex after an infarction. Sex minimally increases the risk of infarction. The duration and the intensity of exertion are sufficient to provoke ischemia in some cases.

Non-ST Segment Elevation Myocardial Infarction (NSTEMI)

Management of NSTEMI differs from STEMI in the following ways:

- No thrombolytic use
- Heparin used routinely (low molecular weight heparin is superior to IV unfractionated heparin)
- Glycoprotein IIb/IIIa inhibitors lower mortality, particularly in those undergoing angioplasty

A 54-year-old man with a history of diabetes and hypertension comes to the ED with crushing, substernal chest pain that radiates to his left arm. The pain has been on and off for several hours, with this last episode being 30 minutes in duration. He has had chest pain on exertion before but this is the first time it has developed at rest. EKG is normal. Aspirin, oxygen, and nitrates have been given. Troponin levels are elevated. Which of the following is most likely to benefit this patient?

a. Low molecular weight (LMW) heparin
b. Thrombolytics
c. Diltiazem
d. Morphine
e. CK-MB level

Answer: **A.** LMW heparin is the only choice here that has been shown to produce lower mortality. Thrombolytics do not lower mortality, unless there is ST elevation or a new LBBB. Positive cardiac enzymes are not an indication for thrombolytics. Other answers that could be right if they were choices are GPIIb/IIIa inhibitors, such as eptifibatide, tirofiban, or abciximab, or the use of angioplasty/PCI.

> **GPIIb/IIIa inhibitors**
> with ACS work best when used in combination with angioplasty and stent placement. Abciximab does not benefit STEMI.

> Thrombolytics are used only if there is ST segment elevation or a new LBBB within 12 hours of the onset of chest pain.

Basic Science Correlate

Mechanism of Heparin

Heparin potentiates the effect of antithrombin. Antithrombin actually inhibits almost every step of the clotting cascade. This is why it does not work with antithrombin deficiency.

Heparin only prevents new clots from forming.

Chronic CAD

Office-based cases of further management will emphasize the same issues of mortality benefit. Treatment is as follows:

- Aspirin and metoprolol, because of their benefit on mortality
- Nitrates for angina pain (have no benefit on mortality)
- ACE inhibitors and ARBs only in further management for stable cases if the question describes congestive failure, systolic dysfunction, or low ejection fraction

> ARBs are used interchangeably with ACE inhibitors, especially if the patient has a cough with ACE inhibitors. Both ACE and ARBs cause hyperkalemia.

Coronary angiography is used to determine who is a candidate for coronary artery bypass grafting (CABG). You do not need to do angiography to diagnose CAD; stress testing can show "reversible ischemia." However, angiography is needed to identify who needs CABG.

You do not need to do angiography to initiate the following:

- Aspirin + metoprolol (mortality benefit)
- Nitrates (pain)
- ACE/ARB (low ejection fraction)

- Clopidogrel, prasugrel, or ticagrelor (acute MI or cannot tolerate aspirin)
- Statins
- If pain persists, add ranolazine

Indications for CABG include:

- Three coronary vessels with >70% stenosis
- Left main coronary artery stenosis >50–70%
- 2 vessels in a diabetic
- 2 or 3 vessels with low ejection fraction

> Systolic dysfunction = heart failure with reduced ejection fraction (**HFrEF**)

> Ranolazine, an anti-angina medication, is added if other medications do not control pain.

Which of the following is the main difference between saphenous vein graft and internal mammary artery graft?

a. Less need for aspirin and metoprolol with internal mammary artery graft
b. Warfarin is needed with saphenous vein graft
c. Internal mammary artery graft remains open for 10 years
d. Heparin is needed for vein graft

Answer: **C.** Vein grafts start to become occluded after 5 years while internal mammary artery grafts are often patent at 10 years. There is no difference in the need for medications.

Lipid Management

The standards for the management of hyperlipidemia are currently in a state of change. Questions on Step 3 will not engage in controversy, so you will be asked only clear-cut questions.

The clear standards are as follows:

- Statins are by far superior to any other drug. Every patient with coronary disease and stroke should be on a statin, and most patients with diabetes should be on a statin.
- If the question says "greater than 7.5% 10-year risk," then a statin is the answer.
- Proprotein convertase subtilisin kexin type 9 (PCSK9) inhibitors reduce LDL but the mortality benefit is not clear.

The goal of treatment in those with CAD is LDL <70 mg/dL. The single strongest indication for lipid-lowering therapy is for a statin in a patient with an ACS.

Statins

Anyone with an ACS syndrome needs to be on a statin.

The concept of "goal-directed" therapy to a specific LDL is not clear at this time. On the exam, if you are asked for LDL goal in a patient with CAD *and* diabetes, the answer is LDL goal at least <70 mg/dL.

These CAD equivalents require a statin for any level of LDL:

- PAD
- Aortic disease
- Carotid disease
- Cerebrovascular disease

Risk factors in lipid management include:

- Tobacco use (cigarette smoking)
- High blood pressure (≥140/90 mm Hg or on blood pressure medication)
- Low HDL cholesterol (<40 mg/dL)
- Family history of early coronary heart disease (female relatives age <65, male relatives age <55)
- Age (males ≥45, females ≥55)

Statins do have some side effects, most commonly liver toxicity. About 2% of patients will stop a statin because of its effect on raising transaminases. Check LFTs routinely.

Rhabdomyolysis is another side effect, less common. There is no routine indication to check CPK level.

Many medications—such as statins, cholestyramine, gemfibrozil, ezetimibe, and niacin, lower LDL—lower triglycerides and total cholesterol, and raise HDL. Which of the following is the most important reason for using statins?

a. Fewer adverse effects
b. Lower cost
c. Greater patient acceptance
d. Greatest mortality benefit
e. Greatest effect on lowering LDL

Answer: **D.** Statins have a greater effect on lowering mortality than any other medications. Recent guidelines will be further clarified over time. Give a statin if the 10-year risk >7.5%. This is very hard to put in Step 3 unless there is a risk calculator in the question.

When is the goal of therapy LDL <70 mg/dL?

a. CHF
b. Diabetes
c. Coronary disease and carotid disease
d. Coronary disease and diabetes
e. Diabetes and hypertension

Answer: **D.** LDL goal can be <70 mg/dL for patients at the very highest risk of infarction, i.e., those who have ACS and those with both coronary disease plus a severe risk factor such as diabetes.

Who gets a statin?
- CAD
- PAD
- Aortic disease
- Carotid disease
- cerebral disease
- Diabetes + LDL >100
- 10-year risk >7.5%

PCSK9 Inhibitors

When a maximum dose of statin is used to control severe hyperlipidemia, yet LDL is still not controlled, consider PCSK9 inhibitors. These are injectable medications which block the clearance of LDL by the liver from the blood.

- PCSK9 inhibitors can bring down enormously elevated levels of LDL in familial hypercholesterolemia.
- Evolocumab and alirocumab massively increase hepatic clearance of LDL but do not clearly lower mortality.

Sex and the Heart

Post MI, patients can resume sexual activity within several days if there are no further symptoms of chest pain or dyspnea. This should coincide with the time that the patient is ready for discharge. The duration of an individual sexual event is only 5–7 minutes, which is less than the duration of a stress test.

A man develops erectile dysfunction after an infarction. What is the most common cause?

a. Metoprolol
b. Nitrates
c. ACE inhibitors
d. Aspirin
e. Anxiety

Answer: **E.** Anxiety is the most common cause of erectile dysfunction postinfarction. Although beta blockers may be the most common medication associated with erectile dysfunction, anxiety is still a more common cause of erectile dysfunction than beta blockers.

A man develops erectile dysfunction postinfarction. You are planning to start sildenafil. Which of the following medications must be stopped?

a. Metoprolol
b. Nitrates
c. ACE inhibitors
d. Aspirin
e. Statins

Answer: **B.** Nitrates are contraindicated when medications such as sildenafil are to be used. If used at the same time, they can cause a dangerous level of hypotension.

Congestive Heart Failure (CHF)

The mechanism that matters for congestive failure has to do with the difference in treatment between systolic dysfunction with a low ejection fraction and diastolic dysfunction and a normal ejection fraction.

There is no clear way to distinguish systolic from diastolic dysfunction from symptoms alone. Clues in the history are hypertension, valvular heart disease, and myocardial infarction.

CHF presents with shortness of breath, particularly on exertion, in a person with any of the following:

- Edema
- Rales on lung examination
- Ascites
- Jugular venous distention
- S3 gallop
- Orthopnea
- Paroxysmal nocturnal dyspnea
- Fatigue

> S3: splash
> S4: bang

Basic Science Correlate

Mechanism of Rales

Increased hydrostatic pressure develops in the pulmonary capillaries from left heart pressure overload. This causes transudation of liquid into the alveoli. During inhalation, the alveoli open with a "popping" sound referred to as rales.

Pulmonary Edema

Pulmonary edema is the worst manifestation of CHF. It is a clinical diagnosis.

More important than any diagnostic testing is to remove volume from the vascular system (and thus from the lungs). Shortness of breath, rales, S3, and orthopnea are more important for establishing the diagnosis than any single test.

CCS Tip: On CCS, move the clock forward no more than 15–30 minutes at a time for acutely unstable ICU or ED patients.

Basic Science Correlate

Mechanism of Carvedilol

Carvedilol is an antagonist of both beta-1 and beta-2 receptors as well as alpha-1 receptors. This makes it anti-arrhythmic, anti-ischemic, and antihypertensive.

All of the following tests should be ordered on the first screen on the CCS portion. Order them with the initial therapy (i.e., with the oxygen, furosemide, nitrates, and morphine).

Initial Test to Be Ordered	What it Shows
Chest x-ray	• Pulmonary vascular congestion • Cephalization of flow • Effusion • Cardiomegaly
EKG	• Sinus tachycardia • Atrial and ventricular arrhythmia
Oximeter (consider ordering arterial blood gases)	• Hypoxia • Respiratory alkalosis
Echocardiogram	• Distinguishes systolic from diastolic dysfunction

A 63-year-old woman comes to the ED with acute, severe shortness of breath; rales on lung exam; S3 gallop; and orthopnea. What is the next step?

a. Chest x-ray

b. Oxygen, furosemide, nitrates, and morphine

c. Echocardiogram

d. Digoxin

e. ACE inhibitors

f. Carvedilol

Answer: **B.** Oxygen, furosemide, nitrates, and morphine are the mainstay of therapy for acute pulmonary edema. Although they are not associated with a concrete mortality benefit, they are the standard of care for pulmonary edema.

Basic Science Correlate

Mechanism of "Cephalization" of Flow

The bases or bottom of the lungs are generally more "full" of blood because of gravity. As fluid builds up in the lungs, it fills the vessels from the bottom to the top, like a cup filling with water. This moves the fluid toward the head, a process called "cephalization."

Mechanism of Dobutamine, Inamrinone, and Milrinone

Inamrinone and milrinone are phosphodiesterase inhibitors. They increase contractility and decrease afterload as vasodilators, yielding much the same effect as dobutamine. Dobutamine is less effective for those on beta blockers. Dopamine increases contractility, but dopamine's alpha-1 agonist activity causes vasoconstriction. This increases afterload.

Mechanism of Respiratory Alkalosis in CHF

Fluid overload causes hypoxia. Hypoxia causes hyperventilation. Hyperventilation decreases pCO_2. Decreased pCO_2 causes alkalosis. Hence, hypoxia causes respiratory alkalosis.

CCS Tip: On CCS, the order in which the tests and treatments are written on the screen does not matter, as long as they are written at the same time. Pulmonary edema is a good example: order all tests at the same time as the treatment.

> Cases of pulmonary edema and myocardial infarction should be placed in the ICU.

Treatment is as follows:

- Acute CHF
  - Preload reduction to control the acute symptoms (high success rate)
  - If no response, positive inotrope (but not proven to lower mortality); also use in a CCS case of pulmonary edema when furosemide, oxygen, nitrates, and morphine are given but patient is still short of breath after clock is moved forward
  - Digoxin is never used for acute treatment; it can be used to slow the rate of a-fib

- Chronic CHF
  - Echocardiogram once patient stabilizes, to establish if there is systolic dysfunction with low ejection fraction or diastolic dysfunction with normal ejection fraction
  - For **systolic dysfunction**
    - ○ ACE inhibitors, ARBs, beta blockers e.g., metoprolol, carvedilol (for any stage of disease); if those are contraindicated, use hydralazine + nitrates (hydralazine acts to reduce afterload)
    - ○ Digoxin to decrease symptoms and frequency of hospitalization (but does not lower mortality in CHF)
    - ○ Mineralocorticoid receptor antagonists (MRAs), e.g., spironolactone, eplerenone, to lower mortality in those with systolic dysfunction
      - Spironolactone if patient originally presents with pulmonary edema; side effects include gynecomastia and erectile dysfunction in men
      - Eplerenone lowers mortality in CHF without anti-androgenic side effects
      - Most common side effect of MRA is hyperkalemia; when mild hyperkalemia is described and you need to lower mortality with an ACE, ARB, MRA, or even beta blockers due to inhibiting the Na/K ATPase, give patiromer (an oral calcium/potassium exchange medication) to allow continued use of those medications
      - Diuretics have not been proven to lower mortality
    - ○ If patient is on ACE inhibitor, beta blocker, MRA, digoxin, and diuretic but is still symptomatic, add hydralazine and nitrates to decrease symptoms
  - For **diastolic dysfunction**, use MRAs (caution not to overuse diuretics); ACE inhibitors have unclear benefit and digoxin is of no benefit.

Positive Inotropic Agents Used Intravenously in the ICU	
• Dobutamine (drug of choice) • Inamrinone • Milrinone	Used as further management of acute pulmonary edema cases after the clock is moved forward 30–60 minutes and there is no response to preload reduction

An 80-year-old woman is admitted to the ICU for acute pulmonary edema. She has rales to the apices and jugulovenous distention. EKG shows ventricular tachycardia. Which of the following is the best therapy?

a. Synchronized cardioversion
b. Unsynchronized cardioversion
c. Lidocaine
d. Amiodarone
e. Procainamide

Answer: A. Synchronized cardioversion is used when VT is associated with acute pulmonary edema. The same answer would be used if the acute pulmonary edema was associated with the onset of a-fib, flutter, or supraventricular tachycardia. Unsynchronized cardioversion is used for ventricular fibrillation or VT without a pulse. Medical therapy such as lidocaine or amiodarone can be used for sustained VT that is hemodynamically stable.

> "Synchronized" = Timing with cardiac cycle

When is **nesiritide** the answer?

- To treat acute pulmonary edema as a part of preload reduction, only if dobutamine or the phosphodiesterase inhibitors inamrinone and milrinone fail; nesiritide is a synthetic version of atrial natriuretic peptide, which decreases symptoms of shortness of breath but is not clearly associated with a reduction in mortality

When is a **brain natriuretic peptide (BNP)** level the answer?

- To establish a diagnosis of CHF if a patient is short of breath; it can help to distinguish between pulmonary embolus, pneumonia, asthma, and CHF
- BNP elevates in CHF but is nonspecific; a normal BNP level will exclude CHF

A patient comes with pulmonary edema. A right heart catheter is placed. Which of the following readings is most likely to be found?

	Cardiac Output	Systemic Vascular Resistance	Wedge Pressure	Right Atrial Pressure
a.	Decreased	Increased	Increased	Increased
b.	Decreased	Increased	Decreased	Decreased
c.	Increased	Decreased	Decreased	Decreased
d.	Decreased	Increased	Decreased	Increased

Answer: A. Pulmonary edema is associated with decreased cardiac output because of pump failure, which results in the backup of blood into the left atrium and an increased wedge pressure. There is also an increased right atrial pressure, which is the same as saying jugular venous distention. Increases in sympathetic outflow will increase systemic vascular resistance in an attempt to maintain intravascular filling pressure. Choice B represents hypovolemic shock, e.g., dehydration. Choice C represents septic shock, which is driven by massive systemic vasodilation, e.g., from gram-negative sepsis. Choice D represents pulmonary hypertension.

> ## Basic Science Correlate
>
> **Mechanism of Increased Wedge Pressure in CHF**
>
> Wedge pressure = Left atrial (LA) pressure
>
> The inflated balloon blocks pressure from behind catheter, making the catheter tip pick up flow from "in front," or downstream. "Downstream" for the pulmonary capillaries means the left atrium.
>
> **LV failure = Increased LA pressure = Increased wedge pressure**

Treatment of Chronic CHF

Once patients with acute pulmonary edema have been stabilized, they should get an echocardiogram to establish whether there is systolic dysfunction with low ejection fraction or diastolic dysfunction with normal ejection fraction.

Long-term management of dilated cardiomyopathy or systolic dysfunction is based on the following:

- ACE inhibitors (or ARBs), beta blockers, and mineralocorticoid receptor antagonist (MRAs) such as spironolactone and eplerenone
- Beta blockers that have proven to lower mortality in CHF are metoprolol, carvedilol, and bisoprolol.
- ACE inhibitors and beta blockers are indicated for CHF patients with systolic dysfunction at any stage of disease.
- If ACE inhibitors or ARBs cannot be used, use hydralazine combined with nitrates (hydralazine acts to reduce afterload).
- If a patient is on ACE inhibitors, beta blockers, MRAs, digoxin, and diuretics but is still symptomatic, add hydralazine and nitrates to decrease symptoms.
- Digoxin is used to decrease symptoms and frequency of hospitalization but has not been proven to lower mortality in congestive failure.
- Diuretics have not been proven to lower mortality.
- MRAs (e.g., spironolactone or eplerenone) lower mortality in those with systolic dysfunction
  - Spironolactone is anti-androgenic. It can cause gynecomastia and erectile dysfunction in men. Eplerenone lowers mortality in CHF without anti-androgenic side effects.
  - The most common side effect of MRA is hyperkalemia; when mild hyperkalemia is described and you need to use a medication that lowers mortality, i.e., ACE, ARB, MRA, or even beta blocker due to inhibiting the Na/K ATPase, give patiromer (an oral calcium/potassium exchange medication) or zirconium to allow continued use of those medications.
- For diastolic dysfunction, use MRA (caution not to overuse diuretics); ACE inhibitors have unclear benefit and digoxin is of no benefit.

The patient is still dyspneic after using ACE inhibitors, beta blockers, diuretics, digoxin, and mineralocorticoid inhibitors. What is the next step?

Answer:

- Sacubitril/valsartan: This combination is used instead of an ACE inhibitor. Sacubitril is added only to an ARB; this neprilysin inhibitor has a mortality benefit for systolic dysfunction.
- Ivabradine: SA nodal inhibitor of "funny channels" that slows the heart rate. Add it to systolic dysfunction if pulse >70 beats/min or beta blockers cannot be used. There is no mortality benefit with ivabradine. Since ivabradine blocks the SA node, it only works if the patient is in sinus rhythm.

> Most likely ivabradine question: What CHF med causes transient excess brightness of vision?

Further management of CHF calls for the following treatments:

Systolic Dysfunction (Low Ejection Fraction)	Diastolic Dysfunction (Normal Ejection Fraction)
• ACEI or ARB • Metoprolol, carvedilol, or bisoprolol • Spironolactone or eplerenone • Diuretics • Digoxin • Hydralazine/nitrates • Sacubitril with valsartan	• MRAs: spironolactone, eplerenone

> The single most important fact about the "further management" of CHF is that ACE/ARB, beta blockers, and spironolactone decrease mortality. Digoxin decreases symptoms but does not lower mortality.

A 69-year-old man is seen in the office for further management of congestive heart failure. He currently has no symptoms and good exercise tolerance. He has been on lisinopril, metoprolol, spironolactone, and furosemide for the last 6 months. His ejection fraction is 23%. Which of the following is most likely to benefit this patient?

a. Intermittent dobutamine therapy
b. Digoxin
c. Cardiac transplantation
d. Implantable cardioverter/defibrillator
e. Chlorthalidone

Answer: **D.** Implantable cardioverter/defibrillators are indicated in dilated cardiomyopathy. The most common cause of death in CHF is sudden death from arrhythmia. Those with ejection fraction below 35% that persists are candidates for implantable defibrillator placement.

When is **biventricular pacemaker** the answer for CHF?

- When there is severe congestive failure with ejection fraction <35% and QRS >120 msec (also called "cardiac resynchronization therapy"). The wider the QRS, the greater the benefit. When QRS >150 msec, there is a greater decrease in mortality and symptom reduction.

When is **warfarin** the answer for CHF?

- When there is a-fib in the presence of a metal valve or mitral stenosis. Otherwise, there is no place for routine anticoagulation with warfarin, no matter how low the ejection fraction may be in CHF.

> If the patient is still short of breath and QRS is wide (>120), then resynchronize with a biventricular pacer.

> **Basic Science Correlate**
>
> **Mechanism of Biventricular Pacemaker**
>
> Wide QRS means ventricles are not beating together. Ventricles not beating together means inefficient forward flow, like trying to hop on one leg. Biventricular pacemaker means both ventricles go back to beating at same time. Effect instant.

Which of the following is an absolute contraindication to the use of beta blockers?

a. Symptomatic bradycardia

b. PAD

c. Asthma

d. Emphysema

e. Diabetes

Answer: **A.** Symptomatic bradycardia is an absolute contraindication for the use of beta blockers. The overwhelming majority of patients with PAD can still use beta blockers. About 70% of asthma patients can tolerate beta blockers. In a patient with a myocardial infarction, the mortality benefit of metoprolol far exceeds the risk of its use when asthma, emphysema, or PAD is present.

Valvular Heart Disease

All valvular heart disease presents with the following:

- Shortness of breath (most common symptom); look for the phrase "worse with exertion or exercise"
- In the history, hypertension, myocardial infarction, ischemia, increasing age, and rheumatic fever (but, with the exception of rheumatic heart disease, are probably too nonspecific to give the diagnosis)
- In young patients, mitral valve prolapse (MVP), hypertrophic obstructive cardiomyopathy (HOCM), mitral stenosis (MS), or bicuspid aortic valves

The following are clues to the diagnosis:

Clue to Diagnosis	Likely Diagnosis
Young female, general population	MVP
Healthy young athlete	HOCM
Immigrant, pregnant	MS
Turner syndrome, coarctation of aorta	Bicuspid aortic valve
Palpitations, atypical chest pain not with exertion	MVP

All valvular heart disease can be expected to have murmurs and rales on lung exam. Possible findings on exam are as follows:

- Peripheral edema
- Carotid pulse findings
- Gallop

For the physical exam, choose the CV exam, chest, and extremities.

Murmurs and the effect of auscultation are often the most difficult part of the valvular heart disease section.

- **Systolic murmurs** are most commonly aortic stenosis (AS), mitral regurgitation (MR), mitral valve prolapse (MVP), and hypertrophic obstructive cardiomyopathy (HOCM).
- **Diastolic murmurs** are most commonly aortic regurgitation (AR) and MS.
- All right-sided murmurs increase in intensity with inhalation, while all left-sided murmurs increase with exhalation.

Murmur intensity increases with...	Exhalation	Inhalation
Side of murmur	Left	Right
Associated disease	Mitral and aortic valve lesions	Both stenosis and regurgitation of tricuspid valves

Cardiac maneuvers predominantly affect the volume of blood entering the heart.

- Squatting and lifting the legs in the air increase venous return to the heart.
  - When you squat, you are squeezing the veins of the legs, which are rather large. This essentially squeezes blood up into the heart, like squeezing a tube of toothpaste.
  - For those too weak to squat suddenly, the physician can lift the legs. This has the same effect, which is to drain blood into the chest from the lower extremities.
- Valsalva maneuver and standing up suddenly decrease venous return to the heart.
  - Valsalva maneuver is exhaling against a closed glottis, like bearing down during a bowel movement or blowing against a thumb stuck in the mouth.
  - This increases intrathoracic pressure, which decreases blood return to the heart.
- Most murmurs increase in intensity with squatting and leg raise. AS, AR, MS, MR, and all right-sided heart lesions will become louder with squatting and leg raising.
- The only murmurs that decrease in intensity (soften) with these maneuvers are MVP and HOCM.

The table shows the effect of venous return on murmurs.

Valvular Lesion	Effect of Change in Venous Return	
	Increase (squat, leg raise)	Decrease (stand, Valsalva)
AS	Increased murmur	Decreased murmur
AR	Increased murmur	Decreased murmur
MS	Increased murmur	Decreased murmur
MR	Increased murmur	Decreased murmur
Ventricular septal defect (VSD)	Increased murmur	Decreased murmur
HOCM	Decreased murmur	Increased murmur
MVP	Decreased murmur	Increased murmur

Handgrip maneuver increases afterload by compressing the arteries of the arm by contracting the muscles of the arm.

- Does not significantly increase venous return to the heart: the veins of the arms are not as large as those of the legs, so compressing them makes little difference in venous return to the heart
- Because it increases afterload, functions in the opposite way of an ACE inhibitor and worsens the murmurs of conditions that would improve with an ACE inhibitor
  - For instance, AR and MR are treated with ACE inhibitors, because afterload reduction increases the forward flow of blood into the aorta. Handgrip will, therefore, worsen AR and MR murmurs by pushing blood backward into the heart. Handgrip will make the murmurs of AR and MR louder and more intense.
  - The same is true for VSD; handgrip worsens the murmur of VSD because more blood now goes from the left ventricle into the right ventricle.
  - Improves (lessens) the murmurs of MVP and HOCM (when the left ventricular chamber is larger or more full)

> What happens to the size of the LV chamber if there is increased afterload?
> - The LV chamber will not empty and thus the LV will be larger.
> - A larger LV chamber relieves or lessens the obstruction in HOCM.

Amyl nitrate is a vasodilator that decreases afterload by dilating peripheral arteries.

- Has the opposite effect of handgrip; i.e., functions like an ACE inhibitor or ARB.
- If handgrip worsens AR and MR, then amyl nitrate improves AR and MR.
- Increases ventricular emptying and thus decreases the size of the LV. Amyl nitrate worsens the murmurs of MVP and HOCM by increasing the obstruction and the degree of prolapse of the valves in MVP.

The effect of handgrip and amyl nitrate on AS can be hard to understand.

- Handgrip softens the murmur of AS. This happens by preventing blood from leaving the ventricle (you can't have a murmur if blood is not moving). If afterload goes up, blood can't eject from the LV, and the AS murmur will soften.

Handgrip and amyl nitrate have little effect on MS, since they generally do not affect ventricular filling (the major component of MS).

Similarly, ACE inhibitors have very little effect on MS.

- In other words, the murmur of AS is based on the gradient between the LV and the aorta; if the LV pressure is greater than the aorta pressure, then the gradient or difference is high. The higher the gradient, the louder the murmur and the more severe the AS.
- Handgrip increases pressure in the aorta, so the gradient or difference between the LV and aorta decreases. Handgrip is like covering up a trombone or trumpet. You can't produce music if you cover the wind instrument with your hand.

- Amyl nitrate has the opposite effect on AS. It decreases afterload and decreases the pressure in the aorta, thus increasing the gradient between LV and aorta and worsening (making louder) the murmur of AS.

Valvular Lesion	Effect on Murmur Volume	
	Handgrip (Increased Afterload)	**Amyl Nitrate (Decreased Afterload)**
AS	Decrease	Increase
AR	Increase	Decrease
MS	Negligible effect	Negligible effect
MR	Increase	Decrease
VSD	Increase	Decrease
HOCM	Decrease	Increase
MVP	Decrease	Increase

Location and Radiation of Murmurs

One of the main clues to the identity of a murmur is the location at which the murmur is heard.

USMLE multimedia will play heart sounds that must be identified.

- AS is heard best at the second right intercostal space and radiates to the carotid arteries. It is classically described as a crescendo-decrescendo murmur.
- Pulmonic valve murmurs are heard at the second left intercostal space.
- AR and tricuspid murmurs, as well as VSD murmurs, are heard at the lower left sternal border.
- MR is heard at the apex and radiates into the axilla. The apex is at the level of the 5th intercostal space, below the left nipple.

USMLE multimedia will show an animation of auscultation at a particular location on the chest wall and then play the sound.

Intensity of Murmurs
- I/VI: only heard with special maneuvers (e.g., Valsalva, handgrip)
- II/VI and III/VI: majority of murmurs; no objective difference between them
- IV/VI: thrill present (a thrill is a palpable vibration you can feel from a severe valve lesion)
- V/VI: can be heard with stethoscope partially off the chest
- VI/VI: stethoscope not needed to hear it

The **best initial test** for valve lesions (on single best answer questions) is an echocardiogram. The **most accurate test** is left heart catheterization. This can also measure pressure gradients (as in AS) most accurately.

In a CCS case, add an EKG and chest x-ray for valvular lesion assessment.

Treatment is as follows:

- **Regurgitant lesions**: vasodilator therapy (ACE inhibitors, ARBs, nifedipine); if handgrip makes it worse, ACE inhibitors are the most effective medical therapy
  - Afterload reduction is not proven to slow progression of regurgitant lesions.
  - If the patient still progresses despite medical therapy, then surgical repair or replacement of the valve should be performed. Valve replacement with a catheter can be done for AS, but cannot be done for regurgitant lesions. Regurgitant lesions can be tightened with clips placed by catheter, but not replaced.

- **Stenotic lesions**: anatomic repair
  - MS: balloon valvuloplasty, even if patient is pregnant
  - Severe AS: aortic valve replacement, even in the very old (well-tolerated); try replacement first via catheter
  - Transcatheter aortic valve replacement (TAVR) has better efficacy and fewer adverse effects than surgical replacement
  - Diuretics can decrease pulmonary vascular congestion with stenotic lesions but are less effective than anatomic repair
  - Valsalva improves murmur = diuretic indicated
  - Amyl nitrate improves murmur = ACE inhibitor indicated

> Order transthoracic echocardiography (TTE) first on CCS. Then order a transesophageal echocardiogram (TEE) if the TTE is not fully diagnostic.

Valvular Lesion	Standing/Valsalva	Diuretics Indicated
AS	Decrease	Yes (replacement best treatment)
AR	Decrease	Yes
MS	Decrease	Yes (balloon best treatment)
MR	Decrease	Yes
VSD	Decrease	Yes
HOCM	Increase	No
MVP	Increase	No

Valvular Lesion	Amyl Nitrate	ACE Inhibitor Indicated
AS	Increase	No
AR	Decrease	Yes
MS	Negligible effect	No
MR	Decrease	Yes
VSD	Decrease	Yes
HOCM	Increase	No
MVP	Increase	No

On CCS, the intensity, radiation, and location of the murmur will automatically be provided with the CV examination. There is no need to ask for them separately.

Aortic Stenosis (AS)

AS most commonly presents with chest pain; syncope and CHF are less common. Patients are older and often have a history of hypertension. CAD will be present in as many as 50% of patients.

Prognosis is as follows:

- Coronary disease: 3- to 5-year average survival
- Syncope: 2- to 3-year average survival
- CHF: 1.5- to 2-year average survival

Basic Science Correlate

Mechanism of Syncope/Angina in AS

In AS, a stiff valve just proximal to the entry point of coronaries blocks blood flow into the vertebral and basilar arteries and carotids. No flow to brain = passing out.

Thus, AS causes LV hypertrophy. LV hypertrophy = increased demand.

AS = blocked flow with increased demand = chest pain

Physical exam is CV exam, chest, and extremities.

AS gives a crescendo-decrescendo systolic murmur. The case may describe delayed carotid upstroke as well.

- Murmur will be heard best at second right intercostal space and radiate to the carotid arteries.
- Murmur will increase in intensity with leg raising, squatting, and amyl nitrate.
- Murmur will decrease with Valsalva, standing, and handgrip.

Normal aortic valve gradient is zero.

Basic Science Correlate

Mechanism of Crescendo/Decrescendo Murmur of AS

The first part of the cardiac cycle is isovolumetric contraction. With isovolumetric contraction, no blood moves. No blood moving = No murmur. Peak flow occurs in mid-systole. Peak flow = Peak noise. Hence, AS yields a diamond-shaped crescendo-decrescendo murmur.

The **best initial diagnostic** test is transthoracic echocardiogram (TTE) (transesophageal echocardiogram (TEE) is more accurate). The **most accurate diagnostic test** is left heart catheterization, which allows the most accurate method of assessing the pressure gradient across the valve.

- Mild disease: gradient <30 mm Hg
- Moderate disease: gradient 30–70 mm Hg
- Severe disease: gradient >70 mm Hg

For CCS cases, also choose an EKG and a chest x-ray, which will show left ventricular hypertrophy.

Treatment is as follows:

- Diuretics (**best initial treatment**), but they do not alter long-term prognosis; use caution because overdiuresis is dangerous
- Valve replacement (superior to balloon dilation): transcatheter aortic valve replacement (TAVR) is preferred to surgical valve replacement
  - TAVR is simply a valve replacement deployed through a catheter
  - TAVR has lower risk of death, stroke, bleeding, and arrhythmia compared with surgery
  - TAVR is not an option for regurgitant lesions
- Valve replacement is well tolerated, even in the elderly
- Bioprosthetic valve (porcine, bovine) will last around 10 years but requires no anticoagulation with warfarin; mechanical valve will last longer but requires warfarin to goal INR 2–3

Aortic Regurgitation (AR)

AR is caused by hypertension, rheumatic heart disease, endocarditis, and cystic medial necrosis. Rarer causes are Marfan syndrome, ankylosing spondylitis, and syphilis.

AR can also be caused by reactive arthritis (previously called Reiter syndrome), an inflammatory arthritis of large joints, inflammation of eyes (conjunctivitis and uveitis), and urethritis.

The most common symptoms include shortness of breath and fatigue.

For the physical examination, choose the CV exam, chest, and extremities.

The murmur of AR is a diastolic decrescendo murmur heard best at the left sternal border. Rarely, there are several unique physical findings (the murmur will increase in intensity with leg raising, squatting, and handgrip):

- Quincke pulse: arterial or capillary pulsations in the fingernails
- Corrigan pulse: high bounding pulses (a "water-hammer pulse")
- Musset sign: head bobbing up and down with each pulse
- Duroziez sign: murmur heard over the femoral artery
- Hill sign: blood pressure gradient much higher in lower extremities

The **best diagnostic test** is TTE. TEE is more accurate. Left heart catheterization is the **most accurate test**.

For CCS cases, also choose an EKG and chest x-ray, which will show left ventricular hypertrophy.

Treatment is ACE inhibitors, ARBs, and nifedipine, though they are not proven to slow the velocity of dilation. For CCS cases, add a loop diuretic such as furosemide.

About AS, the exam may ask the following:

- Which has a higher risk of acute kidney injury and atrial fibrillation? (Answer: surgery)
- Which has a higher risk of need for pacemaker placement? (Answer: TAVR)

Balloon dilate AS only if the patient is too sick to undergo surgery.

Mechanical valves can wear out after 15–20 years.

Bicuspid Aortic Valve

- Usually AS progressing to AR
- Can lead to aneurysm
- Endocarditis increased
- BP control critical
- Monitor with echo
- Repair when >5 cm

Surgery is the answer when ejection fraction drops <55% or the left ventricular end systolic diameter >55 mm—even if patients are asymptomatic.

Basic Science Correlate

Why Does High Pressure Dilate the Aortic Valve?

The law of Laplace says: The wall tension, or force dilating a vessel, is proportionate to the radius of the vessel times the pressure on the inside.

Tension = Radius × Pressure

The wider a vessel is, the faster it will get pulled apart. Hence, the more the aortic ring or aorta is dilated, the faster it will get pulled apart. Likewise, the higher the interior pressure is, the faster the interior will be pulled apart. This force of being "pulled apart," or dilation, is called "wall tension" in the law of Laplace.

ACE and ARB drugs vasodilate peripheral arterioles. Lower pressure = Lower wall tension.

Mitral Stenosis (MS)

The most common cause of MS is rheumatic fever. Look for an immigrant patient (because of the low rates of rheumatic fever in the United States). Also look for a pregnant patient because of the large increase in plasma volume with pregnancy.

Special features of MS are as follows:

- Dysphagia: large left atrium pressing on esophagus
- Hoarseness: pressure on recurrent laryngeal nerve
- Atrial fibrillation leading to stroke

Basic Science Correlate

Mechanism of Increased MS Symptoms in Pregnant Women

Pregnant women have a 50% increase in plasma volume. More volume with the same valve diameter means more pressure, backflow, and symptoms.

Pregnancy also changes the hypothalamic osmolar receptors; ADH levels stay higher during this time, so the collecting duct absorbs more free water.

For the physical exam, choose the CV exam, chest, and extremities.

The murmur of MS is a diastolic rumble after an opening snap, which can be described as an "extra sound" in diastole. The S1 is louder. As the MS worsens, the opening snap moves closer to S2. The murmur will increase in intensity with leg raising, squatting, and expiration.

> **Basic Science Correlate**
>
> **Mechanism of Opening Snap Earlier in Worsening MS**
>
> The mitral valve opens when LA pressure > LV pressure. Worse MS = Higher LA pressure. Higher LA pressure pushes the mitral valve open earlier.

TTE is the **best initial diagnostic test**. TEE is more accurate. Left heart catheterization is the most accurate test. For CCS cases, also choose an EKG and a chest x-ray, which will show left atrial hypertrophy. On chest x-ray, there is straightening of the left heart border and elevation of the left mainstem bronchus. There may also be a description of a double density in the cardiac silhouette (from left atrial enlargement).

The **best initial treatment** is diuretics; they do not alter progression. Balloon valvuloplasty is the **most effective therapy**. Pregnant women can and should be readily treated with balloon valvuloplasty.

> Pregnancy is not a contraindication to valvuloplasty.

> **Basic Science Correlate**
>
> **Mechanism of Balloon Valvuloplasty**
>
> Balloon valvuloplasty works in MS because the stenosis results from excessive fibrosis of the valve. Rheumatic fever causes cardiac endomyocardial and valvular fibrosis. Fibrosis can be stretched by the balloon.
>
> By contrast, AS is calcified, and calcification does not stretch or rip easily with a balloon.
>
> **MS = Balloon fibrosis**
>
> **AS = Remove/replace calcification**

Mitral Regurgitation (MR)

MR is caused by hypertension, ischemic heart disease, and any other condition that leads to dilation of the heart. You cannot have dilation of the heart without the mitral valve leaflets separating. Dyspnea on exertion is the most common symptom.

Choose the CV exam, chest, and extremities.

> S3 gallop is associated with fluid overload states, such as CHF or mitral regurgitation. S3 can be normal in patients age <30.

The murmur of MR is holosystolic and obscures both S1 and S2. MR is heard best at the apex and radiates to the axilla. The murmur increases in intensity with leg raising, squatting, and handgrip. Standing, Valsalva, and amyl nitrate decrease the intensity. S3 gallop is often present.

TTE is the **best initial diagnostic test**. TEE is more accurate.

Treatment is ACE inhibitors, ARBs, and nifedipine. Vasodilators do not delay progression. In a CCS case, add a loop diuretic such as furosemide.

> When anticoagulating for metal valves, aspirin should still be added to full-dose warfarin to prevent clots.

If the left ventricular ejection fraction drops below 60% or left ventricular end systolic diameter >40 mm, consider surgery—even when patients are asymptomatic. Surgery can be valve replacement or repair (i.e., placing clips/sutures on the valve to tighten it). Repair is preferred to replacement. In the mitral position, mechanical valves need warfarin with target INR 2.5–3.5. In the aortic position, target INR is 2–3.

The operative criteria for regurgitant lesions in asymptomatic patients are as follows:

	Aortic Regurgitation	**Mitral Regurgitation**
Ejection fraction	<55%	<60%
Left ventricular end systolic diameter	>55 mm	>40 mm

Ventricular Septal Defect (VSD)

Asymptomatic patients may present with only a holosystolic murmur at the lower left sternal border. Larger defects lead to shortness of breath. The murmur worsens with exhalation, squatting, and leg raise.

The **best initial diagnostic test** is echocardiography, but catheterization (**most accurate diagnostic test**) will determine the degree of left-to-right shunting most precisely.

Mild defects with normal pulmonary artery pressure require no treatment, i.e., they can be left without mechanical closure.

Atrial Septal Defect (ASD)

Small ASDs are asymptomatic. Larger ones may lead to signs of right ventricular failure, such as shortness of breath and a parasternal heave. ASD is associated with fixed splitting of S2 (**frequently tested** point).

> **Basic Science Correlate**
>
> **Mechanism of Fixed Splitting of S2 in ASD**
>
> S2 splitting is caused by different pressures on different sides of heart. Same pressure on both sides means no splitting.
>
> **LA/RA pressure no change in respiration = no change in splitting**

Diagnose with an echocardiogram.

Treatment is a percutaneous or catheter device. Repair is most often indicated when the shunt ratio exceeds 1.5:1.

Splitting of S2		
Wide, P2 Delayed	**Paradoxical, A2 Delayed**	**Fixed**
• RBBB • Pulmonic stenosis • Right ventricular hypertrophy • Pulmonary hypertension	• LBBB • AS • Left ventricular hypertrophy • Hypertension	ASD

Cardiomyopathy

Dilated Cardiomyopathy

Dilated cardiomyopathy presents and is managed in the same way as CHF, previously described. The most common causes are ischemia, alcohol, doxorubicin, radiation, and Chagas disease.

Echocardiography is the **best initial diagnostic test** to determine the ejection fraction and look for wall motion activity. MUGA or nuclear ventriculography is the **most accurate test** to determine ejection fraction.

Treatment is ACE inhibitors, ARBs, beta blockers, and spironolactone.

- Spironolactone and eplerenone are MRAs or aldosterone antagonists given to reduce the work of the heart (not for their diuretic effect)
  - Spironolactone is anti-androgenic and inhibits testosterone
  - Eplerenone does not inhibit androgens
- Digoxin decreases symptoms but does not prolong survival
- Ivabradine is a funny sodium channel blocking the SA node; add if heart rate >70 beats/min after beta blockers have been tried

Hypertrophic Cardiomyopathy

This condition presents with shortness of breath on exertion and an S4 gallop on examination.

The **best diagnostic test** is echocardiography, which shows a normal ejection fraction.

Treatment is MRAs. ACE inhibitors are less clear in their benefit. Digoxin is of no benefit.

> S4 gallop is a sign of left ventricular hypertrophy and decreased compliance or stiffness of the ventricle. S4 gallop does not automatically indicate the need for additional therapy.

Restrictive Cardiomyopathy

Restrictive cardiomyopathy presents with a history of sarcoidosis, amyloidosis, hemochromatosis, cancer, myocardial fibrosis, or glycogen storage diseases. Shortness of breath is the main presenting complaint in all forms of

Amyloid:
- Low-voltage EKG
- Speckled pattern on echo

cardiomyopathy. Kussmaul sign is present: this is an increase in jugular venous pressure on inhalation.

Cardiac catheterization shows rapid x and y descent. EKG shows low voltage. Echocardiography is the mainstay of diagnosis.

Endomyocardial biopsy is the **most accurate diagnostic test** of the etiology.

Treatment is diuretics and correcting the underlying cause.

Takotsubo Cardiomyopathy

This is a rare, sudden systolic dysfunction brought on by extreme emotions. Look for a vignette involving a postmenopausal woman with sudden psychological stress. Takotsubo cardiomyopathy presents like acute myocardial infarction with ventricular dysfunction. Coronary arteries are normal.

Treatment is ACE inhibitors, diuretics, and beta blockers—as in any other ventricular failure. If there is no acute death, the patient recovers in a few weeks.

Pericardial Disease

Pericarditis

On the Step 3 exam, the presentation of pericarditis is most often chest pain that is pleuritic (changes with respiration) and positional (relieved by sitting up and leaning forward). The pain will be described as sharp and brief. Ischemic pain is dull and sore, like being punched.

The vast majority of pericarditis cases are viral. Although any infectious agent, collagen-vascular disease, or trauma can be in the history, remember that Step 3 often provides a clear diagnosis and asks what to do about it.

The only pertinent positive finding is a friction rub, which can have 3 components.

- Only 30% of patients have rub
- No pulsus paradoxus, tenderness, edema, or Kussmaul sign present
- Blood pressure normal, and no jugular venous distention or organomegaly

The **best initial test** is the EKG. ST segment elevation is present everywhere (all leads). PR segment depression is pathognomonic in lead II, but is not always present.

Treatment is an NSAID (naproxen/aspirin/ibuprofen) plus colchicine, which prevents recurrent episodes. If pain persists after 1–2 days, then add oral prednisone.

Pericardial Tamponade

Tamponade presents with shortness of breath, hypotension, and jugular venous distention. On CCS, also examine the lungs, because they will be clear.

Following are the unique features of tamponade:

- Pulsus paradoxus: blood pressure is decreased >10 mm Hg on inhalation
- Electrical alternans: this is alterations of the axis of QRS complex on EKG, manifested as the height of QRS complex

---

Basic Science Correlate

Mechanism of Pulsus Paradoxus

Inhalation increases venous return. Increased venous return expands the RV. Expanded RV compresses the LV. Compressed LV decreases blood pressure. Tamponade compresses the whole heart.

Inhale = Big RV = Smaller LV = BP drop >10 mm Hg

The **most accurate diagnostic test** is echocardiogram. The earliest finding of tamponade is diastolic collapse of the right atrium and right ventricle. (It is normal to have ≤50 mL of pericardial fluid, but there should be no collapse of the cardiac structures.)

- EKG will show low voltage and electrical alternans. Electrical alternans is variation of the height of the QRS complex from the heart moving backward and forward in the chest.
- Right heart catheterization will show "equalization" of all the pressures in the heart during diastole.
- Wedge pressure will be the same as the right atrial and pulmonary artery diastolic pressure.

Treatment is pericardiocentesis. For long-term conditions, do pericardial window placement.

Do not use diuretics, as they are dangerous.

Constrictive Pericarditis

Constrictive pericarditis presents with shortness of breath and the following signs of chronic right heart failure:

- Edema
- Jugular venous distention
- Hepatosplenomegaly
- Ascites

Following are the unique features of constrictive pericarditis:

- Kussmaul sign: Increase in jugular venous pressure on inhalation
- Pericardial knock: Extra diastolic sound from the heart hitting a calcified, thickened pericardium

Diagnostic testing is chest x-ray (shows calcification); EKG (low voltage); and CT and MRI (show thickening of the pericardium).

The **best initial treatment** is a diuretic. The **most effective treatment** is surgical removal of the pericardium (i.e., pericardial stripping).

Aortic Disease

Dissection of the Thoracic Aorta

Dissection of the thoracic aorta presents with the following symptoms:

- Chest pain radiating to the back between the scapula
- Pain described as very severe and "ripping"
- Difference in blood pressure between right and left arms

The **best initial test** is chest x-ray showing a widened mediastinum. The **most accurate test** is CT angiogram.

Treatment is as follows:

- If there is severe chest pain radiating to the back and hypertension, order beta blockers with the first screen, plus an EKG and chest x-ray.
- No matter what the EKG shows, move the clock forward and order any of the following (all are equally accurate): CT angiography, TEE, or MRA.
- After starting beta blockers, order nitroprusside to control the blood pressure.
- Place patient in the ICU and order a surgical consult. Surgical correction is the **most effective therapy**.

Abdominal Aortic Aneurysm (AAA)

Screening with an ultrasound should be ordered in men age 65–75 who are current or former smokers.

> **Basic Science Correlate**
>
> AAAs are detected by ultrasound first and repaired when >5 cm in size. Smaller ones are monitored.
>
> As an aneurysm enlarges, the rate of expansion increases (wider aorta = widens faster). This principle is expressed in the law of LaPlace:
>
> $$\text{Wall tension} = \text{Radius} \times \text{Pressure}$$
>
> The next step is to lower BP. If the aneurysm goes >5 cm, repair with stent or endovascular procedure.

Peripheral Arterial Disease (PAD)

PAD presents with claudication (pain in the calves on exertion). The case may also describe "smooth, shiny skin" with loss of hair and sweat glands, as well as loss of pulses in the feet.

The **best initial diagnostic test** is ankle-brachial index (ABI) (normal ABI ≥0.9). Blood pressure in the legs should be equal to or greater than the pressure in the arms; if the difference is >10%, an obstruction is present.) The **most accurate test** is angiogram.

Treatment is as follows:

- **Best initial therapy**
  - Aspirin
  - ACE inhibitors (best treatment) for blood pressure control
  - Exercise as tolerated
  - Cilostazol
  - Statins for lipid control to target LDL <100 mg/dL
  - CCBs are ineffective for PAD
- Vorapaxar (antiplatelet drug) added to aspirin or clopidogrel
- Beta blockers are not contraindicated with PAD; use if needed for ischemic disease

> Spinal stenosis will give pain that is worse with walking downhill and less with walking uphill or while cycling or sitting. Pulses and skin exam will be normal with spinal stenosis.

> Pain + Pallor + Pulseless = Arterial occlusion

> Acute arterial embolus will be very sudden in onset with loss of pulse and a cold extremity. It is also quite painful. AS and a-fib are often in the history for arterial embolus.

Basic Science Correlate

CCBs do not work in PAD because in PAD the atherosclerotic obstruction is on the inside of the vessel. CCBs dilate the muscular layer, which is exterior to the atherosclerosis in the center. Dilating the outer layer does not expand the inside.

CCS Tip: On CCS, move the clock forward several weeks. PAD is not an emergency! If initial therapies do not work and the pain progresses, or there are signs of ischemia such as gangrene or pain at rest, then perform surgical bypass.

Rhythm Disorders

Atrial Fibrillation (A-Fib)

A-fib presents with palpitations and an irregular pulse in a person with a history of hypertension, ischemia, or cardiomyopathy.

If the initial EKG does not show the answer, a patient in the hospital should be placed on telemetry monitoring. Hemodynamically stable outpatients should undergo Holter monitoring, which is continuous, ambulatory cardiac rhythm monitoring for 24 hours or longer.

CCS Tip: For CCS cases, other tests to order once a-fib is found on EKG are:

- Echocardiography: looking for clots, valve function, and left atrial size
- Thyroid function: T4 and TSH level
- Electrolytes: potassium, magnesium, and calcium level
- Troponin or CK-MB level: may be appropriate in some acute-onset cases

Treatment is as follows:

- **Unstable patients**: immediate synchronized electrical cardioversion
  - Instability is defined as a systolic blood pressure <90 mm Hg, congestive failure, confusion related to hemodynamic instability, or chest pain
  - Cardiovert with the first screen, without waiting for TEE or anticoagulation with heparin
- **Stable patients**: rate control medications to slow ventricular heart rate if >100–110 beats/min
  - Medications include beta blockers (metoprolol, carvedilol), CCBs (diltiazem), or digoxin
  - In the acute setting, i.e., the ED, give intravenously
- Once the rate has been controlled, anticoagulation (**next best step**) should be done in all patients with an atrial arrhythmia persisting beyond 2 days. (If the exam question does not state the duration, treat as if it were persisting >2 days.)
  - Oral anticoagulants: NOACs such as dabigatran, rivaroxaban, edoxaban, and apixaban which have similar or better efficacy than warfarin but no need to monitor INR
- The long-term use of anticoagulation + rate control medication (metoprolol, diltiazem, digoxin) is equal or better than cardioversion with electricity or medication.
- Anticoagulation in atrial arrhythmias: novel oral anticoagulants (NOACs) work by inhibiting either factor Xa (rivaroxaban, apixaban, edoxaban) or inhibiting thrombin with dabigatran. If severe bleeding occurs with warfarin, it is reversible with prothrombin complex concentrate (PCC) or fresh frozen plasma (FFP). PCC is comprised of factors II, VII, IX and X, which are the specific factors inhibited by warfarin. If bleeding occurs with dabigatran, it is reversible with idarucizumab. If bleeding occurs with the Xa inhibitors, it is reversible with andexanet.
  - NOACs prevent more strokes and cause less intracranial bleeding than warfarin. In a-fib they decrease mortality more than warfarin.
  - Warfarin should be used for a-fib when the patient has metallic heart valves or mitral stenosis.

CHA_2DS_2-VASc: (**C**HF, **H**ypertension, **A**ge >75, **D**iabetes, or **S**troke/TIA, **V**ascular disease, **A**ge 65–74, **S**ex) is a scoring system to indicate the need for anticoagulation:

- Score 0 or 1: use aspirin or nothing
- Score ≥2: use apixaban, dabigatran, edoxaban, or rivaroxaban (NOACs)
- When score ≥2, control the rate and anticoagulate with NOACs, which become therapeutic in a few hours (not days, as with warfarin)

Atrial Flutter (A-Flutter)

A-flutter is managed in the same way as a-fib. The only difference is that the rhythm is regular on presentation.

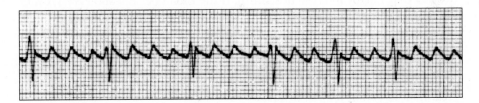

The table shows how to choose the right rate control medication for a-fib and a-flutter.

Beta Blockers (Metoprolol)	Calcium Channel Blockers (Diltiazem)	Digoxin
• Ischemic heart disease • Migraines • Graves disease • Pheochromocytoma	• Asthma • Migraine	• Borderline hypotension

Multifocal Atrial Tachycardia (MAT)

This condition presents like an atrial arrhythmia in association with COPD/emphysema. EKG will show polymorphic P waves, revealing different atrial foci for the QRS complexes.

As the name implies, patients with MAT have tachycardia (heart rate >100 beats/min). MAT manifests as an irregular chaotic rhythm on EKG.

CHA_2DS_2-VASc

C = CHF

H = Hypertension

A_2 = Age >75

D = Diabetes

S_2 = Stroke or TIA

V = Vascular disease

A = Age 65–74

S = Sex category

Stroke/TIA = 2 points

Age >75 = 2 points

Routine cardioversion of a-fib is not indicated.

Even when warfarin is used for a-fib, there is no need to bolus the patient with heparin.

Why? Because a-fib takes months/years to develop a risk of stroke, while full-dose heparin carries a risk of bleeding. Just start the warfarin or NOAC; it is safe.

Idarucizumab reverses dabigatran.

For MAT, if pO_2 <55, give oxygen first.

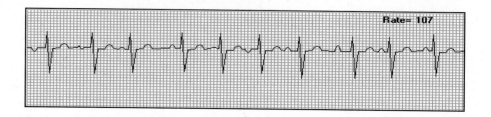

Treatment is oxygen first, then diltiazem. Do not use beta blockers.

Supraventricular Tachycardia (SVT)

SVT presents with palpitations and tachycardia and occasionally syncope. It is *not* associated with ischemic heart disease. SVT has a regular rhythm with a ventricular rate of 160–180 beats/min. If the EKG does not show SVT, order Holter monitor or telemetry to increase the sensitivity of detection.

CCS Tip: On CCS, all cases of dysrhythmia should undergo **transthoracic echo-cardiography (TTE)** after the initial set of orders.

Treatment is as follows:

- Synchronized cardioversion (**best initial management for unstable patients**)
- Vagal maneuvers (carotid sinus massage, ice immersion of the face, Valsalva) (**best initial management for stable patients**)
- If vagal maneuvers do not work, IV adenosine (**frequently tested point**); if adenosine does not work, use beta blocker, diltiazem or digoxin, which will slow the rate and likely convert the rhythm to sinus.
- Best long-term management: radiofrequency catheter ablation

Wolff-Parkinson-White Syndrome (WPW)

WPW presents as SVT that can alternate with VT. The other clue to the diagnosis is worsening of SVT after the use of calcium blockers or digoxin.

The **initial diagnostic test** is EKG, where a delta wave will be found. The **most accurate test** is electrophysiologic study.

Treatment is procainamide, sotalol, or amiodarone if the patient is in SVT or VT due to WPW (avoid amiodarone in structural heart disease). For long-term disease, use radiofrequency catheter ablation.

Basic Science Correlate

Mechanism of WPW

There is an abnormal piece of neutralized cardiac muscle going around the AV node in WPW. This can result in either atrial or ventricular arrhythmia. The slowest conduction in the heart is the AV node. Conduction in the aberrant tract is faster; that is why the PR is short (<120 msec) and there is a delta wave on EKG. CCBs and digoxin block conduction more in the normal AV and force the conduction down the abnormal conduction tract.

Ventricular Tachycardia (VT)

Symptoms include palpitation, syncope, chest pain, or sudden death.

The **best initial diagnostic test** is EKG. You cannot determine whether VT is present without that.

If the EKG does not detect VT, do telemetry monitoring.

The **most accurate diagnostic test** is electrophysiologic studies.

Treatment for persistent VT is as follows:

- Hemodynamically unstable: synchronized cardioversion
- Hemodynamically stable: amiodarone, lidocaine, procainamide, magnesium

Ventricular Fibrillation (V-Fib)

V-fib presents as sudden death.

The **best diagnostic test** is EKG. You cannot tell what caused the loss of pulse without that.

Treatment is always unsynchronized cardioversion (defibrillation) first. Administer in the following order:

1. Continue CPR
2. Reattempt defibrillation
3. Administer IV epinephrine
4. Reattempt defibrillation
5. Administer IV amiodarone or lidocaine
6. Reattempt defibrillation
7. Repeat several cycles of CPR between each shock

Torsade de pointes is VT with an undulating amplitude. Always give magnesium along with medical or electrical therapy.

With V-Fib, do not do intubation first. Dead people are never breathing.

Always do unsynchronized cardioversion first. If you shock them back to life, they are more likely to breathe!

	Unsynchronized	Synchronized
When to deliver electricity	At any point in cycle	Not during the T-wave
Indications	V-fib, pulseless VT	Everything except V-fib and pulseless VT

> ### Basic Science Correlate
>
> **Mechanism of Need for Synchronization**
>
> The T-wave represents the refractory period. An electrical shock delivered during the T-wave can set off a worse rhythm—specifically, asystole and ventricular fibrillation are worse than VT. Do not deliver a shock during the refractory period.

Syncope Evaluation

The management of syncope is based on 3 criteria:

1. Was the loss of consciousness sudden or gradual?
2. Was the regaining of consciousness sudden or gradual?
3. Is the cardiac exam normal or abnormal?

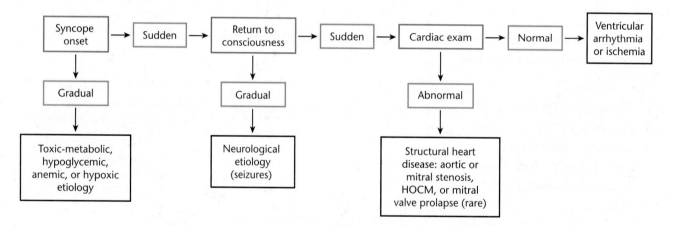

Diagnostic testing is as follows:

- Initial testing: cardiac and neurological exam; EKG; chemistries (glucose); oximeter; CBC; cardiac enzymes (CK-MB, troponin)
- Echocardiogram if murmur is present
- Head CT if:
  - Neurological exam is focal
  - History of head trauma due to syncope
  - Headache is described
  - Seizure is described/suspected (also do EEG)

> Carotid Doppler is not useful in syncope. A patient cannot pass out from a carotid embolus.

Basic Science Correlate

Mechanism of Syncope: Caused by Brainstem Stroke Only

The brainstem controls sleep and wake in the brain. Only stroke or TIA of the posterior circulation can cause syncope. Vertebral/basilar circulation is synonymous with the posterior or brainstem circulation. There is no place in the circulation of the middle cerebral artery that can cause syncope.

CCS Tip: On further management, if the diagnosis is not clear after you move the clock forward to obtain the results of initial tests, order the following:

- Holter monitor on outpatients
- Telemetry monitoring for inpatients
- Repeat check of CK-MB and troponin levels 4 hours later
- Urine and blood toxicology screens

CCS Tip: On further management, particularly if the etiology is not clear, order the following:

- Tilt table testing to diagnose neurocardiogenic (vasovagal) syncope
- Electrophysiological testing

> Exclude cardiac causes of syncope. More than 80% of mortality from syncope is from cardiac causes.

The Holter monitor is a 24–72-hour continuous ambulatory EKG. This is routine for most patients with syncope and sudden loss/sudden regaining of consciousness. If the Holter is negative, continued monitoring can be done for 1–3 months.

Treatment of syncope is based on the etiology. Most cases never get a specific diagnosis.

- First, exclude a cardiac etiology, such as an arrhythmia. Most mortalities due to syncope have a cardiac etiology.
- If a ventricular dysrhythmia is diagnosed as the etiology of syncope, use an implantable cardioverter/defibrillator.

CCS Tip: Bottom line, order the following for syncope:

- EKG
- Enzymes: troponin/CKMB
- Echocardiogram
- Head CT

Infectious Diseases

Introduction to Antibiotics

Staphylococcus aureus: Bone, Heart, Skin, Joint

- **Sensitive staph (MSSA)**
  - IV: oxacillin/nafcillin, or cefazolin (first-generation cephalosporin)
  - Oral: dicloxacillin or cephalexin (first-generation cephalosporin)
- **Resistant staph (MRSA)**
  - **Severe infection**: vancomycin, daptomycin, linezolid, ceftaroline, tigecycline, or telavancin
    - Oritavancin, telavancin, and dalbavancin are long-acting drugs equal to vancomycin
    - Tedizolid is like linezolid in controlling MRSA and also VRE
  - **Minor infection**: trimethoprim/sulfamethoxazole (TMP/SMX), clindamycin, doxycycline, delafloxacin (a quinolone covering skin MRSA and gram-negative bacilli)
- Penicillin allergy
  - Rash: cephalosporins
  - Anaphylaxis: clindamycin or linezolid
  - Severe infection: vancomycin, linezolid, daptomycin, telavancin
  - Minor infection: clindamycin, TMP/SMX, delafloxacin
- Least effective MRSA drugs are clindamycin and tigecycline; never use for blood isolates

> Since so many medications cover MRSA, look for exam questions on side effects:
> - Linezolid causes thrombocytopenia and interferes with MAO inhibitors.
> - Daptomycin causes myopathy and a rising CPK.
> - Tedizolid does not affect platelets or MAO.

> Daptomycin is not effective for lungs. Do not use daptomycin or doripenem for lung infection.

> Telavancin is a vancomycin derivative with similar efficacy.

Basic Science Correlate

- Telavancin, dalbavancin, and oritavancin are bactericidal lipopolysaccharides. They inhibit bacterial cell wall synthesis by binding to the D-Ala-D-Ala terminus of the peptidoglycan in the growing cell wall.
- Ceftaroline, like all cephalosporins, inhibits cell wall growth by binding the penicillin-binding protein.
- Linezolid inhibits protein synthesis.
- TMP-SMX is a folate antagonist.

Streptococcus

The medications above will cover *Streptococcus* as well as *Staphylococcus*.

The following medications are specific for *Streptococcus*:

- Penicillin
- Ampicillin
- Amoxicillin

> If the organism is sensitive, oxacillin, nafcillin, or cefazolin is superior to vancomycin.

Gram-Negative Bacilli (Rods): *Escherichia coli, Enterobacter, Citrobacter, Morganella, Pseudomonas, Serratia*

All of the following medications have equal efficacy for gram-negative bacilli.

Cephalosporins	Penicillins	Monobactam	Quinolones	Aminoglycosides	Carbapenems
Cefepime	Piperacillin	Aztreonam	Ciprofloxacin	Gentamicin	Imipenem
Ceftazidime	Ticarcillin		Levofloxacin	Tobramycin	Meropenem
			Moxifloxacin	Amikacin	Ertapenem
			Gemifloxacin		Doripenem

Extended Spectrum Beta-Lactamases (ESBLs)

ESBLs are enzymes which cause resistance to several classes of antibiotics normally used against gram-negative bacilli, i.e., most beta-lactam antibiotics (penicillins, cephalosporins); the monobactam aztreonam; and possibly aminoglycosides and quinolones.

ESBL-producing organisms are more dangerous than sensitive organisms. They are seen more frequently in hospital-acquired infection than in community-acquired types.

Treatment is as follows:

- Carbapenems, tried first
- If there is resistance to carbapenems, then a cephalosporin-beta lactamase combination (ceftolozane-tazobactam and ceftazidime-avibactam)
- If there is resistance to those agents, then meropenem-vaborbactam
- Polymyxin/colistin (tried last because of toxicity)

Use the following guidelines:

- Carbapenems are excellent antianaerobic medications. They cover streptococci and all sensitive staphylococcus (MSSA). Use for ESBL.
  - The only carbapenem that does not cover *Pseudomonas* is ertapenem.
- Piperacillin and ticarcillin also cover streptococci and anaerobes.
- Levofloxacin, gemifloxacin, and moxifloxacin are excellent pneumococcal drugs.
- Aminoglycosides work synergistically with other agents to treat staph and enterococcus.

- Vancomycin in combination with piperacillin/tazobactam is associated with an increased risk of AKI. Substitute linezolid for vancomycin.
- Tigecycline covers MRSA and is broadly active against gram-negative bacilli. Tigecycline is weaker than other anti-MRSA drugs.
- Polymyxin/colistin is strongly active against multidrug-resistant gram-negative rods.
  - Causes renal and neural toxicity so use last; reserve for carbapenem-resistant gram-negative bacilli (or try ceftolozane-tazobactam and ceftazidime-avibactam)
  - Look for failed therapy for ventilator-associated pneumonia

For pseudomonal lung infection in cystic fibrosis, use inhaled tobramycin or aztreonam. If those drugs are not available, try colistin.

> Gemifloxacin is a quinolone for pneumonia.

> Use delafloxacin for:
> - MRSA of skin/soft tissue
> - Gram-negative rods

Basic Science Correlate

The beta-lactam antibiotics all inhibit the cell wall by binding the penicillin-binding protein. The 4 classes are:

- Penicillin
- Cephalosporins
- Carbapenem
- Monobactam (the only one is aztreonam)

Antibiotics Combined with Beta-Lactamase Inhibitors

Combining beta-lactamase inhibitors with penicillins or cephalosporins broadens their spectrum of coverage. Beta-lactamase inhibitors are:

- Clavulanate
- Sulbactam
- Tazobactam
- Avibactam
- Vaborbactam (inhibitor of carbapenemase)

The additional coverage is against staphylococci and some gram-negative bacilli. (Beta-lactamase inhibitors do not add MRSA coverage. For example, amoxicillin does not cover *Staphylococcus*, but amoxicillin-clavulanate does. Ampicillin does not cover *Staphylococcus*, but ampicillin-sulbactam does [but not MRSA].) Clavulanate and sulbactam add coverage for resistant *Haemophilus* to ampicillin and amoxicillin. This makes these 2 medications a great answer for sinusitis, oral infections including abscess, otitis media, and human or animal bites.

The other combinations are:

- Piperacillin-tazobactam (covers anaerobes)
- Ticarcillin-clavulanate (covers anaerobes)
- Ceftolozane-tazobactam

- Ceftazidime-avibactam
- Meropenem-vaborbactam

Anaerobes

- Gastrointestinal anaerobes (*Bacteroides*)
  - Metronidazole is the best medication for abdominal anaerobes.
  - Carbapenems, piperacillin, and ticarcillin are equal in efficacy for abdominal anaerobes compared to metronidazole.
  - Cefoxitin and cefotetan (in the cephamycin class) are the only cephalosporins that cover anaerobes.
- Respiratory anaerobes (anaerobic strep)
  - Clindamycin is the best drug for anaerobic strep.
- Medications with no anaerobic coverage
  - Aminoglycosides, aztreonam, fluoroquinolones, oxacillin/nafcillin, and all the cephalosporins except cefoxitin and cefotetan

CCS Tip: CCS does not require you to know doses, but you are expected to know the route of administration.

A man is admitted for endocarditis. Blood cultures grow *S. aureus*. Vancomycin is started while awaiting sensitivity testing. He develops red skin, particularly on the neck. What should you do?

Answer: Slow the rate of the infusion. Vancomycin is associated with "red man syndrome," which is red, flushed skin from histamine release. This happens from rapid infusion of vancomycin. There is no specific therapy, and the medication does not need to be switched. Simply slow the rate of infusion to prevent. Telavancin does not cause red man syndrome.

Antiviral Agents

- Acyclovir, valacyclovir, and famciclovir (all equal in efficacy) (herpes simplex, varicella zoster)
- Valganciclovir, ganciclovir, and foscarnet (all equal in efficacy) (cytomegalovirus [CMV], herpes simplex, varicella)
  - Valganciclovir best long-term therapy for CMV retinitis
  - Side effects include neutropenia and bone marrow suppression (valganciclovir and ganciclovir); renal toxicity (foscarnet)
- Sofosbuvir-ledipasvir, elbasvir-grazoprevir, daclatasvir-sofosbuvir, ombitasvir-paritaprevir-dasabuvir, and sofosbuvir
  - All are oral agents for chronic hepatitis C; none is used as a single agent
  - Sofosbuvir and ledipasvir do not need to be combined with interferon; they are all better than interferon and ribavirin (greater efficacy and fewer side effects)
  - Velpatasvir, when combined with sofosbuvir, will cover all the genotypes of hepatitis C; add voxilaprevir to velpatasvir and sofosbuvir in the small percentage of those who fail initial therapy

Adverse Effects

Daptomycin: myopathy

Linezolid: low platelets

Imipenem: seizures

- Oseltamivir, zanamivir, and peramivir (neuraminidase inhibitors): influenza A and B. *Baloxavir* is an endonuclease inhibitor active against influenza
- Ribavirin: hepatitis C (combined with interferon) for those patients who have not responded to other treatments, respiratory syncytial virus; ribavirin causes anemia
- Lamivudine, adefovir, tenofovir, entecavir, telbivudine, and interferon: chronic hepatitis B

> Echinocandin's unique mechanism: 1,3 glucan inhibition in fungi only.

Basic Science Correlate

Mechanisms of Oral Hepatitis C Medications
- Sofosbuvir, dasabuvir: RNA polymerase inhibitor
- Paritaprevir, daclatasvir, ombitasvir: Protease inhibitors that prevent viral maturation by inhibiting protein synthesis

Antifungal Agents

At high doses, all *-azoles* can cause liver toxicity.

- Fluconazole: *Candida* (not *Candida krusei* or *Candida glabrata*), *Cryptococcus,* oral and vaginal candidiasis as an alternative to topical medications; controls fungus
- Itraconazole: equal in efficacy to fluconazole but more difficult to use; rarely the best initial therapy for anything
- Voriconazole: covers all *Candida*; best agent against *Aspergillus* (side effects include visual disturbance)
- Isavuconazole: equivalent to voriconazole; covers *Aspergillus*
- Posaconazole: also covers mucormycosis (Mucorales)
- Echinocandins (caspofungin, micafungin, anidulafungin)
  - Excellent for neutropenic fever (better than amphotericin)
  - Have no significant human toxicity because they inhibit the 1,3 glucan synthesis step, which does not exist in humans
  - Do not cover *Cryptococcus*
- Efinaconazole and tavaborole: topical antifungal agents against onychomycosis but less effective than terbinafine

> Treat Candidemia with fluconazole and caspofungin.

Basic Science Correlate

Mechanism of Antifungal Medications

Azole antifungals inhibit conversion of lanosterol to ergosterol. Ergosterol is the major component of the cell wall of fungi. Disrupting ergosterol damages the cell membrane and increases its permeability, resulting in cell lysis and death.

- **Amphotericin:** effective against all *Candida*, *Cryptococcus*, and *Aspergillus*
  - Last 2 main indications for amphotericin are *Cryptococcus* and mucormycosis
  - *Aspergillus*: voriconazole, isavuconazole, and caspofungin superior to amphotericin
  - Neutropenic fever: caspofungin (echinocandin) superior to amphotericin
  - *Candida*: fluconazole equal in efficacy to amphotericin but has far fewer adverse effects
  - Side effects include renal toxicity (increased creatinine); hypokalemia; metabolic acidosis from distal renal tubular acidosis; fever, shakes, chills

---

Basic Science Correlate

Mechanism of Renal Toxicity of Amphotericin

Amphotericin is directly toxic to the tubules. Distal tubule toxicity results in renal tubular acidosis. Distal renal tubular acidosis gives excess potassium and magnesium loss and hydrogen ion retention. In cases where there is renal toxicity, switch to liposomal amphotericin.

Osteomyelitis

Is the infection in the soft tissue (skin) only, or has it spread into the bone?

Osteomyelitis in adults almost always presents in a patient with diabetes, peripheral arterial disease, or both with an ulcer or soft tissue infection. You can also think about osteomyelitis in patients with direct trauma and a history of orthopedic surgery, but the case with diabetes and peripheral vascular disease is more likely to appear on the exam.

The "What is the next best step?" question is essentially asking if you know how to distinguish a soft tissue infection from a contiguous spread into the bone.

Diagnostic testing is as follows:

- Plain x-ray (**best initial test**)
  - For x-ray to be "abnormal," over 50% of calcium content of the bone must be lost; it may take up to 2 weeks for x-ray to reflect that
  - X-ray used as initial test in same way you would not skip an EKG and go straight to a stress test
- MRI if x-ray is negative and if there is clinical suspicion
- Bone biopsy and culture (**most accurate test**)

> MRI is far superior to a bone scan with nuclear isotope, which is very poor at distinguishing between infection in the bone and infection of the soft tissue above it.

Which of the following is the earliest finding of osteomyelitis on an x-ray?

a. Periosteal elevation

b. Involucrum

c. Sequestrum

d. Punched-out lesions

e. Fracture

Answer: **A.** The earliest finding of osteomyelitis on x-ray is elevation of the periosteum. Involucrum and sequestrum are terms applied to the formation of abnormal new bone in the periosteum and chunks of bone chipped off from the infection. Punched-out lesions are seen in myeloma, not osteomyelitis. Osteomyelitis does not have an association with fracture.

On Step 3, a question might provide an x-ray result in one of 2 ways:

1. Single best answer: The stem of the question simply states, "x-ray of the bone is normal."

2. CCS: You move the clock forward, and the x-ray result will pop up as you pass the time when it says "report available."

A 67-year-old man with diabetes and peripheral arterial disease comes in with pain in his leg for 2 weeks. There is an ulcer with a draining sinus tract. X-ray is normal. What is the next best step?

a. Bone scan

b. CT scan

c. MRI

d. ESR

e. Biopsy

Answer: **C.** If the x-ray is normal, MRI is the next best test to diagnose osteomyelitis. Bone scan does not have the same specificity.

Sedimentation rate is the best way to monitor a response to therapy. Remember that osteomyelitis is most commonly caused by direct contiguous spread from overlying tissue, but hematogenous (blood) infection can also be present as a cause or result of osteomyelitis, so a blood culture is not a bad idea (especially if the patient looks septic).

However, perform the MRI first.

Which test has greater sensitivity, the **MRI or bone scan**?

- MRI and bone scan are equal in sensitivity; they can equally exclude osteomyelitis if they are normal. The MRI, however, is far more specific. A swab of the ulcer for culture is extremely inaccurate. We cannot tell what is growing inside the bone for sure by growing something from the superficial ulcer. Would you allow yourself to be treated for weeks to months with IV antibiotics with only a 50% chance you are treating the right organism?

Never culture the draining sinus tract or swab an ulcer.

> **Basic Science Correlate**
>
> **Diagnostic Testing in Osteomyelitis**
>
> MRI is based on water content. When the bone is infected, it swells and increases water content (within 48 hours of infection). Water changes the spin of hydrogen ions in tissue, which is why MRI and bone scan become abnormal at the same time. Nuclear bone scan is based on osteoblasts depositing technetium in tissue. Osteomyelitis and cancer both destroy and form bone. Bone scan needs new bone formation to light up after 48 hours. CT and x-ray are based on calcium loss; this takes 1–2 weeks.

If 90% of patients have no fever and normal WBC, how do we know **how long to treat**?

- By following the sedimentation rate. If the ESR is still markedly elevated after 4–6 weeks of therapy, further treatment and possible surgical debridement is necessary.

Treatment is as follows:

> To treat osteomyelitis appropriately, perform a bone biopsy/culture.

- *Staphylococcus* (most common cause of osteomyelitis): IV oxacillin or nafcillin for 4–6 weeks; oral therapy cannot be used
- MRSA: vancomycin, dalbavancin, oritavancin, linezolid, ceftaroline, or daptomycin
- Chronic osteomyelitis: debridement (no urgency to treat; get the biopsy, move the clock forward, and treat what is found on the culture)
- Gram-negative bacilli (*Salmonella* and *Pseudomonas*): oral antibiotics (only time they will be effective)
  - You must confirm it is gram-negative with a bone biopsy.
  - The organism must be sensitive to antibiotics.

Skin Infections

Impetigo

Impetigo (most superficial of the bacterial skin infections) is caused by *Streptococcus pyogenes* or *Staph. aureus* infecting the epidermal layer of the skin. Because it is so superficial, there is weeping, crusting, and oozing of the skin.

A specific microbiologic diagnosis is rarely made or necessary. Look for "weeping, oozing, honey-colored lesions."

Treatment is as follows:

- Topical mupirocin or retapamulin (mupirocin has greater activity against MRSA, bacitracin has less efficacy as a single agent)
- Severe disease: Oral dicloxacillin or cephalexin

- Community-acquired MRSA (CA-MRSA): TMP/SMX or doxycycline; clindamycin is sometimes useful; linezolid and delafloxacin are definitely effective.
- Penicillin allergy: What to use?
  - Rash: Cephalosporins are safe.
  - Anaphylaxis: Clindamycin, doxycycline, linezolid, TMP/SMX
  - Severe infection with anaphylaxis: Vancomycin, telavancin, linezolid, daptomycin

Erysipelas

This is a group A (pyogenes) streptococcal infection of the skin. The skin is very bright red and hot because of dilation of the capillaries of the dermis due to locally released inflammatory mediators. As with most bacterial skin infections, a specific microbiologic diagnosis is rarely made.

The face is often the site of the infection.

Blood culture may be positive. In a CCS case, order blood culture but go straight to treatment on the single best multiple-choice answer.

Can erysipelas lead to rheumatic fever?

- No, only pharyngeal infection can lead to rheumatic fever. Skin infection can lead to glomerulonephritis, however.

Treatment is oral dicloxacillin or cephalexin. Topical antibiotics are useless.

If the organism is confirmed as group A beta hemolytic streptococci, you may treat with penicillin VK.

> Skin (erysipelas) goes to kidneys (glomerulonephritis) only.
>
> Throat (pharyngitis) goes to kidneys (glomerulonephritis) and heart (rheumatic fever).

Cellulitis

Look for a warm, red, swollen, tender skin. It is likely to present in the arm or leg but can present anywhere on the skin.

If presented with a case of cellulitis in a leg, make sure you order a lower extremity Doppler to exclude a blood clot. Both clotting and cellulitis can cause a fever.

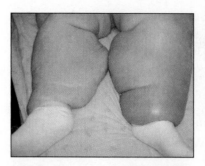

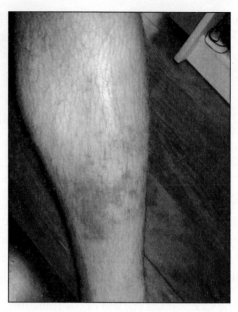

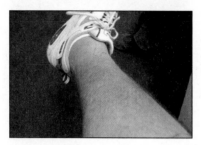

Retapamulin:
- Topical antibiotic
- Only for impetigo

Staphylococcus aureus and *Streptococcus pyogenes* are nearly equal in the cause of cellulitis.

Treatment is as follows:

- **Minor disease**: dicloxacillin, cephalexin, or amoxicillin/clavulanate orally for minor disease
- **Severe disease**: oxacillin, nafcillin, cefazolin, or ampicillin/sulbactam IV
- Penicillin allergy
  - Rash: cephalosporin e.g., cefazolin or ceftaroline
  - Anaphylaxis: vancomycin, linezolid, or daptomycin
  - Minor infections: clindamycin, TMP/SMX

What **skin infection** does *Staphylococcus epidermidis* cause?

- None. *S. epidermidis* is a normal commensal inhabitant of the skin. It lives there and does not cause skin infection. Remember that urticaria is considered immediate IgE-related hypersensitivity like anaphylaxis.

Folliculitis < Furuncles < Carbuncles < Boils

These are aureus-related skin infections beginning at the hair follicle. The only difference between them is size. Folliculitis is the smallest and most minor. Furuncles are larger, carbuncles larger than that, and boils even larger. An "abscess" would be considered the largest.

Diagnosis of these skin infections is based on appearance.

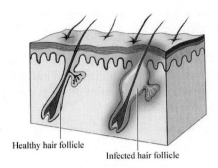

Folliculitis

Antibiotic therapy is identical to that described for cellulitis. Larger infections, such as boils, respond to drainage. As with all other skin infections, the patient can develop post-streptococcal glomerulonephritis but not rheumatic fever.

Fungal Infections of Skin and Nails

Common symptoms in skin infections are severe itching of the scalp, dandruff, and bald patches where the fungus has rooted itself in the skin. In onychomycosis, nails may be thickened, yellow, cloudy, and appear fragile and broken.

KOH preparation is the **best initial test**.

1. Scrape the skin or nail.
2. Place the scraping on a slide with KOH and acid and heat it.
3. The epithelial cells will dissolve and leave the fungal forms behind, visible on the slide.

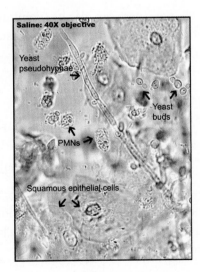

KOH Prep

> **Basic Science Correlate**
>
> Fungi have chitin in their outer wall. Chitin is a polymer that will not break down with KOH. Chitin is what makes up crab and lobster shells. Epithelial cells melt and fungi remain behind in a KOH prep because the chitin in the fungus is tougher than epithelial cells.

Treatment is as follows:

- Topical antifungal medication (if no hair or nail involvement): clotrimazole, miconazole, ketoconazole, econazole, terconazole, nystatin, or ciclopirox
- Oral antifungal medication for scalp (tinea capitis) or nail (onychomycosis)
  - Terbinafine: causes increased LFTs
  - Itraconazole
  - Griseofulvin (for tinea capitis): less effective than terbinafine or itraconazole

Sexually Transmitted Diseases

Screening guidelines are as follows for STDs:

- Women age <25 should be screened yearly for gonorrhea and chlamydia.
- Men who have sex with men should be screened yearly for gonorrhea, chlamydia, and syphilis.
- Everyone, regardless of risk factors, should be tested for HIV.

Urethritis

Look for a urethral discharge. There can also be symptoms of dysuria, such as frequency, urgency, and burning. Discharge without dysuria is still considered urethritis. With dysuric symptoms but not discharge, the patient does not necessarily have urethritis; the patient could just have cystitis (i.e., a UTI).

Diagnostic testing is as follows:

- Nucleic acid amplification tests (NAATs) are comparable to PCR and are highly effective as well. NAAT is done on a voided urine sample.
- Urethral swab for Gram stain, WBC count, and culture are seldom the answer.

Treatment for urethritis and cervicitis is 2 medications: one drug active against gonorrhea and one drug active against chlamydia (because these are very often present in coinfection).

Disseminated gonorrhea gives:

- Polyarticular disease
- Petechial rash
- Tenosynovitis

Gonorrhea medications	Chlamydia medications
• Ceftriaxone IM	• Azithromycin (single dose) • Doxycycline (for a week)
Pregnant patients • Ceftriaxone IM	Pregnant patients • Azithromycin

A patient develops recurrent episodes of gonorrhea. What should he be tested for?

a. Presence of a spleen.
b. HIV.
c. Terminal complement deficiency.
d. Steroid use.
e. Malabsorption.

Answer: **C.** Terminal complement deficiency predisposes a patient to recurrent episodes of *Neisseria* infection. This includes any form, including genital and CNS infection.

Cervicitis

This presents with cervical discharge. The answer is DNA testing in the same way as for urethritis, by nucleic acid amplification testing (NAAT). Speculum examination is not needed; it can be done by self-administered blind vaginal swab. This is just as accurate as a speculum examination. Gram stain and culture is not needed routinely. Culture is done if there is treatment failure to see if there is resistance.

Treatment is the same as for urethritis.

> Nucleic acid amplification test (NAAT) is a "DNA probe." NAAT is the single best test for both gonorrhea and chlamydia.

Pelvic Inflammatory Disease (PID)

Symptoms include lower abdominal pain, tenderness, fever, and cervical motion tenderness. Dysuria and/or vaginal discharge are also possible.

Diagnostic testing is as follows:

- There are no specific blood tests; leukocytosis is a measure of severity
- **Best initial test:** pregnancy test, then DNA probe (NAAT) for chlamydia and gonorrhea; cervical culture and stain are sometimes done
- **Most accurate test** is laparoscopy (rarely needed) for recurrent or persistent infection or when diagnosis is not clear

---

Basic Science Correlate

Leukocytosis in infection is caused by demargination of WBCs from the side of blood vessels. Half of WBCs are in circulation and half are on the walls of endothelial cells. Catecholamines (epi, norepi) and cortisol take WBCs off the margins of blood vessels and put them in circulation, meaning stress alone potentially doubles the WBC count.

A 30-year-old woman comes to the ED with lower abdominal pain and tenderness, fever, leukocytosis, and cervical motion tenderness. What is the next best step in management?

a. Cervical culture
b. Pelvic sonogram
c. Urine pregnancy test
d. Laparoscopy
e. Ceftriaxone and doxycycline

Answer: **C.** With lower abdominal pain or tenderness, it is important to exclude an ectopic pregnancy. Do a urine pregnancy test first and then get a cervical culture and start therapy.

Treatment is as follows:

- Ceftriaxone (IM) and doxycycline (oral) for outpatient
- Cefoxitin (IV) and doxycycline and maybe metronidazole for inpatient (cefotetan can be used instead of cefoxitin)
- Clindamycin and gentamicin for penicillin allergy

Antibiotics that are safe in pregnancy:

- Penicillins
- Cephalosporins
- Aztreonam
- Erythromycin, azithromycin

> NAAT can be done on voided urine for men or self-administered blind vaginal swab for women.

Basic Science Correlate

Mechanism of Infertility and Ectopic Pregnancy in PID
The tubes become scarred and narrowed. Sperm cannot travel in to fertilize the egg. Fertilized eggs get caught and implant in the wrong place—all from loss of ciliary action, fibrosis, and occlusion.

Epididymo-Orchitis

Presents with an extremely painful and tender testicle with a normal position in the scrotum.

Testicular torsion is different in that it presents with an elevated testicle in an abnormal transverse position.

Treatment is ceftriaxone and doxycycline for those age <35, and fluoroquinolone for those age >35.

Ulcerative Genital Diseases

All forms of ulcerative genital disease can be associated with enlarged lymph nodes. Sexual history is not as important as the presence of ulcers.

Chancroid

The ulcer will be painful (*Haemophilus ducreyi*). The **best initial tests** are a swab for Gram stain (gram-negative coccobacilli) and culture (will require specialized medium: Nairobi medium or Mueller-Hinton agar).

Treatment is a single IM shot of ceftriaxone or single oral dose of azithromycin.

Lymphogranuloma Venereum (LGV)

Large tender nodes are present in addition to the ulcer. The enlarged nodes, sometimes called "buboes," may develop a suppurating, draining sinus tract. Diagnostic testing is NAAT of a lymph node aspirate or serology for *Chlamydia trachomatis*.

Treatment is aspiration of the bubo, followed by doxycycline or azithromycin.

Basic Science Correlate

Mechanism of Erythromycin Adverse Effects

Erythromycin is not used for chlamydia for the following reasons:

- Less effective than azithromycin
- Causes severe nausea, vomiting, and diarrhea
- Increases the release of motilin, a hormone which increases GI motility between meals to the point of excess GI motility (which is why it works for hypomotility disorders such as diabetic gastroparesis)

Herpes Simplex Virus (Genital Herpes)

A 34-year-old man comes to the clinic with multiple vesicles on his penis. There is enlarged adenopathy in the inguinal area. What is the next step in management?

a. Tzanck prep
b. Viral culture
c. Valacyclovir
d. Valganciclovir
e. PCR

Answer: C. When there are clear vesicular lesions present, there is no need to do a diagnostic test for herpes—go straight to treatment: acyclovir, valacyclovir, or famciclovir for 7–10 days. For recurrent genital herpes, give chronic suppressive therapy. If the roofs come off the vesicles and the lesion becomes an ulcer of unclear etiology, then the **most accurate test** for herpes is PCR. Tzanck prep has limited accuracy. Valganciclovir is treatment for CMV.

Acyclovir is safe in pregnancy. Use acyclovir in pregnancy if there is evidence of active lesions at 36 weeks.

The PCR test of genital herpes is more sensitive than viral culture. Viral culture, however, is the only way to determine viral sensitivity. If the lesions continue to recur the answer is chronic suppressive therapy with valacyclovir or acyclovir. If the lesion persists despite therapy, get a viral culture. If the herpes is resistant to acyclovir, the answer is foscarnet. The most common wrong answer for treating acyclovir resistant herpes is ganciclovir. If the thymidine kinase is mutated causing acyclovir resistance, there will be resistance to ganciclovir too.

Syphilis

The responsible pathogen is *Treponema pallidum.*

Serological testing for herpes antibody has no clinical utility.

> A man comes to the clinic having had a painless, firm genital lesion for the last several days. The inguinal adenopathy is painless. What is the most accurate diagnostic test?
>
> a. VDRL
> b. RPR
> c. FTA
> d. Darkfield microscopic exam
>
> Answer: **D.** The most accurate test in primary syphilis is darkfield microscopy, which is far more sensitive than a VDRL or RPR (only 75% sensitive, with a 25% false-negative rate).

Primary Syphilis

- Symptoms: chancre, adenopathy
- **Initial diagnostic test**: Darkfield, then VDRL or RPR (75% sensitive in primary syphilis). False positives are caused by SLE, increasing age, and many infections such as endocarditis.
- Treatment: Single IM shot of penicillin. Use doxycycline for the penicillin-allergic. Some patients will develop a Jarisch-Herxheimer reaction, with fever, headache, and myalgia developing 24 hours after treatment for early stage syphilis. It is a benign, self-limited reaction caused by the release of pyrogens from dying treponemal. Treat with aspirin and continue the treatment.

Secondary Syphilis

- Symptoms: rash, mucous patch, alopecia areata, condylomata lata
- **Initial diagnostic test**: RPR and FTA; both are 100% sensitive
- Treatment: Single IM shot of penicillin. Use doxycycline for the penicillin-allergic.

> FTA is more sensitive than VDRL for neurosyphilis.

Tertiary Syphilis

- Neurological involvement: Tabes dorsalis, Argyll-Robertson pupil, general paresis, rarely a gumma or aortitis
- **Initial diagnostic tests**: RPR (75% sensitive in blood) and FTA (95% sensitive), lumbar puncture for neurosyphilis (test CSF with VDRL and FTA) CSF VDRL is only 50% sensitive. FTA is 100% sensitive in CSF.
- Treatment: IV penicillin; if penicillin-allergic, desensitize

> If the patient is allergic to penicillin, desensitization is the answer for:
> - Neurosyphilis
> - Pregnant women

Syphilis by Stage			
Stage	**Primary**	**Secondary**	**Tertiary**
Presentation	Chancre	• Rash • Alopecia • Condylomata lata • Mucous patch	• Neurosyphilis: Tabes dorsalis, general paresis, Argyll-Robertson pupil • Gummas • Aortitis
Test	• Darkfield (most sensitive) • RPR or VDRL (75% positive) • FTA	• RPR or VDRL (99% positive) • FTA (99% positive)	• RPR or VDRL (50% positive in CSF) • FTA (100% sensitive in CSF) • Lumbar puncture
Treatment	1. Single IM penicillin 2. Doxycycline if allergic	1. Single IM penicillin 2. Doxycycline if allergic	1. IV penicillin 2. Desensitization if allergic

Granuloma Inguinale

This is indicated by a rare, beefy red genital lesion that ulcerates.

Diagnostic testing is biopsy or "touch prep," *Klebsiella granulomatis,* "Donovan bodies."

Treatment is doxycycline, TMP/SMX, or azithromycin.

> Neurosyphilis is excluded with a negative CSF FTA.

Warts

All warts (condylomata acuminata, verrucous wart, molluscum contagiosum) are diagnosed by how they look. They are caused by human papillomavirus (HPV).

Treatment is mechanical removal.

- Imiquimod, an immunostimulant, to slough off the wart
- Cryotherapy, laser removal, and trichloroacetic acid to burn/melt off the wart
- Surgical removal (if large)

> **Basic Science Correlate**
>
> Imiquimod stimulates the release of cytokines such as interferon, TNF-alpha, and interleukin-6. It also stimulates natural killer cells to get rid of HPV infected cells and malignant cells that are not melanoma. Imiquimod is indicated for basal cell cancer, actinic keratosis, and minor squamous cell cancer, in addition to venereal warts.

Urinary Tract Infection

Cystitis

Cystitis often presents with urinary frequency, urgency, burning, and dysuria in young, otherwise healthy women. The **best initial test** is urinalysis. The **most accurate test** is urine culture, although that is not typically required for uncomplicated cases.

Treatment is as follows:

- **Uncomplicated cystitis**
  - Fosfomycin, nitrofurantoin, or TMP/SMX orally for 3 days if *E. coli* resistance in that area is low (if resistance >20%, use ciprofloxacin or levofloxacin)
  - Quinolones for more serious infections
- **Complicated cystitis** (presence of an anatomic abnormality, i.e., a stone, obstruction): TMP/SMX or ciprofloxacin for 7 days
- Pain relief: phenazopyridine is a urinary tract anesthetic for bladder infection; pentosan is an anesthetic for interstitial nephritis (both are oral)

> First line in cystitis:
> - Fosfomycin
> - Nitrofurantoin
> - TMP/SMX
>
> Fosfomycin and nitrofurantoin are considered safe in pregnancy and are class B.

A 25-year-old, generally healthy woman comes to the office with burning on urination. There are 50 white cells on the urinalysis. What is the next best step in management?

a. Wait for results of urine culture
b. Urine culture
c. TMP/SMX for 3 days
d. Ciprofloxacin for 7 days
e. Renal ultrasound

Answer: **C.** When there are clear symptoms of cystitis and white cells in the urine, it is not necessary to obtain a urine culture or to wait for results of the culture or a sonogram. For uncomplicated cystitis, go straight to treatment for 3 days. Ultrasound is important in males, as it is unusual for a male patient to have a UTI in the absence of an anatomic abnormality.

> Asymptomatic bacteriuria: Do not treat asymptomatic bacteriuria, unless the patient is pregnant or getting urinary instrumentation.

Pyelonephritis

Pyelonephritis is a more severe disease than cystitis. Symptoms include urinary frequency, urgency, burning, dysuria, and high fever, plus flank pain and tenderness. In general, patients are much more ill than they are with cystitis.

Testing is urinalysis and urine culture to diagnose, as is done for cystitis. Sonogram or CT will help to identify the etiology. Ask, if there a stone? a stricture? a tumor? an obstruction? an anatomic defect which must be corrected so the infection will not recur?

- Dysuria + white cells in urine + suprapubic tenderness = **cystitis**
- Dysuria + white cells in urine + flank pain + fever = **pyelonephritis**

Treatment is a medication for gram-negative bacilli. For outpatient, use ciprofloxacin. For inpatient, use ceftriaxone, ertapenem, quinolones, or ampicillin + gentamicin.

> Urinalysis: For infections, the concern is mainly with the presence of white blood cells (WBCs). Numerous squamous epithelial cells suggest an improperly collected specimen, and unless symptomatic, do not treat.
>
> Leukocyte esterase is derived from granulocytic white blood cells and serves as indirect evidence of the presence of bacteriuria.
>
> Nitrites are indicative of gram-negative bacteria. Protein is very nonspecific in a urinalysis. Protein can be from both infection and glomerular disorders. Red cells are nonspecific as well.

Perinephric Abscess

This is a rare complication of pyelonephritis. Look for a patient with pyelonephritis who does not respond to treatment after 5–7 days. The patient remains febrile and still shows white cells on urinalysis. Perform a sonogram or kidney CT to find the collection.

The **best diagnostic test** is biopsy (the only way to determine a precise microbiologic diagnosis to guide therapy).

Treatment is a quinolone + staphylococcal coverage such as oxacillin nafcillin, or vancomycin, because treatment with antibiotics for gram-negative organisms preferentially selects out for staphylococci.

Prostatitis

This is indicated by frequency, urgency, and dysuria and perineal or sacral pain. The prostate is tender and may be described as "boggy" on examination.

Sexually active men may get prostatitis from GC and chlamydia.

The **best initial diagnostic test** is urinalysis. The **most accurate test** is urine WBCs after prostate massage.

Treatment is ciprofloxacin or TMP/SMX for an extended period (2 weeks for acute and 6 weeks for chronic).

- Prostatitis is like an abscess. Use the same drugs as for cystitis and pyelo-nephritis but extend the length of therapy.
- Fosfomycin can also be used.

HIV/AIDS

Everyone should be tested for HIV.

Following are the "must know" facts about HIV:

- Adverse effects of medications
- Needle-stick injury management
- Pregnancy/perinatal HIV management

When to start therapy?

- Any CD4 count if there is any level of detectable viral load
- Pregnant women: all of them, any stage of pregnancy, any CD4, any viral load
- Needle-stick, when the patient is known to be HIV-positive

Genotyping: Patients should have their HIV tested for sensitivity. This is because 10–20% of patients have resistance at baseline. HIV is not tested by growing it in a lab.

- HIV sensitivity is based on the presence or absence of viral mutations; certain mutations correspond to resistance to certain drugs.
- Pregnancy is the only exception for waiting for genotyping prior to treatment. It is so urgent to start therapy in pregnancy that treatment should be started and altered later if resistance is found.

Start antiretroviral therapy (ART), which is one of the following:

- Lamivudine + abacavir + an integrase inhibitor (e.g., bictegravir)
- Tenofovir + emtricitabine + an integrase inhibitor (single combination pill with all of these)

- When a protease inhibitor such as atazanavir or darunavir is used with tenofovir or emtricitabine, add a small amount of ritonavir to boost the level of the other protease inhibitors.
- When an integrase inhibitor such as bictegravir, dolutegravir, elvitegravir, or raltegravir is used, combine with 2 nucleosides.

The 3-drug combination is considered superior to the combination with efavirenz or a protease inhibitor. The precise combination is not as important as knowing the adverse effects of each medication.

- Efavirenz is more prone to drug resistance and is avoided in those with mental health issues.
- Tenofovir is associated with RTA and Fanconi syndrome; it also causes decreased bone mineral density.
- Abacavir should be used only in those who are negative for the HLA-B*5701 mutation.

Nearly everyone with HIV should be on ART. Two nucleosides and an integrase inhibitor are the standard of care.

- Abacavir can be used instead of tenofovir.
- Before starting abacavir use, test for HLA-B*5701 mutation to predict the risk of skin reaction.

> Cobicistat is contraindicated in pregnancy.

Class	Nucleoside Reverse Transcriptase Inhibitors	Protease Inhibitors	Nonnucleoside Reverse Transcriptase Inhibitors	Integrase Inhibitors
Adverse effects of the class	Lactic acidosis	Hyperglycemia Hyperlipidemia	Drowsiness; avoid with mental illness (efavirenz)	
Individual medications	• Zidovudine: anemia • Didanosine: pancreatitis and peripheral neuropathy • Stavudine: pancreatitis and neuropathy • Lamivudine: none • Abacavir: rash (HLA-B*5701) • Emtricitabine • Tenofovir: renal toxicity/RTA and bone demineralization	• Indinavir: kidney stones • Ritonavir • Lopinavir • Nelfinavir • Saquinavir • Darunavir • Tipranavir • Amprenavir • Atazanavir	Efavirenz Nevirapine Etravirine Rilpivirine Doravirine	Bictegravir Raltegravir Elvitegravir Dolutegravir

Basic Science Correlate

Integrase inhibitors prevent the integration of the genetic material of the HIV virus from being integrated into the CD4 cell chromosome. HIV is an RNA virus. Reverse transcriptase turns it into DNA, and this viral DNA must be integrated into human DNA in order to be reproduced. This is the step blocked by the integrase inhibitor raltegravir.

> **Basic Science Correlate**
>
> Chemokine receptor 5 (CCR5) is the mechanism whereby the HIV virus enters the CD4 cell. CCR5 is the attachment point of the GP120 on the surface of the HIV virus whereby it finds its way into human cells. Maraviroc is an entry inhibitor: Maraviroc blocks the CCR5 receptor.

Prophylaxis

Preexposure Prophylaxis (PrEP)

PrEP is the use of ART in uninfected persons before high-risk events occur, such as needle-sharing or sexual contact. The HIV uninfected person starts using a 2-drug combination of tenofovir and emtricitabine before exposure. This 2-drug treatment is continued daily for a month after the last exposure. If the sexual or needle-sharing exposures continue regularly, PrEP should continue regularly.

> Forms of tenofovir:
> - Disoproxil form (has renal and bone toxicity)
> - Alafenamide form (less toxic)

Tenofovir also treats hepatitis B, so testing for hepatitis B before starting therapy is recommended. The older form of tenofovir is the disoproxil form, which is associated with renal insufficiency, Fanconi syndrome, and bone demineralization. The alafenamide form of tenofovir is not associated with bone or renal damage.

Postexposure Prophylaxis (Needle-Stick Injury)

With any significant exposure to HIV-positive blood via a needle, scalpel, or penetrating injury, the answer is the same: ART for a month. Start within 72 hours of exposure. Use two nucleosides and an integrase inhibitor.

This would also be true for the exposure of mucosal surfaces to HIV-positive blood or after unprotected sexual contact with a person known to be HIV-positive. Do not use abacavir, because you need to start therapy immediately and you do not have HLA-B*5701 testing available.

Pneumocystis jiroveci Pneumonia (PCP) (<200 CD4 cells)
- TMP/SMX is the best prophylaxis for PCP by far.
- If TMP/SMX causes a rash, switch to atovaquone or dapsone. (Dapsone cannot be used if there is G6PD deficiency.)
- Aerosolized pentamidine has the poorest efficacy and is rarely used. There is the most amount of breakthrough.

Mycobacterium Avium-Intracellulare (MAI) (<50 CD4 cells)
- Use azithromycin once a week orally.

> **Basic Science Correlate**
>
> **Mechanism of Ritonavir**
>
> Ritonavir inhibits hepatic p450 systems—the route through which protease inhibitors are metabolized. A small amount of ritonavir blocks metabolism of the other protease inhibitors, allowing higher blood levels with less frequent dosing.

Pregnancy/Perinatal

- If the patient is already on ART, then simply continue the same therapy.
- Mother-to-child transmission with fully suppressive ART is <1%. Every HIV-positive pregnant woman should be on HIV medications regardless of the stage of her pregnancy or her CD4 count. Do not wait for the second trimester of pregnancy to start therapy.

If the mother's viral load is undetectable at the time of delivery, there is no need for intrapartum zidovudine for the mother. The baby will receive oral zidovudine for several weeks even if the mother is undetectable.

> Start HIV+ pregnant women on HIV medications in the first trimester and continue.

- Dolutegravir is not used in the first trimester of pregnancy because of teratogenicity.
- Cobicistat is not used in pregnancy because it changes the pharmacokinetics of the other ART, bringing it to subtherapeutic levels.
- Use the integrase inhibitor raltegravir in pregnancy, or protease inhibitors.
- Emtricitabine and tenofovir are safe in pregnancy.
- Do not wait for results of genotyping to start ART in pregnancy so that treatment is not delayed.

> All HIV+ pregnant women at any CD4 or viral load need treatment.

Opportunistic Infections

Pneumocystis Pneumonia (PCP)

PCP presents with shortness of breath, dry cough, hypoxia, and increased LDH. The **best initial test** is chest x-ray, which will show increased interstitial markings bilaterally. The **most accurate test** is bronchoalveolar lavage.

Treatment includes:

- IV TMP/SMX
- If there is a rash, use IV pentamidine or the combination of clindamycin and primaquine.
- Atovaquone for mild pneumocystis
- Dapsone (not intravenous) for prophylaxis, not for treatment
- Steroids if PCP is severe (pO_2 <70 or A-a gradient >35)

Toxoplasmosis

Look for headache, nausea, vomiting, and focal neurologic findings. The **best initial test** is a head CT with contrast showing "ring" or contrast-enhancing lesions.

Treat with pyrimethamine and sulfadiazine for 2 weeks and repeat the CT scan. (Atovaquone can be used instead of pyrimethamine.)

- If the lesions are smaller, that is confirmative of toxoplasmosis.
- If the lesions are unchanged in size, then perform a brain biopsy, since this is most likely lymphoma.

Cytomegalovirus (CMV)

Look for HIV with <50 CD4 cells and blurry vision. Perform a dilated ophthalmologic examination. CMV is diagnosed by the appearance of the lesions on examination.

Treatment is ganciclovir or foscarnet. Caution that ganciclovir can cause low WBC, while foscarnet can elevate creatinine. Give the medication intravenously if the infection is immediately sight-threatening.

Maintenance therapy is with oral valganciclovir lifelong, unless the CD4 goes up with ART. If the CD4 rises, you can stop the CMV medications.

Cryptococcus

Echinocandins such as caspofungin do not cover *Cryptococcus*.

Look for HIV and <50 CD4 cells with fever and headache. Neck stiffness and photophobia are not always present. Lumbar puncture will show an increase in the level of lymphocytes in the CSF. The India ink stain has a 60% sensitivity. The **most accurate test** is a cryptococcal antigen test, which is over 95% sensitive and specific.

Treat initially with amphotericin and 5-FC, followed by fluconazole. The fluconazole is continued lifelong unless the CD4 count rises. If the CD4 count rises, all opportunistic infection treatment and prophylaxis can be stopped. The only treatment that cannot be stopped is the antiretrovirals.

Progressive Multifocal Leukoencephalopathy (PML)

Look for HIV and <50 CD4 cells with focal neurologic abnormalities. The **best initial test** is a head CT or MRI. The lesions do not show ring enhancement and there is no mass effect. PCR of CSF for JC virus is most accurate.

There is no specific therapy available for PML. Treat with ART. When the CD4 count rises, PML will resolve.

Mycobacterium Avium-Intracellulare (MAI)

Look for HIV and <50 CD4 cells, plus wasting with weight loss, fever, and fatigue. Anemia is frequent from invasion of the bone marrow. Increased alkaline phosphatase and GGTP with a normal bilirubin are characteristic of hepatic involvement.

Diagnostic testing is blood culture (least sensitive), bone marrow (more sensitive), and liver biopsy (most sensitive).

Treatment is azithromycin (or clarithromycin), rifampin, and ethambutol. Rifabutin is sometimes added.

Infective Endocarditis

Clinically, endocarditis is diagnosed by meeting Duke criteria (2 major and 5 minor criteria). The diagnosis of endocarditis is made by the presence of 2 major, 1 major and 3 minor, or 5 minor criteria.

Duke Criteria for Endocarditis	
Major	**Minor**
Two positive blood cultures with • *Staphylococcus aureus* • Viridans streptococci, *Streptococcus bovis/epidermis*, enterococci, gram-negative rods, *Candida* HACEK organisms are generally culture-negative. • *Haemophilus aphrophilus/parainfluenzae* • *Actinobacillus actinomycetemcomitans* • *Cardiobacterium hominis* • *Eikenella corrodens* • *Kingella kingae*	Fever (>38.0°C [>100.4°F])

Abnormal echocardiogram:
• Intracardiac mass or valvular vegetation
  OR
• Abscess
  OR
• New partial dehiscence of prosthetic valve
	Presence of risk factors:
	• IV drug use (IDU)
	• Presence of structural heart disease
	• Prosthetic heart valve
	• Dental procedures involving bleeding
	• History of endocarditis

	Vascular findings: • Janeway lesions • Septic pulmonary infarcts • Arterial emboli • Mycotic aneurysm • Conjunctival hemorrhage
	Immunological findings: • Roth spots • Osler nodes • Glomerulonephritis
	Microbiologic findings • Positive blood culture but does not meet major criteria

Look for a patient with a risk such as the following:

- Prosthetic heart valve
- Injection drug use
- Dental procedures that cause bleeding
- Previous endocarditis
- Unrepaired or recently repaired cyanotic heart disease

When there is fever and a new murmur or change in a murmur, the "best next step" in management is to perform blood cultures first. If the blood cultures are positive, then perform an echocardiogram to look for vegetations.

Other physical findings are rarely seen but are useful in establishing the diagnosis of endocarditis if the blood cultures are negative:

- Roth spots (retina)
- Janeway lesions (flat, painless in hands and feet)
- Osler nodes (raised, painful, and pea shaped)
- Splinter hemorrhages (under fingernails)

Diagnostic testing is as follows:

	Transthoracic Echocardiogram (TTE)	Transesophageal Echocardiogram (TEE)
Sensitivity	60%	90–95%
Specificity	90–95%	90–95%
	If TTE is negative, then proceed to TEE.	

> **Fever + murmur** means **possible endocarditis.**
>
> Do blood cultures. If you get 2 positive blood cultures + positive echo, you have endocarditis.

The most common causes of culture-negative endocarditis are not the HACEK group of organisms; the most common causes are *Coxiella* and *Bartonella* (together, 80% of cases). *Clostridium septicum* is even more frequently associated with colonic pathology than *Streptococcus bovis*.

Empiric treatment is vancomycin and gentamicin (or ceftriaxone) in combination for 4–6 weeks. This will cover the most common organisms, which are *S. aureus*, MRSA, and viridans group streptococci.

- You do not need to cover empirically for fungi or resistant gram-negative rods, since these are less common.
- Colonoscopy for *S. bovis* or *Clostridium septicum*; both are associated with colonic pathology.
- Valve replacement for anatomic defects (valve rupture, abscess. prosthetic valves, fungal endocarditis, and embolic events once antibiotics have been started), which are hard or impossible to correct with antibiotics alone.

> Most common culture-negative endocarditis:
> - *Bartonella*
> - *Coxiella*

> Daptomycin is an alternative to vancomycin in MRSA endocarditis.

Endocarditis Prophylaxis

The only **cardiac defects** that need prophylaxis are the following:

- Prosthetic valves
- Unrepaired cyanotic heart disease
- Previous endocarditis
- Transplant recipients who develop valve disease

The only **procedures** that need prophylaxis are the following:

- Dental procedures that cause bleeding: The prophylactic antibiotic to use for dental procedures is amoxicillin. For penicillin-allergic patients, clindamycin is the drug of choice.
- Respiratory tract surgery
- Surgery of infected skin

The following procedures do not need prophylaxis:

- Dental fillings
- All flexible scopes
- All OB/GYN procedures
- All urinary procedures, including cystoscopy

The following cardiac defects do **not** need prophylaxis:

- Aortic stenosis or regurgitation
- Mitral stenosis or regurgitation
- Atrial or ventricular septal defects
- Pacemakers and implantable defibrillators
- Mitral valve prolapse, even if there is a murmur
- HOCM (IHSS)

What is the drug to give as prophylaxis?

- For dental/oral procedures, amoxicillin; if rash with penicillin, then cephalexin; if anaphylaxis to penicillin, then azithromycin, clarithromycin, or clindamycin
- For skin procedures, cephalexin; if allergic to penicillin, then vancomycin

Tropical, Fungal, and Animal-Borne Diseases

Tropical Diseases and Parasites

Dengue

- Viral, mosquito-borne (*Aedes* sp.) in tropics, giving fever
- Dengue translates as "severe bone pain"; headache, retro-orbital pain
- Platelets drop, giving petechiae, second episode associated with hemorrhage
- Capillaries leak
- Diagnose with ELISA serology
- No treatment; vaccine is available
- Hydrate

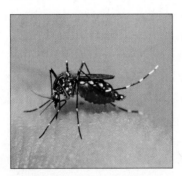

Aedes mosquito, transmitter of dengue, chikungunya, and yellow fever (source: WikiCommons)

Ebola

- Hemorrhagic fever (RNA filovirus)
- Infection requires direct contact with body fluids (blood, feces, vomit)
- Not airborne/respiratory (**most likely question on the exam**)
- Diagnose with serology or PCR
- No specific therapy or vaccine

Chikungunya

- Virus transmitted by *Aedes* mosquito
- Headache, fatigue, fever
- Special characteristic: joint pain/arthralgia, half presenting with rash
- Diagnose with serology and PCR
- No specific therapy or vaccine

Zika

- *Aedes* mosquito, Flavivirus
- Fever, rash, conjunctivitis
- Causes microcephaly when pregnant women are infected
- No specific therapy or vaccine; acetaminophen and fluids for symptoms
- Associated with Guillain-Barré syndrome

Crimean-Congo Hemorrhagic Fever

- Presents with headache, high fever, back pain, and vomiting. Red eyes, a flushed face, a red throat, and petechiae (red spots) on the palate are common.
- Special characteristics: bleeding from puncture sites, petechiae, ecchymoses. Bleeding can be fatal!
- Viral etiology (RNA), transmitted by ticks
- Diagnose with ELISA and PCR.
- Treatment: no clearly effective antiviral, no vaccine
- Ribavirin effective in labs and tried in people; if asked, answer ribavirin.

Leishmaniasis

- Protozoan spread by sandflies (look for "returning Iraqi veteran" in the exam question)
- Skin/mucosal or "visceral" form of liver, spleen, and fever
- Diagnose with direct visualization on aspirates of liver, spleen, marrow, or white cells. PCR and culture confirm direct visualization.
- Treatment: liposomal amphotericin, miltefosine, or antimonials (stibogluconate). Miltefosine works on cutaneous, mucosal, and visceral leishmaniasis.

Echinococcus

- Animal source: dogs and sheep shedding eggs
- Eggs ingested by human
- Spreads to liver, lung, and brain forming hydatid cysts
- Detect cysts with sonogram, CT, MRI; confirm with ELISA
- Aspiration of cyst can spread it accidentally
- Treatment: albendazole and injecting alcohol into cysts

Bedbug (*Cimex*) Bites

- Presentation:
  - Pink macules that become papules, plaques, and hives
  - Intensely pruritic
  - Symptoms appear minutes to days after a bite.
- Bedbugs are red-brown, wingless insects that live in the dark, emerging at night for a blood meal.
- Treatment: no anti-infective exists; insecticides like DEET keep the bugs away; kill bedbugs by heating all bedding, clothing, and furniture to 50°C (122°F)
- Symptom control: **antihistamines and topical corticosteroids**

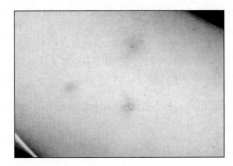

Bedbug (*Cimex*) Bites

Middle Eastern Respiratory Syndrome (MERS)

- Presentation: fever, dry cough, and potentially fatal respiratory distress
- Causative organism: *Coronavirus*
- History of recent travel in the Middle East, especially Saudi Arabia
- Transmission (airborne) can be from household or nosocomial contact
- Treatment: no effective anti-infective therapy

Cholera

- Presentation:
  - Massive watery, nonbloody ("rice-water") diarrhea, vomiting, and muscle cramps
  - Sunken eyes and loose skin
  - Hypokalemia and acidosis (50% mortality without treatment)
  - Massive hydration solves most cases; administer 10% of body weight over first 2–4 hours and continue eating food
- Prevention: vaccination for travel to cholera-affected areas, not for most tourists
- Treatment is fluid and electrolyte replacement; azithromycin or doxycycline for extremely severe cases.

Fungal and Atypical Respiratory Diseases

Nocardia

> *Nocardia* gives branching, gram-positive filaments that are weakly acid fast.

This involves immunocompromised people (leukemia, lymphoma, steroid use, HIV). Respiratory/pulmonary disease may disseminate to any organ, with skin and brain being the most common.

Diagnostic testing includes chest x-ray (**best initial test**) and culture (**most accurate test**).

Treatment is TMP/SMX or imipenem.

Actinomyces

Actinomyces is a part of normal mouth flora. Trauma, such as a tooth extraction, can put it into the facial area, thorax, and abdomen.

The host has a normal immune system. There is a history of facial or dental trauma, which inoculated these organisms into the cervicofacial area.

Diagnose with Gram stain and confirm with anaerobic culture. Like *Nocardia*, *Actinomyces* is a branching, filamentous bacterium.

Treatment is penicillin.

Histoplasmosis

This is a lung disease that can present as a viral syndrome. It is also associated with bat droppings (guano) from caves. Look for wet areas, such as river valleys.

Physical exam will show palate and oral ulcers and splenomegaly. The disseminated disease enters the bone marrow and causes pancytopenia.

Anything tuberculosis can do, histoplasmosis can do.

Diagnostic testing includes:

- Histoplasmosis urine and serum antigen are the **best initial tests**.
- Biopsy with culture is **most accurate test** for both histoplasmosis and tuberculosis.

Acute pulmonary disease is transient and requires no treatment. Disseminated disease is treated with amphotericin, followed by itraconazole.

Coccidioidomycosis

This is an acute respiratory illness that occurs in very dry areas like Arizona. It causes joint pain (common) ("desert rheumatism") and erythema nodosum.

Sputum culture and serology are the **most accurate tests**.

Treatment is fluconazole for moderate disease, and amphotericin for severe disease. Echinocandins such as caspofungin are not effective.

Blastomycosis

This is an acute pulmonary disease in the rural southeast. Look for broad budding yeast.

Bone and skin lesions are common. Diagnosis confirmed by culture.

Treatment is antifungal agents: itraconazole for mild disease and amphotericin for severe disease.

Sporotrichosis

- Fungus living in soil and plants (e.g., in rose gardens)
- Acquired from direct inoculation
- Leads to cutaneous nodules and is diagnosed by culture
- Treatment is itraconazole

Fungal Infections

Mucormycosis (Zygomycosis)

- Immunocompromised host, particularly diabetics in DKA
- Deferoxamine increases the risk by mobilizing iron
- Eats through nasal canals, through eyes, and into brain, killing the patient
- Hard to grow in culture, seen on biopsy
- Surgical emergency! Resect necrotic face.
- Treatment: amphotericin IV
- Follow-up therapy: posaconazole or isavuconazole

Aspergillus

- **Allergic bronchopulmonary** aspergillosis
  - Found in asthmatics and cystic fibrosis patients: coughing brown mucous plugs, abnormal x-ray
  - Confirm with *Aspergillus* precipitin antibodies and IgE in serum or skin test
  - Eosinophil count often elevated
  - Treatment: oral prednisone (inhaled is most common wrong answer)
  - Itraconazole or voriconazole orally
- **Invasive** *Aspergillus*
  - Found in severely immunocompromised patients, particularly in neutropenia and leukemia
  - Rapidly progressive, severe lung infiltrates on x-ray and CT
  - Diagnose with biopsy (sputum lacks sensitivity)
  - Serum galactomannan assay, beta-D-glucan level, or PCR (2 positive tests have >95% specificity)
  - Treatment: voriconazole, isavuconazole, or caspofungin
  - Amphotericin is the most common wrong answer

> Isavuconazole covers:
> - *Aspergillus*
> - Mucormycetes
> - Candida

Candida auris

- Fungal infection of the bloodstream
- Immunocompromised host
- Diagnosis: isolated from blood cultures
- Treatment: sensitive to echinocandins (e.g., caspofungin, micafungin) but resistant to fluconazole and voriconazole

Animal-Borne Diseases

Leptospirosis

In the history, there is exposure to animals, and the patient has eaten food contaminated by the urine of infected animals. This disease is a spirochete.

Animal exposure + jaundice + renal = **leptospirosis**

- Symptoms include fever, abdominal pain, and muscle aches; severe disease leads to altered mental status.
- Diagnose with serology. Look for CPK elevation.
- Treatment is ceftriaxone or penicillin.

Tularemia

In the history, there is contact with rabbits in the summer. Look for a hunter or someone who has touched a small, furry animal. The pneumonic (lung) form of the disease is rapidly fatal.

- There is an ulcer at the site of contact and enlarged lymph nodes. Conjunctivitis is another clue.
- Diagnose with serology. Note that taking a culture is dangerous, as spores can cause severe pneumonia in lab personnel.
- Treatment is doxycycline.

Cysticercosis

This disease is often transmitted by infected pork that is ingested. Infection is most likely in those who have eaten pork in endemic areas such as Mexico, South America, Eastern Europe, or India.

- CT scan of the head will show thin-walled cysts, which are most often calcified.
- Treatment is albendazole; if there are no active lesions and patient presents only with calcifications and seizures, only anti-epileptic therapy is needed.
- Many people have had cysticercosis in the past. After the active infection is gone, all that remains is calcification.

Trichinellosis

In the history, there is ingestion of undercooked meats, most often pork.

- Initial infection presents with diarrhea, abdominal pain, and vomiting; later symptoms include swelling of the face, muscle pains, rash.
- Diagnose with increased eosinophils, increased CPK and confirm with ELISA or muscle biopsy.
- Treatment is albendazole or mebendazole.
- Prevent future cases by fully cooking meat.

Plague

In the history, there is rodent exposure in the American Southwest region.

- Lung form of the disease (pneumonic plague) can be fatal in 24 hours.
- Early symptoms include sudden-onset high fever, intense headache, severe myalgia; later symptoms include massively enlarged lymph nodes (buboes).
- Testing is gram-negative rods on smear of node aspirate (**best initial test**) and culture (**most accurate test**).
- Treatment is gentamicin or doxycycline.

Strongyloides

- Causative organism is a nematode (roundworm).
- Presentation: skin involvement, respiratory and GI symptoms
- Further symptoms:
  - Itchy lesions, particularly on the feet (wear shoes where the organism entered)
  - Eosinophilic pneumonia (coughing up the organism from the lymphatics)
  - Nausea, diarrhea (from swallowing what was coughed up)
  - Hyperinfection syndrome everywhere in the immunocompromised
  - Worms/larvae (not eggs) seen in stool and bronchoscopy
- Treatment is ivermectin or albendazole.

> *Strongyloides* infection can present as asymptomatic eosinophilia or death from hyperinfection.

Brucellosis

Brucella needs long periods to grow. In the history, there is exposure to unpasteurized milk or uninspected meat from outside the United States; "returning war veteran."

- Symptoms include fever for weeks/months, hepatosplenomegaly, endocarditis, osteomyelitis, meningitis, chronic joint pain.
- Diagnose with culture (blood, CSF, urine, marrow) and serology.

Chagas Disease (American Trypanosomiasis)

In the history, there is travel to South America. This can also be spread by blood transfusion or organ transplantation.

- Early symptoms: fever, lymphadenopathy headache, local swelling at eye (which resolves)
- Symptoms decades later: heart, esophagus, and colon dysfunction (30% of patients)
- Diagnosis: organisms visible on blood smear
- Treatment is benznidazole or nifurtimox for early disease
- Untreated disease dilates organs: look for dilated cardiomyopathy, esophageal dysmotility, and colonic dilation and dysmotility

Anthrax

- Gram-positive, spore-forming rod occurring in sheep, cattle, horses, goats
- Presentation:
  - Cutaneous: painless, black eschar at site of contact; often self-limited
  - GI: ulcerative lesion gives abdominal pain, vomiting, and diarrhea and may perforate.
  - Inhalational: wide mediastinum with hemorrhagic lymphadenitis and pleural effusion; can be rapidly fatal
- Diagnosis: culture showing boxcar-shaped, encapsulated rods
- Treatment is quinolone or doxycycline.

Bartonella

- Catscratch disease (*B. henselae*)
  - Presentation: enlarged, tender regional lymph nodes
  - Diagnosis is clinical, supported by serology.
  - Treatment is not usually needed, but azithromycin speeds resolution; hepatosplenic disease or neuroretinitis definitely needs doxycycline or azithromycin + rifampin.
- Endocarditis (*B. quintana*)
  - In the history, there is homelessness or flea bites.
  - Diagnose with serology/PCR.
  - Treatment is doxycycline.

Tick-Borne Diseases

Lyme Disease

For the Step 3 exam, camping and hiking are markers for the presence of ticks.

- The cause is a spirochete named *Borrelia burgdorferi*, which is carried by the Ixodes genus (deer) tick.
- The exam question may say something about vacationing in the Northeast or Midwest (Connecticut, Delaware, Maine, Maryland, Massachusetts, Minnesota, New Hampshire, New York, New Jersey, Pennsylvania, Wisconsin).
- Only 20% of those with Lyme disease recall getting a tick bite, because it is so small.
- The rash is shaped like a target with a pale center and a red ring on the outside.

Long-term manifestations/complications of Lyme are as follows:

- Joint involvement (most common late manifestation)
- Cardiac (most common is AV conduction block/defect)
- Neurologic (most common is 7th cranial nerve palsy [Bell palsy])

Diagnostic testing includes serology, such as IgM, IgG ELISA, Western blot, or PCR.

Treatment is as follows:

- Oral doxycycline, amoxicillin, or cefuroxime for rash, joint, Bell palsy
- IV ceftriaxone for CNS or cardiac involvement

> A 43-year-old man presents with a target-shaped rash that has developed over the last several days. He was on a camping trip in the woods last week in Maine. What is the next best step in management?
>
> a. Serology for IgM
> b. ELISA
> c. Western blot
> d. Doxycycline
> e. Ceftriaxone
>
> Answer: **D.** A rash suggestive of Lyme is enough to indicate treatment. A 5-cm-wide target-shaped rash, particularly with a history of camping/hiking, is enough to indicate the need for antibiotic treatment with doxycycline. A characteristic rash is more specific than serology. Ceftriaxone is used for CNS or cardiac Lyme.

The proper term for Lyme is erythema migrans, but this term has no precise meaning.

Camping/hiking + target-shaped rash = Lyme disease

There is no "chronic" Lyme disease.

7th cranial nerve palsy is not CNS.

Babesiosis

Babesiosis is transmitted by the same *Ixodes* (deer) tick that transmits Lyme. As a result, it is also common in the northeast. Presentation includes hemolytic anemia, which is severe in asplenic individuals.

> **Basic Science Correlate**
>
> Asplenic patients have more Babesia because a functional spleen removes infected cells from circulation. When Babesia infects a red cell, it further deforms the cell. The spleen detects this deformity and removes the cell before Babesia can reproduce.

Diagnostic testing is a peripheral blood smear looking for tetrads of intraerythrocytic ring forms (Maltese crosses) or a PCR.

Treatment is azithromycin and atovaquone.

Ehrlichia/Anaplasma

Ehrlichia is transmitted by the lone star tick (*Amblyomma americanum*). *Anaplasma* is transmitted by the *Ixodes* tick. There is no rash. Instead, there are elevated LFTs (ALT and AST), thrombocytopenia (decreased platelets), and leukopenia (decreased white blood cells).

Diagnostic testing is a peripheral blood smear looking for "morulae" (inclusion bodies in the white cells) or PCR.

Treatment is doxycycline.

Malaria

Malaria is rarely domestic. Look for a traveler recently returning from an endemic area with hemolysis. GI complaints are always present.

Diagnostic testing is blood smear.

Treatment is as follows:

- Mefloquine or atovaquone/proguanil for mild disease
- Mefloquine or atovaquone/proguanil for acute disease
- Artemisinins for severe disease (parasitemia >5-10%; renal insufficiency; metabolic acidosis; hypoglycemia; and CNS manifestations)
  - Artesunate, an artemisinin derivative, is the single most effective medication for severe malaria
  - Compared with quinine, artesunate clears parasitemia faster and has no cardiac precautions (quinine, given as quinidine, causes QT prolongation)
- Quinine/doxycycline or artesunate for very severe disease

Prophylaxis of malaria is with atovaquone/proguanil given daily or mefloquine given weekly (caution those taking mefloquine of the neuropsychiatric side effects, sinus bradycardia, and QT prolongation).

Daily doxycycline can be used for prophylaxis if there is resistance to all other agents.

For both acute treatment and prophylaxis of malaria, the same drugs can be used:
- Mefloquine
- Atovaquone/proguanil

Test for G6PD before using primaquine!

Allergy and Immunology 5

Anaphylaxis

Anaphylaxis is a hypersensitivity/allergic reaction that is potentially life-threatening. The most common causes are food (e.g., peanuts, shellfish); insect stings/bites; and medication (e.g., penicillin, allopurinol, sulfa-containing drugs).

Anaphylaxis presents as hemodynamic instability with hypotension and tachycardia, as well as difficulty breathing.

Treatment for anaphylaxis has not changed for decades. The best initial therapy is to administer all of the following:

- Intramuscular epinephrine in a 1:1,000 concentration
- Corticosteroids
- H1-inhibiting antihistamine, e.g., diphenhydramine or hydroxyzine

CCS Tip: You are not required to know doses on the CCS, but you must know the **route of administration** and **type of medication**. Thus, you must know to give the epinephrine **intramuscularly.**

> **Basic Science Correlate**
>
> Epinephrine will cause vasoconstriction through alpha-1 receptor stimulation. The beta-2 receptor stimulation effect dilates bronchi. Corticosteroids need 4–6 hours to work, and they increase vasoconstriction by up-regulating alpha-1 receptors. Steroids also inhibit leukotriene release.

> IVIG has trace IgA. It can cause anaphylaxis in IgA-deficient patients.

A patient comes to the ED with shortness of breath, facial swelling, and lip swelling 30 minutes after a bee sting. There was no response to epinephrine auto-injection in the field. Six hours after a bolus of steroid and diphenhydramine, the patient is still short of breath and has lip swelling. Where should the patient be placed?

Answer: This patient should be placed in the ICU. If the patient comes with anaphylaxis from any cause, the placement of the patient for CCS is based entirely on the response to therapy that occurs after treatment. In this case, the source of the allergic reaction, an insect sting, is irrelevant. What matters is that after moving the clock forward, the symptoms do not resolve. Any persistent lip, facial, or hemodynamic involvement after initial therapy should send the patient to the ICU.

Angioedema

Angioedema is a sudden swelling of the face, palate, tongue, and airway in association with minor trauma to the face or hands or the ingestion of ACE inhibitors. There is no urticaria, wheezing, or pruritus.

Other symptoms include stridor and abdominal pain. The question may describe a person hit in the face with a pillow or wood chips hitting the arm.

The hereditary form of angioedema occurs from deficiency of C1 esterase inhibitor.

> **Why is there abdominal pain in angioedema?**
>
> Because the bowel wall swells just like the face.

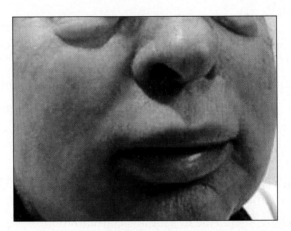

Angioedema Face

The diagnosis of angioedema arising from C1 esterase deficiency is based on low levels of C2 and C4 in the complement pathway. They are chronically depleted because of the deficiency of the C1 esterase inhibitor.

Elevated white cell count is not specific.

Treatment is as follows. The ICU may be required.

- C1 inhibitor plasma-derived concentrate (**best initial treatment for severe laryngeal involvement**); alternative is recombinant C1 inhibitor
- Icatibant (bradykinin receptor antagonist); lanadelumab is an antibody against kallikrein (ecallantide inhibits kallikrein)
- Ecallantide and icatibant (**drugs of choice for acute hereditary angioedema**)
  - Antihistamines, glucocorticoids, and epinephrine are **not** effective in acute bradykinin-mediated hereditary angioedema
  - They are effective in anaphylaxis but not in C1 esterase inhibitor deficiency
- Infusion of fresh frozen plasma (for acute episodes) if C1 inhibitor, ecallantide, and icatibant are not available
- Androgens (danazol and stanozolol) (**for chronic disease**); raise C1 esterase inhibitor levels

> Ecallantide, an inhibitor of kallikrein, treats acute angioedema. Kallikrein makes bradykinin. Ecallantide blocks bradykinin production.

- Prophylaxis may be needed (use C1 inhibitor, ecallantide, or icatibant); surgical and dental procedures can precipitate angioedema episodes in susceptible patients
- Steroids are not helpful

A man comes in with neurosyphilis. He has a history of life-threatening anaphylaxis to penicillin. He also has a history of essential tremor and is on propranolol. He has asthma and is on an inhaled beta agonist and inhaled steroids. Which of the following is most appropriate?

a. Use ceftriaxone instead of penicillin
b. Stop propranolol prior to desensitizing him
c. Bolus with oral steroids prior to penicillin use
d. Add long-acting beta agonists to treatment

Answer: **B.** Neurosyphilis is only effectively treated with penicillin. The patient must be desensitized. Prior to desensitization it is important to stop propranolol and all beta blockers. This is because epinephrine may have to be used in the event of anaphylaxis when you desensitize the patient. Bolusing with steroids in inappropriate, because anaphylaxis is treated first with epinephrine.

Primary Immunodeficiency Syndromes

Common Variable Immunodeficiency (CVID)

CVID presents in both men and women and may present only in adulthood.

Both CVID and X-linked agammaglobulinemia present with recurrent episodes of sinopulmonary infections, such as bronchitis, sinusitis, pneumonia, and pharyngitis.

In addition, CVID causes the following:

- A sprue-like abdominal disorder
- Malabsorption, steatorrhea, and diarrhea
- Lymph nodes, adenoids
- Spleen may be enlarged

The machinery to make immunoglobulins is intact. The nodes and both B and T cells are present, but they do not make enough antibody. Hence total IgG levels are low.

Treatment is infusion of IV immunoglobulins.

X-Linked Agammaglobulinemia (Bruton)

This presents in male children with recurrent sinopulmonary infections.

Lymph nodes, adenoids, and the spleen are diminished in size or absent. B cells are missing, as are the immunoglobulins.

Treatment is infusion of IV immunoglobulins.

IgA Deficiency

With IgA deficiency (most common primary immunodeficiency), many people are asymptomatic.

- Possible recurrent sinopulmonary infections
- A sprue-like malabsorption syndrome
- Increased incidence of atopic conditions
- Possible anaphylaxis when receiving blood from donors who are not IgA deficient

Treat the infections as they arise. IV immunoglobulins will not work since it has little IgA in it. IVIG can actually be dangerous in IgA-deficient patients because the small amount of IgA in it will cause anaphylaxis.

Hyper IgE Syndrome

Hyper IgE syndrome presents with recurrent skin infections caused by *Staphylococcus*.

Treat the infections as they arise.

A 3-year-old boy comes in with recurrent sinopulmonary infections. On oral exam there are no nodes palpated in the cervical area and no tonsils seen. The child has been treated for an infection nearly every 1–2 months since birth. There are no skin infections. What is the most likely diagnosis?

a. Hyper IgE syndrome
b. IgA deficiency
c. X-linked agammaglobulinemia
d. Common variable immunodeficiency

Answer: **C.** X-linked agammaglobulinemia is exclusively in male children, whereas common variable immunodeficiency presents in adults. The absence of skin infection in this case goes strongly against hyper IgE syndrome. Patients are best managed with IV immunoglobulin infusions on a regular basis and with antibiotics for infections as episodes arise.

Endocrinology 6

Diabetes

The strongest indication for screening for diabetes is hypertension.

Diagnosis is made with one of the following:

- Two fasting glucose ≥126
- One random glucose ≥200 with symptoms (polyuria, polydipsia, polyphagia)
- Abnormal glucose tolerance test (2-hour glucose tolerance test with 75 g glucose load)
- Hemoglobin A1c >6.5%

> HgA1c >6.5% will be a diagnosis of diabetes.

Diabetes	Type 1	Type 2
Onset	Juvenile	Adult
Body type	Thin	Obese
Diabetic ketoacidosis	Frequent	Rare
Treatment	Insulin	Lifestyle management, oral agents, or insulin

Basic Science Correlate

Mechanism of Type 2 Diabetes

Adipose tissue must have insulin to permit entry of glucose and free fatty acids (FFAs). Excess fat creates a deficiency of insulin. Insulin receptors are a tyrosine kinase, which is neither a peptide nor a steroid hormone receptor. Tyrosine kinase is also a mechanism for many forms of protein production.

Type 2 Diabetes

Treatment is as follows. First, lifestyle change and medical therapy are tried.

- Diet, exercise, and weight loss (**best initial therapy**); 25% of cases can be controlled with exercise and weight loss alone
- Metformin (**best initial medical therapy**), particularly beneficial in obese patients
  - Blocks gluconeogenesis
  - No risk of hypoglycemia
  - Does not cause weight gain (sulfonylurea medications cause weight gain because they increase the release of insulin)
  - **Contraindicated** with renal insufficiency (the metformin may accumulate and increase the risk of lactic acidosis) and with contrast agents for any radiologic or angiographic procedure (contrast agent may lead to acute renal failure and, thus, the metformin may accumulate)
- Sulfonylureas (glyburide, glimepiride, and glipizide) work by causing the increased release of insulin from the pancreas. Hypoglycemia and SIADH are side effects.
- Dipeptidyl peptidase IV (DPP-IV) inhibitors (sitagliptin, linagliptin, alogliptin, and saxagliptin) are used as second agent to metformin; they block metabolism of incretins such as glucagon-like peptide (GLP).
- Thiazolidinediones (rosiglitazone, pioglitazone) increase peripheral insulin sensitivity. They may worsen congestive heart failure; do not use with CHF.
- Alpha-glucosidase inhibitors (acarbose, miglitol) block the absorption of glucose at the intestinal lining; side effects include diarrhea, abdominal pain, bloating, and flatulence, similar to lactose intolerance.
- Insulin secretagogues (nateglinide and repaglinide) work similarly to sulfonylureas; they are short acting and can cause hypoglycemia.
- SGLT inhibitors (canagliflozin, dapagliflozin, empagliflozin); side effects include UTI

- Rosiglitazone is contraindicated with CHF.
- Liraglutide helps weight loss.

DPP-IV inhibitors (saxagliptin, linagliptin, alogliptin, and sitagliptin) increase insulin release and block glucagon.

A 65-year-old Hispanic man is seen in the office for follow-up. He was placed on metformin for type 2 diabetes several months ago after not responding to diet modifications and exercise. Despite maximal doses of metformin, his blood glucose today is >150 mg/dL and HgA1c above 7%. What is the next best step in management?

a. Add sitagliptin
b. Add insulin subcutaneously
c. Add insulin pump
d. Add rosiglitazone
e. Add acarbose or miglitol
f. Switch to a sulfonylurea

Answer: **A.** If type 2 diabetes cannot be controlled with metformin, add a second medication. A sulfonylurea or DPP-IV inhibitor such as sitagliptin is the most effective and safest option. If the patient had originally been given a sulfonylurea but was not adequately controlled, add metformin. There are several options before having to start insulin.

> **Basic Science Correlate**
>
> The incretins are also called glucagon-like peptides (GLPs) and glucose insulinotropic peptides (GIPs, previously known as gastric inhibitory peptide).
>
> - Incretins increase insulin release and decrease glucagon secretion from the pancreas.
> - DPP-IV metabolizes GLP and GIP; inhibiting DPP-IV maintains high levels of GLP and GIP.
> - GLP is a confusing misnomer: glucagon raises glucose and FFA levels. GLP decreases glucagon.

> **Basic Science Correlate**
>
> **Mechanism of Diarrhea with Glucosidase Inhibitors**
>
> When acarbose and miglitol block glucose absorption, the sugar remains in the bowel, available to bacteria. When bacteria eat the glucose, they cast off gas and acid. Using glucosidase inhibitors is like making a person lactose intolerant.

If lifestyle change and medical therapy do not sufficiently control the level of glucose, then switch the patient to **insulin.**

- A long-acting insulin (e.g., insulin glargine), injected 1x/day is given with a very short-acting insulin at mealtime
- GLP analogs (injections) (exenatide, liraglutide, lixisenatide, dulaglutide) increase insulin and decrease glucagon; they promote weight loss and lower glucose
- Long-acting insulin: glargine 1x/day; degludec (extremely long half-life; less frequent hypoglycemic episodes); detemir; NPH (2x/day)
- Short-acting insulin: aspart; lispro; glulisine (given at mealtime; lasts 2 hours versus regular insulin which is given at mealtime but lasts up to 6 hours)

If insulin does not sufficiently control the diabetes, add **metformin**.

> GLP analogs (e.g., exenatide) slow gastric emptying and promote weight loss.

> Degludec = less hypoglycemia

Type 1 Diabetes (Juvenile Onset)

Type 1 diabetes always results from underproduction of insulin. The pancreas is destroyed during childhood on an autoimmune/genetic basis.

Patients are thin and do not respond to weight loss, exercise, or oral hypoglycemic agents. Sulfonylureas do not work because there is no functioning pancreas to stimulate to increase insulin release.

Patients with this condition are more prone to developing diabetic ketoacidosis because of severe insulin deficiency.

Diabetic Ketoacidosis (DKA)

DKA presents as an extremely ill patient with hyperventilation as compensation for the metabolic acidosis (low bicarbonate). The patient also has a "fruity" odor of the breath from acetone and possibly confusion from the hyperosmolar state.

Testing is as follows:

- Serum bicarbonate and anion gap (**best initial tests**) to determine the severity of illness
  - If glucose is high, this does not tell you that the patient has become acidotic; the patient may just have hyperglycemia
  - A low serum bicarbonate implies an elevated anion gap (the marker for severe DKA)
- Ketones: beta hydroxybutyrate can also be obtained as a marker of ketone production; as you correct the ketoacidosis, the beta hydroxybutyrate level should decrease

Lab findings in DKA are as follows:

- Hyperglycemia (>250)
- Hyperkalemia
  - Initially there will be hyperkalemia; if there is no insulin, potassium builds up outside the cell
  - As you treat the DKA, the hyperkalemia will quickly translate into hypokalemia; for this reason it is important to supplement with potassium
- Decreased sodium bicarbonate
- Low pH, with low pCO_2 as respiratory compensation
- Elevated acetone, acetoacetate, and beta hydroxybutyrate
- Elevated anion gap
- Pseudohyponatremia caused by high glucose

> Very high glucose artificially reduces sodium level.

> Acidosis = hyperkalemia
>
> Alkalosis = hypokalemia

Basic Science Correlate

Hyperkalemia is from transcellular shift of potassium out of the cell in exchange for hydrogen ions going into the cell. The cells "suck up acid" as a way of compensating for the severe metabolic acidosis and release potassium in exchange. Also, insulin drives potassium into cells with glucose.

> **Basic Science Correlate**
>
> **Mechanism of Increased Anion Gap**
>
> In order to use glucose as fuel, most cells need insulin. In the absence of insulin, glucose can't enter, and cells look for an alternate fuel source. The alternate fuel is FFA and ketones. Ketones are negatively charged acids, so using them as fuel drives down the level of bicarbonate.

Treatment is as follows:

- On the initial screen, order both the labs (chemistry, ABG, acetone level) and fluids (bolus of normal saline).
- Once the high glucose and the low serum bicarbonate are found, order IV insulin. CCS does not require you to know doses, and, in fact, there is no way for you to write in a dose.
- High glucose + low bicarb = DKA → give bolus saline and IV insulin
- As you move the clock forward, you will notice that the potassium level drops into the normal range. (Insulin drives potassium into cells, and as the acidosis corrects, potassium drops.) Once the potassium level drops, add potassium to the IV fluids.

> In a patient with DKA, the total body level of potassium is low. Chronic hyperkalemia depletes the body of potassium.

Complications of Diabetes

In a CCS case, you might see a case of follow-up management which addresses complications of diabetes.

- Hypertension: goal in diabetes is BP at least <140/90 mm Hg (same as for general population); BP control is critical in diabetes to prevent long-term complications to the heart, eye, kidney, and brain (lower goals are unclear at this time)
- Lipid management: LDL goal in diabetes is at least <100 mg/dL, but when patient has both CAD and diabetes, goal is at least <70 mg/dL
  - The lower the LDL, the better.
  - If a statin isn't effective, add ezetimibe.
- Retinopathy: perform a dilated eye exam yearly in diabetics to detect proliferative retinopathy
  - If present, perform laser photocoagulation.
  - If severe proliferative retinopathy, use a VEGF inhibitor, ranibizumab, or bevacizumab.
- Nephropathy: order a urine microalbumin, which detects minute amounts of albumin in the urine
  - Give ACE inhibitors if any form of protein is present—no matter how small.
  - Give ACE inhibitors for proteinuria even if blood pressure is normal. ARBs have the same indication.
  - Give ACE inhibitors as first-line hypertensive agents in diabetics.

- Neuropathy: perform a foot examination yearly for diabetic neuropathy; if neuropathy is already present, go straight to treatment
  - Use gabapentin or pregabalin.
  - Tricyclic antidepressants and carbamazepine are less effective.
- Erectile dysfunction (ED): there is no routine screening test for ED except to ask about its presence.
  - Treat with sildenafil and other phosphodiesterase inhibitors as usual.
  - Remember, no sildenafil with nitrates.
  - ED is an early sign of serious vascular disease; if a diabetic presents with it, do a stress test to exclude coronary disease.
- Gastroparesis: major stimulant for gastric motility is *stretch*; with long-standing diabetes, there is impaired ability to perceive stretch in the GI tract and impaired motility
  - Look for "bloating," constipation, abdominal fullness, and diarrhea.
  - Treat with metoclopramide or erythromycin (erythromycin increases the release of "motilin," a promotility GI hormone).
  - Diagnosis can be confirmed with a gastric-emptying scan, but that is often unnecessary.
  - If medical therapy fails, place a gastric pacemaker.

Basic Science Correlate

Mechanism of Glomerular Damage

Uncontrolled diabetes removes the negative charge from the filtration slits of the glomerular basement membrane. Normally, negative charges repel the filtration of albumin, which is also negatively charged. Loss of negative charges allows albumin to pass through the glomerulus.

ACE inhibitors decrease intraglomerular hypertension by dilating the efferent arteriole. This protects the glomerulus from the damage caused by intraglomerular hypertension.

Basic Science Correlate

Mechanism of Neuropathy in Diabetes

Nerves have a supply of blood vessels. Diabetes damages small blood vessels, starving off the nerves.

A 63-year-old man with long-standing diabetes comes to the office with a "pins and needles" sensation in both his feet. He is also chronically bloated and constipated. On review of systems, you find he cannot maintain erection sufficiently to complete intercourse. Urinalysis shows microalbuminuria. LDL is 147 mg/dL. What is the next step in management?

a. HgA1c
b. Nerve conduction studies
c. Hydralazine and sildenafil
d. Ramipril, erythromycin, atorvastatin, and pregabalin
e. Gastric-emptying study and penile tumescence studies

Answer: **D.** Prescribe ACE inhibitors for the proteinuria, erythromycin for the diabetic gastroparesis and to increase GI motility, atorvastatin to decrease LDL to <100 mg/dL, and pregabalin for diabetic neuropathy. No further diagnostic tests are required when you see this collection of abnormalities.

Thyroid Disease

The table shows the clinical presentation of hypo- and hyperthyroidism.

	Hypothyroidism	**Hyperthyroidism**
Weight	Gain	Loss
Intolerance	Cold	Heat
Hair	Coarse	Fine
Skin	Dry	Moist
Mental	Depressed	Anxious
Heart	Bradycardia	Tachycardia, tachyarrhythmias such as atrial fibrillation
Muscle	Weak	Weak
Reflexes	Diminished	
Fatigue	Yes	Yes
Menstrual changes	Yes	Yes

Basic Science Correlate

Thyroid hormone controls the metabolic rate of almost every cell in the body. Low thyroid hormone means reduced use of glucose and FFAs as fuel. This is why glucose intolerance and hyperlipidemia occur in hypothyroidism.

Low thyroid = Decreased metabolic rate = Weight gain

Hypothyroidism

Hypothyroidism arises most often from "burnt out" Hashimoto thyroiditis. It presents as a slow, tired, fatigued patient with weight gain.

The **best initial tests** are T4 (decreased) and thyroid-stimulating hormone (TSH) (elevated).

Treatment is T4 or thyroxine replacement. T4 will be converted in the local tissues to T3 as needed.

Hyperthyroidism

All forms of hyperthyroidism give an elevated T4, and almost all forms give a decreased TSH.

Hyperthyroidism Presentation and Treatment				
	Graves	**Silent**	**Subacute**	**Pituitary adenoma**
Physical findings	Eye, skin, and nail findings	None	Tender gland	None
Radioactive iodine update (RAIU)	Elevated	Low	Low	Elevated
Treatment	Radioactive iodine ablation	None	Aspirin	Surgical removal

Graves Disease

Graves disease is a type of hyperthyroidism. In addition to the findings of hyperthyroidism already described, it has several unique physical findings:

- Ophthalmopathy: exophthalmos (eyes are bulging) and proptosis (lid is retracted)
- Dermopathy: thickening and redness of the skin just below the knee
- Onycholysis (10% of cases): separation of the nail from the nailbed
- Elevated RAIU

Basic Science Correlate

Mechanism of Ophthalmopathy

The levator palpebrae superioris is the muscle that lifts the eyelid, innervated by the third cranial nerve. Hyperthyroidism stimulates the beta receptors of the third cranial nerve. High thyroid levels pull up the eyelid by stimulating the levator muscle. Graves disease also deposits mucopolysaccharides behind the eye. This pushes the eye forward, causing the exophthalmos.

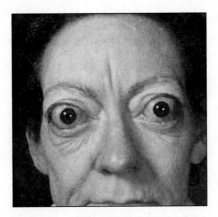

Ophthalmopathy

Treatment is as follows:

- Methimazole or propylthiouracil (PTU) acutely to bring the gland under control
  - Methimazole has fewer side effects but is not safe in pregnancy.
  - PTU is safe in pregnancy.
- Then, radioactive iodine to ablate the gland
- Propranolol to treat the sympathetic symptoms, such as tremors and palpitations

---

Basic Science Correlate

Mechanism of PTU and Methimazole

PTU and methimazole inhibit thyroperoxidase. Peroxidase will do the following:

1. Oxidize iodine
2. Put iodine on the tyrosine molecule to make monoiodotyrosine and diiodotyrosine
3. Couple up mono- and diiodotyrosine to make T4 and T3

PTU and methimazole inhibit all of these steps in thyroid hormone synthesis.

"Silent" Thyroiditis

This condition is an autoimmune process with a nontender gland and hyperthyroidism. There are no eye, skin, or nail findings.

Unlike Graves disease, the RAIU level is low since this is not a hyperfunctioning gland; it is just "leaking." Antibodies to thyroid peroxidase and antithyroglobulin antibodies may be present.

There is no treatment.

Subacute Thyroiditis

This condition has a viral etiology (we think!) and presents with a tender gland.

Diagnostic testing shows the following:
- RAIU (decreased)
- T4 (elevated)
- TSH is decreased, but that is not specific to this form of hyperthyroidism

Treatment is aspirin for pain relief.

Pituitary Adenoma

Pituitary adenoma (rare) is the only cause of hyperthyroidism with an elevated TSH.

RAIU is elevated because excess TSH creates a hyperfunctioning gland.

Treatment is MRI of the brain and removal of the adenoma.

Exogenous Thyroid Hormone Abuse

T4 is elevated and TSH is low. However, the thyroid gland will atrophy to the point of nonpalpability on examination.

Thyroid "Storm"

Thyroid "storm" is an acute, severe, life-threatening hyperthyroidism.

Treatment is as follows:
- Iodine to block uptake of iodine into the thyroid gland and block the release of hormone
- PTU or methimazole to block production of thyroxine
- Dexamethasone to block peripheral conversion of T4 to T3
- Propranolol to block target organ effect

PTU blocks conversion of T4 to T3.

Goiter

You cannot determine etiology only from the presence of a goiter. An enlarged gland can be associated with hyperthyroidism, hypothyroidism, or normal function of the thyroid.

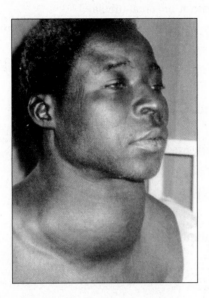

Solitary Thyroid Nodule

Perform a fine needle aspiration. The wrong answers for excluding cancer are radioactive iodine scan and ultrasound (which is used to help place the needle).

If the nodule is cancer, it must be removed surgically, and TSH/T4 must be done prior to biopsy. Do not biopsy lesions with elevated thyroid function.

The most common thyroid cancer is papillary, but the most deadly is anaplastic.

Calcium Disorders

Hypercalcemia

The most common cause of hypercalcemia is primary hyperparathyroidism. An enormous number of people are walking around with hyperparathyroidism with no symptoms. Other causes of hypercalcemia include:

- Malignancy: produces a parathyroid hormone–like particle
- Granulomatous disease: sarcoid granulomas actually make vitamin D
- Vitamin D intoxication
- Thiazide diuretics increase tubular reabsorption of calcium
- Tuberculosis
- Histoplasmosis
- Berylliosis forms granulomas
- Lithium
- Vitamin A toxicity

> **Basic Science Correlate**
>
> **Mechanism of Parathyroid Hormone (PTH) Effect**
> - Reabsorbs calcium at distal tubule
> - Excretes phosphate at proximal tubule
> - Activates vitamin D from 25 to the 1,25 dihydroxy form
> - Reabsorbs both calcium and phosphate from bone

Hyperparathyroidism

The vast majority of cases present as asymptomatic hypercalcemia. Target organ damage is as follows:

- Kidney stones
- Osteoporosis/osteomalacia/fractures
- Confusion
- Constipation and abdominal pain

> **Basic Science Correlate**
>
> **Mechanism of Neural Inhibition in Hypercalcemia**
> High calcium levels make it harder for excitable tissue such as nerves to depolarize. High calcium moves the threshold for depolarization away from the resting membrane potential. Bowels are a long muscular tube. High calcium inhibits smooth muscle contraction.
>
> Low calcium = Hyperexcitable

Diagnostic testing is parathyroid hormone (PTH) level (elevated) with hypercalcemia.

When are **sestamibi** and **nuclear imaging** the correct answer for hyperparathyroidism?

- When you need to know which gland to remove
- Sestamibi allows proper localization of adenomatous gland; since 80% of hyperparathyroidism arises from a solitary adenoma, scanning helps identify the location

Treatment is surgical removal.

Remember: Hyperparathyroidism may be a part of multiple endocrine neoplasia (MEN) syndrome. The nature of cases is as follows:

- Solitary adenoma: 80%
- Four-gland hyperplasia: 19%
- Cancer: 1%

When is **surgical removal of the parathyroid gland** the answer to a question about hyperparathyroidism?

- For any symptomatic disease ("stones, bones, psychic moans, GI groans"); renal insufficiency no matter how slight; very elevated serum calcium (>12.5); age <50; and osteoporosis

Acute, Severe Hypercalcemia

This condition presents with the following:

- Confusion
- Constipation
- Polyuria and polydipsia from nephrogenic diabetes insipidus
- Short QT syndrome on the EKG
- Renal insufficiency, ATN, kidney stone

Treatment is as follows:

- Hydration: high volume (3–4 liters) of normal saline
- Bisphosphonate (pamidronate or zoledronate) is very potent but takes a week to work. It inhibits osteoclasts.
- Furosemide (only after hydration has been given). Loop diuretics increase calcium excretion by the kidney if urine is not being produced through hydration alone.
- If hydration and furosemide do not control the calcium and you need something faster than a bisphosphonate, give calcitonin.
- If the etiology is granulomatous disease, use steroids.

> Diuretics are not needed if hydration increases urine output.

> **Basic Science Correlate**
>
> **Mechanism of Volume Depletion in Hypercalcemia**
> High calcium levels inhibit the effect of ADH on the collecting duct, inducing nephrogenic diabetes insipidus. High calcium filtration also promotes osmotic diuresis.

Hypocalcemia

Hypocalcemia may be caused by the following:

- Surgical removal of parathyroid glands
- Hypomagnesemia: magnesium is needed to release PTH from the gland
- Vitamin D deficiency
- Acute hyperphosphatemia: phosphate binds with the calcium and lowers it
- Fat malabsorption: binds calcium in the gut
- PTH resistance: pseudohypoparathyroidism that accompanies short fourth finger, round face, and mental retardation

> PPIs can decrease calcium and magnesium absorption.

Severe hypocalcemia presents with the following:

- Seizures
- Neural twitching (Chvostek sign, Trousseau sign)
- Arrhythmia-prolonged QT on EKG

Treatment is calcium replacement. If there is vitamin D deficiency or hypoparathyroidism, add vitamin D.

Adrenal Disorders

Cushing Syndrome (Hypercortisolism)

Any form of hyperadrenalism or hypercortisolism, no matter what the cause, has a common clinical presentation:

- Fat redistribution: truncal obesity, "moon face," buffalo hump, thin arms and legs
- Easy bruising and striae: loss of collagen from cortisol thins the skin
- Hypertension: from fluid and sodium retention (look for hypokalemia in hyperaldosteronism)
- Muscle wasting
- Hirsutism: from increased adrenal androgen levels

> **Basic Science Correlate**
>
> Cortisol increases glucose levels by increasing gluconeogenesis. Cortisol breaks down proteins so the freed amino acids can be used to make sugar. Specifically, bone and skin proteins are broken down and made into sugar. This leads to bruising, striae, muscle wasting, and osteoporosis.

There are 3 sources of Cushing disease:

	Pituitary Tumor	**Ectopic ACTH Production**	**Adrenal Adenoma**
ACTH	High	High	Low
High-dose dexamethasone	Suppression	No suppression	No suppression
Specific test	MRI Petrosal vein sampling	Scan chest and abdomen	Scan adrenals
Treatment	Removal	Removal	Removal

Lab abnormalities are as follows:

- Hyperglycemia, hyperlipidemia
- Osteoporosis
- Leukocytosis
- Metabolic alkalosis caused by increased urinary loss of H^+ (acid)

Basic Science Correlate

Mechanism of Metabolic Alkalosis

Cortisol has both mineralocorticoid or aldosterone effects on the kidney. Excess adrenal steroids increase hydrogen ion excretion at the alpha-intercalated cell of the late distal/early collecting duct. Hypokalemia results from potassium excretion through the principal cell.

Testing is as follows:

- 1 mg overnight dexamethasone suppression test (**best initial test**) (a normal person will suppress the 8:00 a.m. level of cortisol if given dexamethasone at 11:00 p.m. the night before)
  - Normal test excludes hypercortisolism of all kinds
  - Abnormal test can still be falsely elevated from various stress, e.g., depression or alcoholism
- 24-hour urine cortisol (**most accurate test**) to confirm that an overnight dexamethasone suppression test is not falsely abnormal (adds specificity to the overnight test); if overnight test is abnormal (fails to suppress), get the 24-hour urine cortisol to confirm hypercortisolism (Cushing syndrome)
- Late-night salivary cortisol: normal should be low

Note that these diagnostic tests diagnose the presence of Cushing syndrome, but they do not determine etiology or cause. To identify that, test the adrenocorticotropic hormone (ACTH) level.

- **ACTH low:** origin is in the adrenal gland; scan the gland with a CT or MRI and remove the adenoma that you find
- **ACTH high:** origin is in the pituitary gland or from the ectopic production of ACTH

The next step is a high-dose dexamethasone suppression test.

- If ACTH is suppressed, the origin is the pituitary. Scan the pituitary and remove the adenoma if it is visible.
- If ACTH is not suppressed, the origin is an ectopic production of ACTH or a cancer that is making ACTH. Scan the chest for lung cancer or carcinoid, and remove the cancer if possible.

24-hour urine cortisol gives fewer false-positives than 1 mg overnight testing.

Why bother with all this complex testing for Cushing syndrome? Why not just scan the brain and adrenals and remove what you find?

Answer: Many people have incidental adrenal and pituitary lesions. If you start with a scan, you might remove the wrong part of the body, and you cannot put it back!

A man with hypercortisolism is found to have an elevated ACTH that suppresses with high-dose dexamethasone. MRI of this pituitary shows no visible lesion. What is the next best step in management?

a. Remove the pituitary
b. Repeat the dexamethasone suppression test
c. Ketoconazole
d. Petrosal venous sinus sampling
e. PET scan of the brain

Answer: **D.** MRI and CT of the brain lack both sensitivity and specificity in diagnosing endocrine disorders. It is important to confirm the identity of an adrenal disorder functionally before scanning is done. This patient has high cortisol with high ACTH, indicating the pituitary or an ectopic source of hyperadrenalism. The ACTH levels suppress with high-dose dexamethasone, indicating a pituitary adenoma, which is the cause of Cushing syndrome in almost 50% of cases. If the tests point to a pituitary source but the scanning is indeterminant, inferior petrosal sinus sampling is used to confirm it. Petrosal sinus sampling is also used to localize the lesion, as well to see which half of a pituitary should be removed.

Treatment is removal of the underlying cause.

When the pituitary lesion causing Cushing cannot be removed or there is still residual hyperfunctioning, use pasireotide (a somatostatin analogue). In these patients, mifepristone (a cortisol receptor antagonist) can control the hyperglycemia of hypercortisolism.

Addison Disease (Adrenal Insufficiency)

Most cases of Addison disease are of autoimmune origin. It presents with the following:

- Fatigue, anorexia, weight loss, weakness with hypotension
- Thin patient with hyperpigmented skin

Laboratory abnormalities are as follows:

- Hyperkalemia with a mild metabolic acidosis (due to inability to excrete H^+ or K^+ because of the loss of aldosterone)
- Hyponatremia
- Possible hypoglycemia and neutropenia (glucocorticoids increase glucose and white cell levels)

> **Basic Science Correlate**
>
> Glucocorticoids increase glucose by blocking the uptake at peripheral tissues such as muscle, fat, and lymph. Glucocorticoids also have a permissive effect on glucagon, increasing its ability to break down glycogen from the liver. Glucocorticoids increase gluconeogenesis and break down protein for amino acid substrate.

The **most accurate diagnostic tests** are as follows:

- Cosyntropin (synthetic ACTH) stimulation test, where cortisol is measured before and after the administration of cosyntropin
  - If there is no rise in cortisol level, there is adrenal insufficiency
  - If there is a rise in cortisol level, there is no insufficiency
- CT scan of the adrenal gland

Treatment is as follows:

- Steroid replacement for acute addisonian (hypoadrenal) crisis: draw a cortisol level and give fluids + hydrocortisone (provides both glucocorticoid and mineralocorticoid activity)
- Prednisone for stable (nonhypotensive) patients
- Fludrocortisone (steroid highest in mineralocorticoid content) for adrenal insufficiency with continued hypotension after prednisone treatment; also, for use when renin is elevated

> Hydrocortisone provides both glucocorticoid and mineralocorticoid effects on the kidney.

Hyperaldosteronism

This condition presents with hypertension, hypokalemia, and metabolic alkalosis.

> Hypertension + Low renin + Low potassium = Hyperaldosteronism

Basic Science Correlate

The hypokalemia may lead to motor weakness from the inability to have normal motor contraction with the low potassium level. Nephrogenic diabetes insipidus can occur from hypokalemia. Hence, the case may feature "polyuria and polydipsia"; however, in primary hyperaldosteronism, the glucose level will be normal.

Diagnostic testing is as follows:

- Low renin
- Hypertension
- Elevated aldosterone level despite salt loading with normal saline

Confirm diagnosis with a CT scan of the adrenal glands.

Treatment is surgical resection for a solitary adenoma, and spironolactone or eplerenone for hyperplasia.

Pheochromocytoma

Symptoms include headache, palpitations, tremors, anxiety, and flushing. However, these symptoms are relatively nonspecific. Blood pressure that elevates during episodes is the only clue.

> Pheochromocytoma = Episodic hypertension

The **best initial tests** are high plasma and urinary catecholamine level or plasma-free metanephrine or urine metanephrine level.

Pheochromocytoma is part of MEN II.

The **most accurate test** is CT or MRI of the adrenal glands. MIBG (iobenguane) scan, a nuclear isotope scan which identifies occult collections of pheochromocytoma, can detect metastatic disease.

Treatment is as follows:

- First, phenoxybenzamine (alpha blockade) to control blood pressure; without alpha blockade, the blood pressure can significantly rise intraoperatively
- After an alpha blocker, use propranolol
- Then, surgical or laparoscopic resection
- Metastatic disease cannot be treated surgically

Congenital Adrenal Hyperplasia (CAH)

All types of CAH have elevated ACTH and low aldosterone and cortisol. They are treatable with prednisone, which inhibits the pituitary.

- 21 hydroxylase deficiency (most common type)
  - Hirsutism caused by increased adrenal androgens and hypotension
  - Diagnose with increased 17 hydroxyprogesterone level
- 11 hydroxylase deficiency
  - Hirsutism caused by increased adrenal androgens and hypertension
- 17 hydroxylase deficiency
  - Hypertension with low adrenal androgen level

	Hypertension	Virilization
21	No	Yes
11	Yes	Yes
17	Yes	No

Basic Science Correlate

In CAH, hypertension is caused by increased 11-deoxycorticosterone, which acts like a mineralocorticoid. Because 11- and 17-hydroxylase deficiencies involve an increased level of 11-deoxycorticosterone, there is hypertension. Virilization is caused by increased adrenal androgens, DHEA, and androstenedione.

Prolactinoma

Prolactinoma (most common pituitary lesion) presents differently in men and women:

- **Men**
  - Erectile dysfunction, decreased libido, and occasionally gynecomastia
  - Presents late
  - Signs of mass effect of a tumor, such as headache and visual disturbance
- **Women**
  - Presents early due to amenorrhea and galactorrhea in the absence of pregnancy

> **Basic Science Correlate**
>
> Prolactin inhibits GNRH. If there is no GNRH, the body cannot release LH and FSH.

Prolactinoma should be investigated only under the following conditions:

- Have excluded pregnancy and drugs (metoclopramide, phenothiazines, tricyclic antidepressants) as causing the high prolactin
- Prolactin level very high (>200)
- Have excluded other causes of hyperprolactinemia
  - Hypothyroidism: high thyrotropin-releasing hormone level stimulates prolactin
  - Nipple stimulation, chest wall irritation
  - Stress, exercise

The **most accurate diagnostic test** is very high prolactin level with MRI of the brain.

Treatment is a dopamine-agonist agent such as cabergoline or bromocriptine. Most prolactinomas respond to these agents. Cabergoline has fewer adverse effects than bromocriptine.

> On the Step 3 exam, if both cabergoline and bromocriptine are among the answer options, choose cabergoline.

For the small number of patients in whom medical therapy does not work, surgical removal is done.

Acromegaly

Acromegaly is the excess production of growth hormone (GH) from a growth hormone-secreting adenoma in the pituitary. It presents with enlargement of the head (hat size), fingers (ring size), feet (shoe size), nose, and jaw. In addition, there is intense sweating from enlargement of the sweat glands.

It also causes the following:

- Joint abnormalities: due to unusual growth of the articular cartilage
- Amenorrhea: GH is frequently cosecreted with prolactin
- Cardiomegaly and hypertension
- Colonic polyps
- Diabetes (common): resistant to treatment because GH acts as an anti-insulin

Diagnostic testing for acromegaly starts with insulin-like growth factor (IGF) because it has a long half-life (**best initial test**).

GH (**most accurate test**) is not done first because it has a short half-life and has maximum secretion in the middle of the night during deep sleep. Normally GH should be suppressed by glucose. GH raises glucose because it is a stress hormone. If glucose is high, that should suppress the level of GH. Suppression of GH by giving glucose excludes acromegaly.

MRI will show a lesion in the pituitary, but it is essential to know the function of a pituitary tumor before anatomic visualization happens with an MRI.

Basic Science Correlate

IGF is "insulin-like" because it works through the tyrosine kinase receptor, which is also how GH builds protein. GH has a direct effect of increasing glucose and free fatty acids (FFAs). The protein effect results entirely from the increase in DNA polymerase brought about by IGF stimulation of tyrosine kinase. Insulin also helps build proteins.

Treatment is as follows:

- Surgical resection with transsphenoidal removal (cures 70% of cases)
- Octreotide or lanreotide (somatostatin has some effect in preventing the release of GH)
- Cabergoline (dopamine agonist inhibits GH release)
- Pegvisomant (a GH receptor antagonist)

Hormones of Reproduction

Amenorrhea

Primary amenorrhea is caused by a genetic defect, as in the following:

- Turner syndrome: short stature, webbed neck, wide-spaced nipples, and scant pubic and axillary hair. The XO karyotype prevents menstruation.

- Testicular feminization: a genetically male patient who looks, feels, and acts as a woman. Socially, the patient is female. The absence of testosterone receptors results in no penis, prostate, or scrotum. The patient does not menstruate.
- Müllerian agenesis

Secondary amenorrhea is caused by the following:

- Pregnancy, exercise, extreme weight loss, hyperprolactinemia
- Polycystic ovary syndrome (PCOS) (an idiopathic disorder that presents as infertility and hirsutism):
  - Obesity, amenorrhea, and hirsutism are associated with large cystic ovaries.
  - There are increased adrenal androgens.
  - The reasons androgen levels such as DHEA increase is unknown. The mechanism of diabetes and glucose intolerance is likewise unknown.
  - Treatment is metformin. Treat the virilization with spironolactone, which has anti-androgenic effects.
- Premature ovarian insufficiency

> Testicular feminization presents as a girl who does not menstruate. The girl has breasts but no cervix, tubes, or ovaries, and she is missing the top third of the vagina. She also does not have a penis, prostate, or scrotum.

Male Hypogonadism

Klinefelter Syndrome

Patients are tall men with the following characteristics:

- Insensitivity of the FSH and LH receptors on their testicles
- XXY on karyotype
- Very high FSH and LH
- No testosterone produced from the testicles

Treatment is testosterone.

Kallmann Syndrome

This is a problem originating at the hypothalamus, so there is low GnRH, FSH, and LH.

Symptoms include anosmia with hypogonadism; anosmia is the key to the diagnosis.

Pulmonology 7

Obstructive Lung Disease

Asthma

Asthma presents with shortness of breath and expiratory wheezing. In severe cases, there is use of accessory muscles and an inability to speak in complete sentences.

Severe asthma exacerbation has the following features:

- Hyperventilation/increased respiratory rate
- Decrease in peak flow
- Hypoxia
- Respiratory acidosis
- Possible absence of wheezing

Diagnostic testing for severe asthma is as follows:

- If symptomatic with acute shortness of breath but diagnosis unclear
  - Pulmonary function tests (PFTs) (**best initial test**), both before and after inhaled bronchodilators; asthma and reactive airway disease are confirmed with increased FEV_1 >12%
  - Methacholine stimulation; asthma is confirmed with decreased FEV_1 >20% after methacholine
- If asymptomatic:
  - Methacholine stimulation testing looks for a decrease in FEV_1 in response to synthetic acetylcholine; methacholine will decrease FEV_1 if the patient has asthma
  - Diffusion capacity of carbon monoxide (DLCO), a good test of interstitial lung disease, in which it is decreased; asthmatic patients may have an increased DLCO from hyperventilation

Treatment for **severe asthma** is as follows (on CCS, order with first screen):

- Inhaled bronchodilators (albuterol): no maximum dose
- Inhaled ipratropium
- Bolus of steroids (methylprednisolone): need 4–6 hours to be effective
- Oxygen if saturation <90%

> To wheeze, one must have airflow. If the asthma exacerbation is severe, there may not be any wheezing. This is an ominous sign.

> All patients with shortness of breath should receive the following:
> - Oxygen
> - Continuous oximeter
> - Chest x-ray
> - Arterial blood gas (ABG)

- Magnesium
- ICU for those with respiratory acidosis and CO_2 retention; for persistent respiratory acidosis, intubate and give mechanical ventilation

The following have no benefit for acute asthma exacerbation:

- Theophylline
- Cromolyn and nedocromil
- Montelukast
- Inhaled corticosteroids
- Omalizumab (anti-IgE)
- Salmeterol and other LABAs such as formoterol
- Epinephrine: subcutaneously administered epinephrine has no benefit in addition to inhaled bronchodilators
- Terbutaline (less effective than inhaled albuterol)

> - If there is an indication for beta blockers that decreases mortality in an asthmatic, then use the beta blocker.
> - The efficacy of beta blockers for mortality (MI, CHF) is more important than adverse effects (asthma, COPD).

Basic Science Correlate

Omalizumab is an IgG against IgE. Decreasing IgE decreases activation and release of mast cells.

Treatment for **nonacute asthma** is as follows:

1. Inhaled bronchodilator (albuterol or levalbuterol)(**best initial therapy**)
2. If symptoms are not controlled, add a chronic controller medication, e.g., an inhaled steroid
3. If symptoms are still not controlled, add a long-acting inhaled beta agonist (LABA), e.g., salmeterol, formoterol, olodaterol, or indacaterol; alternatives to LABA are theophylline, leukotriene receptor antagonists (LTRAs), and cromolyn
4. Oral steroids are used as a last resort because of adverse effects

> LABAs are never to be used alone.

Treatment for **exercise-induced asthma** is an inhaled bronchodilator prior to exercise. Choose albuterol first.

The table shows alternate long-term controller medications besides inhaled steroids.

> Mepolizumab and reslizumab inhibit interleukin-5.

Cause	Medication
Extrinsic allergies, such as hay fever	Cromolyn or nedocromil
Atopic disease	Montelukast
COPD	Tiotropium, ipratropium
High IgE, no control with cromolyn	Omalizumab (anti-IgE antibody)
High eosinophils (IL-5 inhibitor)	Mepolizumab, reslizumab
IL-5 receptor blocker	Benralizumab

When is **bronchial thermoplasty** the answer?

- When severe asthma persists despite maximum medical therapy and patient is often on steroids; thermoplasty delivers radiofrequency energy to airway walls by heating it and ablating the smooth muscle

---

Basic Science Correlate

Because they are inhaled, ipratropium and tiotropium inhibit muscarinic receptors predominantly on respiratory mucosae. Antimuscarinic activity dries the secretions of goblet cells, decreases bronchoconstriction, and inhibits excess fluid production in bronchi. These agents are especially effective in COPD.

A young man comes to the clinic for evaluation of intermittent episodes of shortness of breath. Currently he is not short of breath. What is the best test to determine a diagnosis of reactive airway disease?

a. Chest x-ray
b. Diffusion capacity of carbon monoxide (DLCO)
c. High-resolution CT scan
d. Methacholine stimulation testing
e. Pre- and postbronchodilation PFTs

Answer: **D.** Methacholine stimulation testing looks for a decrease in FEV_1 in response to synthetic acetylcholine. Methacholine will decrease FEV_1 if the patient has asthma. Chest x-ray is not specific enough to be the most accurate test. DLCO is a good test for interstitial lung disease. High-resolution CT evaluates interstitial lung disease and bronchiectasis. Pre- and postbronchodilation PFTs are appropriate only when the patient is short of breath.

Chronic Obstructive Pulmonary Disease/Emphysema

Chronic obstructive pulmonary disease (COPD) is common in long-term smokers. Symptoms include increasing shortness of breath and decreased exercise tolerance.

CCS Tip: On CCS, move the clock forward 15–30 minutes and reassess the patient. Oxygen administration in COPD may worsen the shortness of breath by eliminating hypoxic drive.

Do not intubate patients with COPD for CO_2 retention alone. These patients often have chronic CO_2 retention. Intubate only if there is a worsening drop in pH indicative of a worse respiratory acidosis. Serum bicarbonate is often elevated due to metabolic alkalosis as compensation for chronic respiratory acidosis.

Order ABG for cases of COPD. ABG is critical in acute shortness of breath from COPD because there is no other way to assess for CO_2 retention.

For mild respiratory acidosis, answer CPAP or BiPAP and move the clock forward 30–60 minutes. If the CO_2 retention and hypoxia are improved, the patient is spared from intubation.

The Step 3 exam often emphasizes chronic conditions which require "further management." Although one should perform a complete physical examination in these cases, the important findings are as follows:

- Physical findings
  - Barrel-shaped chest
  - Clubbing of fingers
  - Increased anterior-posterior diameter of the chest
  - Loud P2 heart sound (sign of pulmonary hypertension)
  - Edema as a sign of decreased right ventricular output (the blood is backing up due to pulmonary hypertension)
- Lab testing
  - EKG: right axis deviation, right ventricular hypertrophy, right atrial hypertrophy
  - Chest x-ray: flattening of the diaphragm (due to hyperinflation of the lungs), elongated heart, and substernal air trapping
  - CBC: increased hematocrit is a sign of chronic hypoxia; reactive erythrocytosis from chronic hypoxia is often microcytic; erythropoietin level not necessary
  - Chemistry: increased serum bicarbonate is metabolic compensation for respiratory acidosis
  - ABG: should be done even in office-based cases to assess CO_2 retention and the need for chronic home oxygen based on pO_2 (you expect the pCO_2 to rise and pO_2 to fall)
- PFTs
  - FEV_1: decreased
  - FVC: decreased from loss of elastic recoil of the lung
  - FEV_1/FVC ratio ($<70\%$): decreased
  - Total lung capacity from air trapping: increased
  - Residual volume: increased
  - DLCO: decreased (due to destruction of lung interstitium)

Long-acting muscarinic antagonists:
- Tiotropium
- Umeclidinium
- Aclidinium
- Glycopyrrolate

In moderate to severe cases of COPD, patients may become members of the 50/50 club—the pCO_2 is 50 mm Hg and the pO_2 is also 50 mm Hg. Here's an example ABG for a patient with COPD:
- pH: 7.35
- pCO_2: 49
- pO_2: 52
- HCO_3: 32

Basic Science Correlate

Mechanism of Right Heart Enlargement in COPD

Hypoxia in the lungs causes capillary constriction, in which precapillary sphincters in the lungs constrict to shunt blood away from hypoxic areas of the lung. Since the hypoxia of COPD is global throughout the lung, this diffuse vasoconstriction increases pressure in the right ventricle and right atrium. Over time, the result is hypertrophy of both chambers, leading to cor pulmonale, or right heart failure.

Treatment of COPD is as follows:

- **Acute COPD (shortness of breath)**
  - Oxygen and arterial blood gas (ABG)
  - Chest x-ray
  - Inhaled albuterol and ipratropium
  - Bolus of steroids (e.g., methylprednisolone)
  - Chest, heart, extremity, and neurological examination
  - If fever, sputum, and/or a new infiltrate on chest x-ray, ceftriaxone and azithromycin for community-acquired pneumonia

- **Chronic COPD**
  - Anti-muscarinic agent: tiotropium, ipratropium, umeclidinium, aclidinium, or glycopyrrolate, which dilates smooth muscle in bronchi and dries secretions (causes dry mouth)
  - SABA: albuterol inhaler
  - LABA (never use alone): olodaterol, salmeterol, vilanterol, formoterol, or indacaterol
  - Inhaled corticosteroids
    - Can add to LABAs for long-term control
    - However, are less effective in COPD than in asthma because COPD is less "reactive" and the very definition of asthma is "reactive airway disease"
  - Pneumococcal vaccine: 13 polyvalent to start, 23 polyvalent a year later
  - Influenza vaccine: yearly; inactivated injections only
  - Smoking cessation
  - Home oxygen if pO_2 <55 or oxygen saturation <88%; start at pO_2 <60 or saturation <90% if there is cor pulmonale (RV hypertrophy) or elevated hematocrit
  - If still no improvement with agents above: phosphodiesterase inhibitors (roflumilast) or theophylline to relax smooth muscle

> Almost all patients with COPD can tolerate beta-1-specific blockers.

> Inhaled steroids cause dysphonia and thrush.

> - LAMAs: tiotropium, umeclidinium, aclidinium, glycopyrrolate
> - LABAs (never use alone): salmeterol, olodaterol, indacaterol, formoterol, vilanterol

Which of the following lowers mortality in COPD?

a. Smoking cessation
b. Home oxygen therapy (continuous)

Answer: Both of these therapies reduce mortality in COPD.

Basic Science Correlate

COPD generates CO_2 retention. CO_2 retention generates respiratory acidosis. Chronic respiratory acidosis increases new bicarbonate generation at the distal tubule of the kidney.

COPD = Bicarbonate increase

Sleep Apnea

Look for an obese patient complaining of daytime somnolence. The patient's sleep partner will report severe snoring.

In addition, there will be hypertension, headache, erectile dysfunction, and a fat neck.

- **Obstructive** sleep apnea from fatty tissues of the neck blocking breathing (95% of cases)
- **Central** sleep apnea, which is decreased respiratory drive from the CNS (5% of cases)

Diagnostic testing is a sleep study, polysomnography. The patient is observed for periods of apnea lasting >10 seconds each. Oxygen saturation is also monitored.

Mild sleep apnea is 5–20 apneic periods per hour, while **severe** sleep apnea is >30.

Treatment is as follows:

- Obstructive sleep apnea
  - Weight loss
  - Continuous positive airway pressure (CPAP) or BiPAP
  - If not effective, consider surgical resection of the uvula, palate, and pharynx
- Central sleep apnea
  - Avoidance of alcohol and sedatives
  - CPAP
  - Acetazolamide, which causes a metabolic acidosis and may help drive respiration
  - Medroxyprogesterone, a central respiratory stimulant

Basic Science Correlate

Mechanism of Acetazolamide

Acetazolamide is an inhibitor of carbonic anhydrase. This enzyme is needed for reabsorption of bicarbonate that has been filtered at the glomerulus. In the absence of carbonic anhydrase, the bicarbonate is urinated off and the body becomes acidotic. Acidosis acts as a stimulant to the medulla to drive respiration.

Alpha-1 Antitrypsin Deficiency

This is a genetic disorder that presents with a combination of cirrhosis and COPD. Look for a case of COPD at an early age (age <40) in a nonsmoker who has bullae at the bases of the lungs.

Diagnostic testing is as follows:

- Chest x-ray: findings of COPD (bullae, barrel chest, flat diaphragm)
- Blood tests: low albumin level and elevated prothrombin time (caused by cirrhosis)
- Alpha-1 antitrypsin: low
- Genetic testing

Alpha 1 antitrypsin deficiency often gives chronic liver disease.

Treatment is alpha-1 antitrypsin infusion. Also, vaccinate for hepatitis A and B.

Bronchiectasis

Bronchiectasis is caused by an anatomic defect of the lungs, usually from an infection in childhood (CF 50%). This results in profound dilation of bronchi.

It presents as chronic resolving and recurring episodes of lung infection giving a very high volume of sputum that can be measured by the cupful. Hemoptysis and fever occur as well. Clubbing is seldom present.

Chest x-ray shows dilated bronchi with "tram tracking," which are parallel lines consistent with dilated bronchi. The **most accurate diagnostic test** is high-resolution CT scan of the chest.

There is no curative treatment. Treat the infectious episodes as they occur.

- Chest physiotherapy with "cupping and clapping" will help dislodge secretions.
- Rotating antibiotics are tried to avoid the development of resistance.

Interstitial Lung Disease

Interstitial Lung Disease (ILD)

ILD can be idiopathic, such as a form of pulmonary fibrosis secondary to occupational or environmental exposure and medications (e.g., TMP-SMX/sulfamethizole or nitrofurantoin).

If no cause is found, the diagnosis is idiopathic pulmonary fibrosis (IPF) by exclusion.

> Nitrofurantoin is associated with lung fibrosis.

Cause	Disease
Asbestos	Asbestosis
Glass workers, mining, sandblasting, brickyards	Silicosis
Coal worker	Coal worker's pneumoconiosis
Cotton	Byssinosis
Electronics, ceramics, fluorescent light bulbs	Berylliosis
Mercury	Pulmonary fibrosis

ILD is a long-term disease and is often punctuated by episodes of bronchitis and pneumonia. Symptoms include shortness of breath with a dry, nonproductive cough and chronic hypoxia.

Physical findings are the following:

- Dry, "Velcro" rales
- Loud P2 heart sound as a sign of pulmonary hypertension
- Clubbing
- No fever or systemic findings

Diagnostic testing includes:

- Chest x-ray: interstitial fibrosis
- High-resolution CT scan: shows more detail on interstitial fibrosis
- EKG shows pulmonary hypertension with right atrial and right ventricular hypertrophy
- Lung biopsy
- PFTs: all decreased proportionately (decreased FEV_1, FVC with normal ratio, total lung capacity, and DLCO)

PFT Results: ILD					
FEV_1	FVC	FEV_1/FVC Ratio	Total Lung Capacity	Residual Volume	Diffusion Capacity of Lungs for Carbon Monoxide
↓	↓	Normal to ↑	↓	↓	↓

Basic Science Correlate

Pulmonary hypoxia causes vasoconstriction of the lungs. Chronic vasoconstriction causes increased pressure in the pulmonary artery. Pulmonary hypertension kills patients.

> The most common type of cancer in asbestosis is lung cancer, not mesothelioma.

Treatment: no specific treatment to reverse ILD

- For long-term treatment: for those who do respond to steroids, switch to azathioprine to get patient off steroids; for those who do not respond to steroids or azathioprine, give trial course of cyclophosphamide
- In hard-to-treat/unclear cases, the Step 3 exam often asks about adverse effects of medication; the adverse effect of hemorrhagic cystitis with cyclophosphamide is clearer than what therapy is certain to help the lung disease
- If biopsy shows an inflammatory infiltrate, use trial courses of steroids (the only form of ILD that responds to steroids with certainty is berylliosis because it is a granulomatous disease)

- Pirfenidone and nintedanib slow the progression of IPF. Pirfenidone is an antifibrotic agent that inhibits collagen synthesis, and nintedanib is a tyrosine kinase inhibitor that blocks fibrogenic growth factors and inhibits fibroblasts.
- There is definitely no therapy for silicosis, mercury vapor-induced fibrosis, asbestosis, or byssinosis.

BOOP/COP

Bronchiolitis obliterans organizing pneumonia (BOOP) (or cryptogenic organizing pneumonia [COP]), is a rare bronchiolitis or inflammation of the small airways with a chronic alveolitis of unknown origin (although a few cases are associated with rheumatoid arthritis).

BOOP/COP has many similarities to ILD, but with a few differences:

- Presentation more acute than ILD (weeks to months)
- There are cough, rales, and shortness of breath, but there are also systemic findings of fever, malaise, and myalgias (absent from ILD)
- No occupational exposure in the history

Diagnostic testing includes:

- Chest x-ray: bilateral patchy infiltrates
- Chest CT: interstitial disease and alveolitis
- Open lung biopsy (**most accurate diagnostic test**)

Treatment is steroids. Antibiotics will have no effect.

BOOP/COP	ILD
Fever, myalgias, malaise (clubbing uncommon)	No fever, no myalgias
Symptoms present over days to weeks	$\geq$6 months of symptoms
Patchy infiltrates	Interstitial infiltrates
Steroids effective	Rarely responds to steroids

Sarcoidosis

Sarcoidosis is seen in African-American women age <40 with cough, shortness of breath, and fatigue over a few weeks to months. Physical examination shows rales.

Although this disease can involve many organs, the vast majority of cases present with lung findings only.

Rare physical findings and presentation include the following:

- Eye: uveitis that can be sight-threatening
- Neural (seventh cranial nerve involvement most common)
- Skin: lupus pernio (purplish lesion of the skin of the face), erythema nodosum

- Cardiac: restrictive cardiomyopathy, cardiac conduction defects
- Renal and hepatic involvement: occurs without symptoms
- Hypercalcemia (rare) secondary to vitamin D production by the granulomas of sarcoidosis

Diagnostic testing includes:

- Chest x-ray (**best initial test**) always shows enlarged lymph nodes; there may also be interstitial lung disease in addition to nodal involvement
- Lung or lymph node biopsy (**most accurate diagnostic test**) shows noncaseating granulomas
- Calcium and ACE levels may be elevated but these are not specific enough to lead to specific diagnosis
- Bronchoalveolar lavage shows increased numbers of CD4 helper cells

Steroids are the undisputed treatment.

Pulmonary Hypertension

Primary pulmonary hypertension presents as an idiopathic cause of shortness of breath, often in young women, from overgrowth and obliteration of pulmonary vasculature, leading to decreased flow out of the right ventricle.

Pulmonary hypertension can occur secondary to the following:

- Mitral stenosis
- COPD
- Polycythemia vera
- Chronic pulmonary emboli
- Interstitial lung disease

Physical findings are as follows:

- Loud P2
- Tricuspid regurgitation
- Right ventricular heave
- Raynaud phenomenon

Diagnostic testing includes:

- Transthoracic echocardiogram (TTE) shows right ventricular hypertrophy and enlarged right atrium
- EKG shows the same findings as well as right axis deviation
- Right heart catheterization (Swan-Ganz catheterization) (**most accurate diagnostic test**) with increased pulmonary artery pressure

Treatment is as follows:

- Endothelin inhibitors which prevent growth of the pulmonary vasculature (bosentan, ambrisentan, and macitentan)

- Prostacyclin analogs which act as pulmonary vasodilators (epoprostenol and treprostinil); selexipag is the first oral prostacyclin agonist
- Calcium channel blockers (weak efficacy)
- Sildenafil
- Riociguat which increases nitric oxide by stimulating guanylate cyclase and increases vasodilation by generating cGMP

Pulmonary Embolism (PE)

PE presents with the sudden onset of shortness of breath and clear lungs in patients with risk factors for deep venous thrombosis (DVT). The following are risk factors for DVT:

- Immobility
- Malignancy
- Trauma
- Surgery, especially joint replacement
- Thrombophilia, such a factor V mutation, lupus anticoagulant, or protein C and S deficiency

There are no specific physical findings for PE.

Diagnostic testing is as follows:

- Chest x-ray
  - Mostly commonly normal
  - Atelectasis is most common abnormality
  - Wedge-shaped infarction and pleural-based humps are rare
- EKG
  - Sinus tachycardia is most common finding
  - Nonspecific ST-T wave changes are most common abnormality
  - Right axis deviation and right bundle branch block are rare
- ABG shows hypoxia with increased A-a gradient and mild respiratory alkalosis

Basic Science Correlate

PE blocks blood flow. Blood flow block causes a severe pressure increase in the pulmonary artery and right ventricle. The increase in pressure from increased pressure in PE, not as much the hypoxia-induced vasoconstriction of COPD. Right heart strain occurs only with the most severe, large emboli that kill.

Right heart strain + Hypotension = Thrombolytics

A patient who recently had hip fracture repair develops the sudden onset of shortness of breath. His pulse is 110 per minute and BP 128/74 mm Hg. The chest is clear to auscultation. Chest x-ray is normal and EKG shows sinus tachycardia. ABG shows pH 7.48, pCO_2 28, pO_2 75. What is the next best step in management?

a. Apixaban
b. V/Q scan
c. CT angiogram
d. D-dimers
e. Lower extremity Doppler
f. Intravenous heparin

Answer: **A.** When the case so clearly suggests a pulmonary embolus with sudden onset of shortness of breath and clear lungs in a patient with a risk factor, the first thing to do after the chest x-ray and blood gas is to start anticoagulation. Do not wait for the results of V/Q scan or spiral CT to start anticoagulation. IV unfractionated heparin has no role in PE. Hemodynamically stable patients are treated with a NOAC.

Confirmatory testing is as follows:

- CT angiogram to confirm the presence of a PE (sensitivity and specificity >95%); test of choice if x-ray is abnormal; do it after x-ray, EKG, and ABG

- V/Q scan: to be accurate, the chest x-ray must be normal (i.e., the less normal the x-ray, the less accurate the V/Q scan)
  - Only a truly normal scan excludes a PE
  - Of patients with low-probability scan, 15% still have a PE
  - Of patients with high-probability scan, 15% do not have a PE
  - V/Q is done only with an absolute contraindication to CT angiogram
  - V/Q is the **most accurate test** for chronic thromboembolic disease
  - Riociguat treats chronic thromboembolic disease

- Lower extremity Doppler: excellent test if it is positive; in that case, no further testing is necessary
  - Problem is that 30% of PEs originate in pelvic veins, and the Doppler scan is normal even in the presence of a PE
  - Thus, the sensitivity of lower extremity Doppler is about 70%

- D-dimer testing (95–98% sensitive with poor specificity): if this is negative, PE is extremely unlikely. The best use of D-dimer testing is in a patient with a low probability of PE in whom you want a single test to exclude PE.

- Angiography (**most accurate test for PE**): invasive, with a significant risk of death [0.5%]), so rarely the best answer

Treatment is as follows:

- Hemodynamically stable patients
  - NOACs (rivaroxaban, apixaban) (**preferred treatment**): equal in efficacy to warfarin with less intracranial bleeding and without the need for INR monitoring; initial treatment with LMW heparin not required
  - Low-molecular-weight heparin: enoxaparin followed by warfarin for 3–6 months (use after heparin administration)

> Riociguat treats chronic thromboembolic disease and increases vasodilatory nitrous oxide.

> Bleeding from dabigatran is reversed with idarucizumab.

- Venous interruption filter for those with a contraindication to anticoagulation
- Hemodynamically unstable patients (i.e., hypotensive)
  - Thrombolytics
  - If cannot use thrombolytics, remove mechanically; in the same way that it works in a stroke, a catheter can retrieve a clot in PE and open flow.

> Right heart strain such as acute right axis deviation is strongly indicative of dangerous disease.

A 45-year-old man comes to the ED after a car accident resulting in a liver hematoma. On hospital day 3, he becomes suddenly short of breath. Chest x-ray is normal, and he is diagnosed with a pulmonary embolus. What is the next best step in management?

a. Angiography
b. Embolectomy
c. Heparin
d. Inferior vena cava filter

Answer: **D.** When a patient has a pulmonary embolism and there is a contraindication to anticoagulation, a vena cava interruption filter should be placed. This patient has a liver hematoma, so a filter should be placed. Use fondaparinux if there is heparin-induced thrombocytopenia (HIT).

Basic Science Correlate

D-dimers are a metabolic breakdown product of fibrin. Plasmin chops up fibrin into D-dimers, but it is only effective with fresh, new clots that have formed over the last day. Older clots have been stabilized with factor XIII or clot stabilizing factor, which make them impervious to dissolution by plasmin.

D-dimers = plasmin chopped up fresh clot

Basic Science Correlate

Thrombolytics activate plasminogen to plasmin. Plasmin dissolves only fresh clots, not clots stabilized by factor XIII. This is part of why thrombolytics are only useful within 12 hours post-MI. In PE, clots are older than the coronary clots of MI, but when they have formed is unclear. This is why there is no precise time frame for using thrombolytics in PE.

Pleural Effusion

Diagnostic testing is as follows:

- Chest x-ray (**best initial test**): do decubitus films next with patient lying on one side to see if fluid is freely flowing
- Chest CT may add further detail
- Thoracentesis (**most accurate test**)

- Pleural fluid testing:
    - Gram stain and culture
    - Acid-fast stain
    - Total protein (also order serum protein)
    - LDH (also order serum LDH)
    - Glucose
    - Cell count w/differential
    - Triglycerides
    - pH

Treatment is as follows:

- Small pleural effusions: no treatment needed but use diuretics for those caused by CHF
- Large effusions, especially those caused by infection (empyema): place a chest tube for drainage (main criterion is low pH <7.20)
    - If effusion is recurrent from a cause that cannot be corrected, perform pleurodesis
    - If pleurodesis fails, perform decortication, an operative procedure (the stripping off of the pleura from the lung so it will stick to interior chest wall)

Exudate	Transudate
Cancer and infection	Congestive failure
Protein level high (>50% of serum level)	Protein level low (<50% of serum level)
LDH level high (>60% of serum level)	LDH level low (<60% of serum level)

Basic Science Correlate

Pleurodesis is the infusion of an irritative agent, such as bleomycin or talcum powder, into the pleural space. This inflames the pleura, causing fibrosis so the lung will stick to the chest wall. When the pleural space is eliminated, the effusion cannot reaccumulate.

Lung Infection

Pneumonia

Pneumonia presents with fever, cough, and often sputum. Severe illness also presents with shortness of breath.

The most likely organisms involved are *Pneumococcus* for community-acquired pneumonia (CAP), and Gram-negative bacilli for hospital-acquired pneumonia (HAP).

Symptoms for CAP, HAP, and VAP (ventilator-acquired pneumonia) include fever, cough, sputum, and abnormalities on chest x-ray.

HAP and VAP are more likely than CAP to present with severe hypoxia and be caused by resistant gram-negative bacilli and MRSA.

Diagnostic testing is as follows:

- Chest x-ray (**best initial test**): all cases of respiratory disease (fever, cough, sputum) should have a chest x-ray and oximeter ordered with first screen
  - If there is shortness of breath, order oxygen with first screen
  - If there is shortness of breath and/or hypoxia, order an ABG
  - Urine antigen test routinely for pneumococcus and legionella
- Sputum Gram stain and culture (**most accurate test**) but most cases do not get a specific microbiologic diagnosis; outpatient treatment does not need sputum stain/culture

The pneumonia severity index (PSI) is used to risk-stratify patients with pneumonia. For the Step 3 exam, you do not need to memorize the criteria, but know that elderly, hypoxic patients with or without fever should be admitted.

Depending on the severity of the hypoxia, decide whether to do outpatient or inpatient monitoring. Then, if inpatient, decide whether ICU or no ICU.

Treatment of pneumonia is as follows:

- **Outpatient** pneumonia
  - Macrolide (azithromycin or clarithromycin)
  - Respiratory fluoroquinolone (levofloxacin, moxifloxacin)
  - Doxycycline
- **Inpatient** pneumonia
  - Ceftriaxone and azithromycin
  - Fluoroquinolone as a single agent

Treatment for HAP/VAP is 2 antibiotics against gram-negative bacilli and an anti-MRSA medication. Combine a gram-negative agent (e.g., cefepime, piperacillin/tazobactam, or carbapenem) with a second gram-negative agent (e.g., a quinolone or gentamicin with an anti-MRSA drug such as vancomycin or linezolid). Do not use daptomycin in the lung; it is inactivated by surfactant.

Vaccination is given as follows:

- Give pneumococcal vaccine at age 65.
- Give 13 polyvalent first and 23 polyvalent a year later.
- If immunocompromised (smoker; COPD/asthma; steroid use), give pneumococcal vaccine at any age. Also give 13 polyvalent first and then 23 polyvalent 8 weeks later.

> VAP presents with:
> - Fever
> - Hypoxia
> - New infiltrate
> - Increasing secretions

> PPI use increases the risk of hospital-acquired pneumonia.

> A positive sputum culture is not pneumonia.

> Expect to treat all CAP empirically.

Which of the following conditions has the strongest indication for admission?

a. Respiratory distress

b. Tachycardia

c. Confusion

d. Fever

e. Leukocytosis, hyponatremia, hyperglycemia

Answer: A. Patients age >65 with chronic disease of the lungs, liver, or kidney are more prone to respiratory failure. Other risks for a poor prognosis are diabetes, HIV, steroid use, and lack of a spleen. Hypotension or hypoxia as single features compels admission to the hospital.

Specific Associations

Presentation	Cause
Recent viral syndrome	*Staphylococcus*
Alcoholics	*Klebsiella*
Gastrointestinal symptoms, confusion	*Legionella*
Young, healthy patients	*Mycoplasma*
Persons present at the birth of an animal	*Coxiella burnetii*
Arizona construction workers	*Coccidioidomycosis*
HIV with <200 CD4 cells	*Pneumocystis (PCP)*

> Doripenem should not be used in pneumonia.

An HIV-positive man comes to the ED with shortness of breath and a dry cough. His LDH is elevated and chest x-ray shows bilateral interstitial infiltrates. His pO_2 is 65. What is the next best step in management?

a. Sputum induction

b. Respiratory isolation

c. Trimethoprim/sulfamethoxazole and prednisone

d. Pentamidine

e. Bronchoalveolar lavage

Answer: C. PCP is best managed with trimethoprim/sulfamethoxazole, which is more effective than pentamidine. Sputum induction is not as important as starting treatment (also, it is positive in only 50–70% of cases). Steroids are indicated if pO_2 <70 or A-a gradient >35. Bronchoalveolar lavage needs to be done and is the most accurate test, but it is more important to start specific therapy.

Tuberculosis

Tuberculosis (TB) is seen in specific risk groups, e.g., immigrants, HIV-positive patients, homeless patients, prisoners, and alcoholics. Symptoms include fever, cough, sputum, weight loss, and night sweats.

Diagnostic testing includes:

- Chest x-ray (**best initial test**)
- Sputum acid-fast stain and culture to confirm the presence of TB (**most accurate diagnostic tests**)
- PCR is extremely sensitive and fast

Treatment is as follows:

- Once the acid-fast stain is positive, start treatment with 4 antituberculosis medications (6 months of treatment is standard of care)
  - Isoniazid for 6 months
  - Rifampin for 6 months
  - Pyrazinamide for 2 months
  - Ethambutol for 2 months
- However, all of these medications can lead to liver toxicity. Stop if the transaminases reach 5 × the upper limit of normal:
  - Isoniazid: peripheral neuropathy
  - Rifampin: red/orange-colored bodily secretions
  - Pyrazinamide: hyperuricemia
  - Ethambutol: optic neuritis
- The following conditions require >6 months of treatment:
  - Osteomyelitis
  - Meningitis
  - Miliary tuberculosis, cavitary tuberculosis
  - Pregnancy

Latent Tuberculosis

Diagnostic testing is as follows:

- Interferon gamma release assay (IGRA) (**best initial test**)
  - Requires only one visit for a blood test
  - Less prone to reading errors than PPD, i.e., more specific
  - Give no false-positives with previous BCG infection
  - Have 90% sensitivity for previous TB exposure
  - A positive test confers only a 10% lifetime risk of TB (same for PPD)
- PPD (screening test for those in risk groups). Positive test is as follows:
  - 5 mm: close contacts, steroid users, HIV-positive, TNF users
  - 10 mm: those in risk groups described
  - 15 mm: those without increased risk
  - Requires 2 visits: one to implant the PPD and another 48–72 hours later to read the test (by observing skin induration, if any)
  - More prone to reading errors than IGRA

If a patient has never been tested or it has been several years since the last test, do 2-stage testing: if the first test is negative, perform a second test in 1–2 weeks to make sure the first test was truly negative.

> Isoniazid alone is used for 9 months to treat a positive PPD. This reduces the 10% lifetime risk of developing TB to 1% risk. Once a PPD or IGRA is positive, the test should never be repeated.

> Prior Bacille-Calmette Guerin (BCG) administration has no effect or influence on the treatment recommendations for latent TB. In other words, it does not matter if a patient has had BCG in the past; the patient must still take isoniazid if PPD is positive.
>
> If BCG is an answer choice on the Step 3 exam, it is always wrong.

Treatment is as follows:

- Treat latent TB (detected by PPD or IGRA) with 9 months of INH (the shortest course is isoniazid + rifapentine 1x/week for 3 months)
- Pyridoxine (vitamin B6) whenever isoniazid is used
- If positive PPD or IGRA (does not mean active infection)
  - Isoniazid (INH)
  - Chest x-ray to confirm no active occult disease; if chest x-ray is abnormal, perform sputum staining for TB, and if that is positive, proceed with full-dose, 4-drug therapy
  - Anti-TNF before treating with isoniazid for 9 months beforehand, if there is a compelling need. It is not right to let people suffer 9 months of a fistula in order to avoid a small risk of TB re-activation.

Allergic Bronchopulmonary Aspergillosis (ABPA)

ABPA presents as an asthmatic patient with worsening asthma symptoms.

- Coughing up of brownish mucous plugs with recurrent infiltrates
- Peripheral eosinophilia
- Elevated serum IgE
- Visible central bronchiectasis

Diagnostic testing includes *Aspergillus* skin testing, and levels for IgE, circulating precipitins, and *A. fumigatus*-specific antibodies.

Treatment is oral corticosteroids and itraconazole for refractory disease.

Inhaled steroids are the most common wrong answer. They do not help ABPA.

Nontuberculous Mycobacteria (NTM)

These organisms do NOT transmit from person to person.

In HIV-negative cases, *Mycobacterium avium-intracellulare* complex (MAI/MAC) presents as cough/sputum in an older person with COPD.

Because a single positive sputum sample is considered colonization, answer "treatment" only if:

- MAI grows repeatedly, and
- There are both chest symptoms and abnormal x-ray

Look for fibrocavitary disease. Treatment is azithromycin (or clarithromycin) and rifampin (or rifabutin) and ethambutol.

Rapidly Growing Mycobacteria

- *M. abscessus (chelonae)* and *M. fortuitum* occur in skin and soft tissue, especially following surgery or trauma.
  - Grow in 5–10 days
  - Normally live in water and soil
  - On the exam, a question might ask about a colonized water line in a dental unit.
- *M. kansasii* presents with lung disease similar to TB and, in 90% of cases, cavitary lung disease. Treatment is the same as for MAI.

Acute Respiratory Distress Syndrome

Acute respiratory distress syndrome (ARDS) is a sudden and severe respiratory failure syndrome caused by diffuse lung injury secondary to an overwhelming systemic injury:

- Sepsis
- Aspiration of gastric contents
- Shock
- Infection (pulmonary or systemic)
- Lung contusion
- Trauma, burns
- Toxic inhalation
- Pancreatitis
- Near drowning

Diagnostic testing is as follows:

- Chest x-ray shows diffuse patchy infiltrates that become confluent; may suggest congestive failure
- Wedge pressure normal
- pO_2/FIO_2 ratio <300, with FIO_2 expressed as a decimal (e.g., room air is 0.21, and if pO_2 is 100/0.21, the ratio is 476)
  - Mild: 200–300
  - Moderate: 100–200
  - Severe: <100

Treatment is as follows:

- Ventilatory support with low tidal volume of 6 mL per kg
- PEEP to keep the alveoli open
- Prone positioning of patient's body
- Possible use of diuretics and positive inotropes, e.g., dobutamine
- Transfer patient to ICU

Steroids do not help ARDS.

Mechanism of PEEP

Positive-end expiratory pressure (PEEP) keeps the alveoli open, and when they are expanded, more surface area is available for gas exchange. Without PEEP, there is more atelectasis and less surface area for gas exchange.

Pulmonary Artery Catheterization

Also called Swan-Ganz catheterization.

Use the measurements when a case is described and the question says: Which of the following will most likely be found in this patient?

Type	Cardiac Output	Wedge Pressure	Systemic Vascular Resistance (SVR)
Hypovolemia	Low	Low	High
Cardiogenic Shock	Low	High	High
Septic Shock	High	Low	Low

Rheumatology 8

Arthritis

Rheumatoid Arthritis

Rheumatoid arthritis (RA) is often seen in women age >50. Patients have joint pain and morning stiffness that is symmetrical and in multiple joints of the hands lasting for more than 1 hour in the morning, experienced for at least 6 weeks. There is often a prodrome of malaise and weight loss, but this is not enough to make a clear diagnosis.

Diagnosis requires ≥4 of the following conditions:

- Morning stiffness lasting >1 hour
- Positive rheumatoid factor (RF) or anti-CCP
- C-reactive protein (CRP) or ESR
- Inflammatory arthritis in ≥3 joints—the more joints involved, the more likely the diagnosis. The proximal interphalangeal (PIP) and metacarpophalangeal (MCP) joints are frequently involved.
- Duration of symptoms: >6 weeks

Neither an abnormal x-ray nor the presence of skin nodules is necessary to establish a diagnosis of RA. Eliminating an abnormal x-ray as a criterion for diagnosis allows earlier treatment with DMARDs.

RA is diagnosed with physical findings, joint problems, and lab tests. There is no single diagnostic criterion to confirm the diagnosis.

There is no single treatment for the disease.

Joint findings in RA are the following:

- Metacarpophalangeal (MCP) swelling and pain
- Boutonniere deformity: flexion of the proximal interphalangeal (PIP) with hyperextension of the distal interphalangeal (DIP)
- Swan neck deformity: extension of the PIP with flexion of the DIP
- Baker cyst (outpocketing of synovium at the back of the knee)
- C1/C2 cervical spine subluxation: check via x-ray or CT before intubation
- Knee: commonly involved but multiple small joints are involved more commonly over time

> Other findings in RA include:
> - Cardiac: pericarditis, valvular disease
> - Lung: pleural effusion with a very low glucose, lung nodules
> - Blood: anemia with normal MCV
> - Nerve: mononeuritis multiplex
> - Skin: nodules

The sacroiliac joint is spared in rheumatoid arthritis.

Felty syndrome consists of the following:

- Rheumatoid arthritis
- Splenomegaly
- Neutropenia

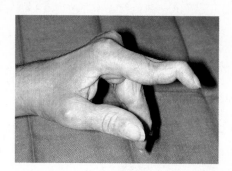

New alternate diagnostic criteria for RA include:

- Synovitis (a single joint is enough to diagnose RA)
- RF or anti-CCP
- ESR or CRP
- Prolonged duration (beyond 6 weeks)

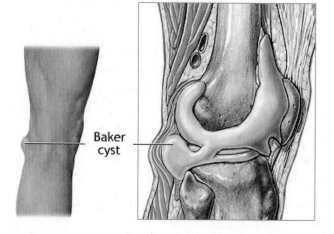

Baker cyst

Normocytic, normochromic anemia is very characteristic of RA.

CCS Tip: In addition to x-rays, RF, and anti-CCP, also order a CBC, sedimentation rate, and C-reactive protein. If the case describes a swollen joint with an effusion, also do an aspiration of the joint to establish the initial diagnosis.

Treatment is RA is usually an NSAID plus a disease-modifying antirheumatic drug (DMARD) (**standard of care**). Start the DMARD as soon as the diagnosis is made.

There is no therapeutic difference among the NSAIDs, and ibuprofen may be used for any of the rheumatological diseases described. NSAIDs will not delay progression of the disease.

- Methotrexate (**most widely used and best-tolerated**); side effects are bone marrow suppression, pneumonitis, and liver disease
  - Alternate DMARDs include anakinra (IL-1 receptor antagonist); tocilizumab, sarilumab (IL-6 receptor antagonists; add to methotrexate if it is ineffective)
  - Rituximab (anti-CD-20 antibody)
  - Leflunomide (pyrimidine antagonist similar to methotrexate with less toxicity)
  - Abatacept (inhibits T-cell activation)
- Anti-TNF biological agents (infliximab, adalimumab, etanercept, certolizumab, golimumab): block the activity of tumor necrosis factor (TNF)
  - Can use in combination with methotrexate; if methotrexate fails, add an anti-TNF agent

DMARDs are started to prevent x-ray abnormalities.

  - Test for hepatitis B and TB before starting

- Safe in pregnancy
- If TNF treatment fails, check TNF level:
  - If level is adequate and there is insufficient TNF effect, look for antibodies against a particular drug
  - If there are antibodies, switch to a different drug in same class
  - If there are no antibodies, switch immediately to another medication in another class
- Tofacitinib: oral Janus kinase inhibitor used in severe RA that is not responsive to methotrexate
- Hydroxychloroquine: used in mild disease; patient will require a regular eye exam to check for retinopathy
- Sulfasalazine (same drug used in the past for UC) to suppress bone marrow
- Steroids such as prednisone are a bridge to DMARD therapy. They are not disease-modifying, but they do enable quick control of the disease and allow time for the other DMARDs to take effect. Avoid their long-term use if possible. Steroids would be the answer for an acutely ill patient with severe inflammation.

A 34-year-old woman presents with pains in both hands for the last few months and stiffness that improves as the day goes on. Multiple joints are swollen on exam. X-ray of the hands shows some erosion. What is the single most accurate test?

a. Rheumatoid factor
b. Anti-cyclic citrullinated peptide (anti-CCP)
c. Sedimentation rate
d. ANA
e. Joint fluid aspirate

Answer: **B.** Anti-cyclic citrullinated peptide (anti-CCP) is the single most accurate test for rheumatoid arthritis (RA). It is >95% specific for RA, and it appears earlier in the course of the disease than the RF. RF is present in only 75–85% of patients with RA (it can also be present in other diseases, so it is rather nonspecific). There is nothing specific on joint aspiration to determine a diagnosis of RA.

Which of the following will have the lowest glucose level on pleural effusion?

a. CHF
b. Pulmonary embolus
c. Pneumonia
d. Cancer
e. RA
f. Tuberculosis

Answer: **E.** Rheumatoid arthritis has the lowest glucose level of all the causes of pleural effusion.

Osteoarthritis

Osteoarthritis (OA) (**most common joint abnormality**) is associated with aging and increased use of a joint.

Symptoms include:

- Morning stiffness <30 minutes in duration
- Crepitus on moving the joint
- Affects the distal interphalangeal (DIP) joints (unlike RA, which does not affect the DIPs)
  - Heberden nodes: DIP osteophytes
  - Bouchard nodes: PIP osteophytes

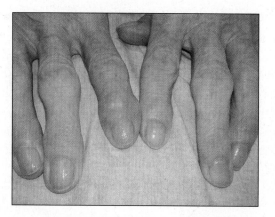 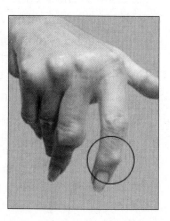

Heberden Nodes

X-ray of the joint is the **best initial test**. There is no specific diagnostic test.

For CCS, all of the following should be ordered.

- ANA
- ESR
- RF
- Anti-CCP

All other inflammatory markers will be normal. Joint fluid will have a low leukocyte count <2,000/mm^3.

Treatment is acetaminophen or NSAIDs. NSAIDs have greater efficacy than acetaminophen but also greater side effects such as ulcer, hypertension, and renal toxicity. On the exam you should not be asked to choose between them. Weight loss and exercise help, but chondroitin sulfate does not.

The table compares osteoarthritis with rheumatoid arthritis.

	OA	RA
Morning stiffness	<30 minutes	>1 hour
DIP	Yes	No
PIP	Yes	Yes
MCP	No	Yes
RF, anti-CCP	No	Yes
Joint fluid leukocyte count	<2,000	5,000–50,000

> Glucosamine is a wrong answer. Glucosamine = placebo

> Duloxetine is useful for the pain of knee osteoarthritis.

If the question describes inadequate pain control with acetaminophen, then the answer is clearly NSAIDs. If NSAIDs do not adequately control the pain or there are contraindications to use (such as renal insufficiency or uncontrolled ulcer disease), the answers are:

- Duloxetine: SSRI/SNRI treats chronic musculoskeletal pain
- Topical diclofenac: NSAID with less toxicity; use with renal insufficiency
- Capsaicin: topical medicine, also for neuropathic pain
- Intraarticular injections: steroids and hyaluronic injections help

> A middle-aged woman presents with osteoarthritis of the hands and damage to the cartilage. She reports pain with intermittent flares of tenderness and swelling, inflammation, and warmth of the distal joints that is abrupt in onset. X-ray shows joints shaped like a "seagull wing," with central erosions. RF and CCP are negative. What is the diagnosis?
>
> Answer: Erosive osteoarthritis

Diffuse Idiopathic Spontaneous Hyperostosis (DISH)

DISH is a type of OA. Look for an older patient with thoracic-level back pain that improves with stretching and movement.

Radiographic diagnosis requires the presence of new bone formation bridging 4 consecutive vertebral bodies in the thoracic spine. Disc spaces are normal, and both degenerative disc disease and significant facet joint changes are absent.

Seronegative Spondyloarthropathies

This group of inflammatory arthritic conditions consists of:

- Ankylosing spondylitis
- Reactive arthritis (formerly known as Reiter syndrome)
- Psoriatic arthritis
- Juvenile idiopathic arthritis (adult-onset Still disease)

These conditions all have the following characteristics:

- Negative test for RF
- Predilection for the spine
- Sacroiliac joint involvement
- Association with HLA–B27

Ankylosing Spondylitis (AS)

AS presents in young males (age <40) with spine or back stiffness (peripheral joint involvement is less common). The pain is worse in the morning after inactivity at night and is relieved by leaning forward. This can lead to kyphosis and diminished chest expansion. Rare findings are these:

- Uveitis (30%)
- Aortitis (3%)
- Restrictive lung disease (2–15%)

Diagnostic testing is as follows:

- X-ray of sacroiliac (SI) joint (**best initial test**)
- If that is negative, MRI (will detect edematous, inflammatory changes years before an x-ray in AS) (**most accurate diagnostic tes**t)
- RF will be negative
- HLA B27 testing when there are characteristic symptoms plus negative SI joint x-ray and equivocal MRI (HLA-B27 is present in 8% of the general population and not necessary to confirm a diagnosis of AS)

A 27-year-old man presents with months of back pain that is worse at night. He has diminished expansion of this chest on inhalation and flattening of the normal lumbar curvature. What is the most accurate of these tests?

a. X-ray
b. MRI
c. HLA-B27
d. ESR
e. Rheumatoid factor

Answer: **B.** MRI of the sacroiliac (SI) joint is more sensitive than an x-ray. The x-ray should be done first and, if negative, do the MRI. HLA-B27 is rarely useful to establish diagnosis, but when x-ray is negative and MRI is equivocal it can be helpful.

Treatment is NSAIDs. When NSAIDs do not control pain, use a TNF inhibitor such as infliximab or adalimumab. When TNF agents are not sufficient, use an IL-17 antagonist such as secukinumab.

Steroids do not work.

Methotrexate does not work well on the spine and sacroiliac joints.

Reactive Arthritis

Reactive arthritis (formerly known as Reiter syndrome) presents with an asymmetric arthritis with a history of urethritis or gastrointestinal infection. There may be constitutional symptoms, such as fever, fatigue, or weight loss.

- Arthritis: may be monoarticular, oligoarticular, or more diffuse
- Genital lesions: circinate balanitis (around head of penis); urethritis or cervicitis in women
- Conjunctivitis
- Keratoderma blennorrhagicum: a skin lesion characteristic of reactive arthritis

There is no specific diagnostic test. Look for the triad of knee (joint), pee (urinary), and see (eye) problems with a history of *Chlamydia, Shigella, Salmonella, Yersinia,* or *Campylobacter.*

Treatment is NSAIDs. If no response, use an intra-articular injection of steroids. Use sulfasalazine for chronic arthritis. Antibiotics do not treat the arthritis.

Psoriatic Arthritis

Psoriatic arthritis presents as joint involvement with a history of psoriasis. RF is absent. The sacroiliac spine is involved, as it is in all seronegative spondyloarthropathies. The following are key features of psoriatic arthritis:

- Nail pitting
- Distal interphalangeal (DIP) involvement (Remember: RA involves the proximal joint.)
- "Sausage-shaped" digits (dactylitis)
- Enthesitis: inflammation of tendinous insertion sites

No single test is specific for psoriatic arthritis.

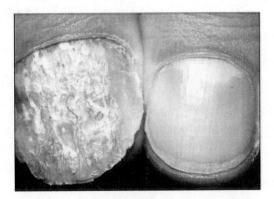

Psoriasis involvement of the nail produces pitting and yellowing, which can be mistaken for onychomycosis.

No single test is specific for psoriatic arthritis.

Treatment is NSAIDs. For resistant disease, use methotrexate.

- Infliximab and the other anti-TNF agents
- Secukinumab (IL-17 antagonist)
- Ustekinumab, an inhibitor of IL-12 and IL-23, treats both psoriasis and psoriatic arthritis
- Abatacept (T-cell inhibitor) treats both RA and psoriatic arthritis
- Apremilast: phosphodiesterase inhibitor orally

Basic Science Correlate

Mechanism of Anti-TNF Reactivation of TB

Most TB is reactivation TB. Old TB is encased off in granulomas. Granulomas are held together by TNF. When you start a TNF inhibitor, it breaks open granulomas and the TB escapes to reactivate.

Juvenile Idiopathic Arthritis

Juvenile idiopathic arthritis (JIA), also called juvenile rheumatoid arthritis (JRA) or adult-onset Still disease, can be a difficult diagnosis to recognize. It presents with:

- Fever
- Salmon-colored rash
- Polyarthritis
- Lymphadenopathy
- Myalgias

Additional minor criteria are hepatosplenomegaly and elevated transaminases.

There is no specific diagnostic test. JRA is characterized by the following:

- Very high ferritin level
- Elevated white blood cells
- Negative RF and negative ANA (essential to establish the diagnosis)

Treatment is NSAIDs. If no response, give steroids. Those with persistent symptoms need IL-1 inhibitors such as anakinra or anti-TNF medications to get off steroids.

Whipple Disease

Although it causes diarrhea, fat malabsorption, and weight loss, the most common symptom of Whipple disease is joint pain. Look for multisystem disease with CNS and ocular symptoms.

Biopsy of the bowel showing PAS positive organisms using PCR of stool is the **most specific test**.

Treatment with TMP/SMX is curative. CNS involvement will require IV ceftriaxone.

Systemic Lupus Erythematosus (SLE)

There are 11 criteria for lupus; **4 are needed** to confirm the diagnosis.

Diagnostic Criteria for SLE	
Skin	• Malar rash • Photosensitivity rash • Oral ulcers rash • Discoid rash
Arthralgias	Present in 90% of patients; nonerosive
Blood	Leukopenia, thrombocytopenia, hemolysis; any blood involvement counts as 1 criterion
Renal	Varies from benign proteinuria to end stage renal disease
Cerebral	Behavioral change, stroke, seizure, meningitis
Serositis	Pericarditis, pleuritic chest pain, pulmonary hypertension, pneumonia, myocarditis
Serology	• ANA (95% sensitive) • Double-stranded (DS) DNA (60% sensitive) Each serologic abnormality counts as 1 criterion, so if a person has joint pain, a rash, and both an ANA and DS DNA, he would have 4 criteria.

> Rash + Joint pain + Fatigue = Lupus

> **Drug-induced lupus** may be caused by hydralazine, procainamide, or isoniazid. Anti-histone antibodies and a positive ANA will always be seen. Complement level and anti-DS DNA will be normal.
>
> There is never renal or CNS involvement.

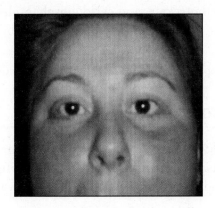

Malar Rash

Diagnostic testing is as follows:

- **Best initial test**: ANA
- **Most specific test**: Anti-DS DNA (60–70%) or anti-Sm (Smith) (10–20%)
- Anti-SM is the only test more specific for lupus than anti-DS DNA
- Ribosomal P: CNS lupus

Additionally, the following are found in SLE:

- Joint x-ray: normal; lupus causes joint pain without destruction of the synovium
- Anemia of chronic disease is more common than hemolysis
- In a lupus flare, complement levels diminish and anti-DS DNA elevate

> **SLE on CCS:** Complement levels, anti-Sm, and anti-DS DNA should be performed on all patients.

What is the best test to follow the severity of a lupus flare-up?

Answer: **Complement levels** (drop in flare-up) and **anti-DS DNA** (rise in flare-up).

As part of prenatal care, a woman with lupus is found to have a negative test for anticardiolipin antibodies, but she is positive for anti-Ro (SSA) antibody. What is the baby at risk for?

Answer: Heart block. The presence of anti-Ro or anti-SSA antibodies is a risk for the development of heart block.

The following are other findings in lupus that are not part of specific diagnostic criteria:

- Fatigue
- Hair loss
- Antiphospholipid syndrome
- Elevated sedimentation rate

Treatment is as follows:

- Hydroxychloroquine (all patients with SLE); 80% of patients achieve control
- Acute flare-ups: prednisone and other glucocorticoids
- NSAIDs for joint pain; if no response, try hydroxychloroquine (also for rash)
- Azathioprine, methotrexate, and cyclophosphamide for disease relapse upon cessation of steroids; if no response, use belimumab, a B-cell inhibitor
- Steroids and mycophenolate mofetil (cyclophosphamide) for nephritis

> The anemia of chronic disease is more common than hemolysis in SLE.

> Belimumab inhibits B cells as treatment of SLE.

Sjögren Syndrome

Look for a woman (9:1 female predominance) with dry eyes, dry mouth, and a sensation of "sand under the eyelid." There is often loss of taste and smell from profound mouth dryness. (You need saliva to wet the food so you can taste it.)

Look for loss of teeth at an early age, because saliva is critical for preventing dental cavities.

Diagnostic testing is as follows:

- Lip biopsy (**most accurate diagnostic test**)
- Schirmer test: decreased wetting of paper held to the eye shows decreased lacrimation

- Serologic testing:
  - ANA: 95% sensitive but least specific
  - RF: 70% sensitive
  - Anti-Ro/SSA: 50–65% sensitive but fairly specific
  - Anti-La/SSB: 30–65% sensitive but fairly specific

> Sjögren syndrome is associated with lymphoma.

CCS Tip: When you see anti-Ro (SSA) or anti-La (SSB), think Sjögren syndrome. They are present in a small number of people with lupus and can help diagnose ANA-negative lupus.

Treatment requires keeping the eyes and mouth moist. Non-salivary involvement is managed like SLE, with anti-malarials (hydroxychloroquine) and sometimes steroids/methotrexate.

- Pilocarpine and cevimeline increase acetylcholine, which increases oral and ocular secretions.
- Sour candy increases salivary production the most.

Basic Science Correlate

Acetylcholine stimulation massively increases secretions from the salivary glands. Pilocarpine directly stimulates acetylcholine receptors everywhere and increases the effect of acetylcholine. Cevimeline is specific to the salivary glands.

Scleroderma (Systemic Sclerosis)

Scleroderma presents with 3 main symptoms:

- Skin: commonly women, with tight, fibrous thickening of the skin that gives a tight face and tight, immobile fingers known as "sclerodactyly"
- Raynaud phenomenon (a 3-phase vascular hyperreactivity): the skin of the fingers become white, then blue, then red
  - Can be quite painful
  - Possible digital ulceration from infarction of the skin
  - Possible abnormal giant capillaries in the nail folds
- Joint pain: pain is mild and symmetrical

> Tight Skin + Heartburn + Raynaud = Scleroderma

Diffuse scleroderma also presents with the following:

- Lung: fibrosis and pulmonary hypertension (leading cause of death)
- GI: wide-mouthed colonic diverticula and esophageal dysmotility, leading to reflux and Barrett esophagus; primary biliary cirrhosis in 15% of patients
- Heart: restrictive cardiomyopathy and premature coronary disease
- Renal: may lead to malignant hypertension

There is no single diagnostic test. ANA is present in 95% of cases but is non-specific. Antitopoisomerase (anti-Scl 70) is present in only 30% of patients.

Treatment for scleroderma is by organ system.

- ACE inhibitors for renal involvement and hypertension
- Bosentan (endothelin antagonist), prostacyclin analogs (epoprostenol, treprostinil, iloprost), or sildenafil for primary pulmonary hypertension
- CCBs for Raynaud
- PPIs for GERD
- Cyclophosphamide for lung fibrosis

Penicillamine is not effective in delaying progression of this disease. Progressive skin-thickening is treated with methotrexate or mycophenolate.

> ACE inhibitors are so good for hypertension and scleroderma they are even used in pregnancy.

> Interstitial lung disease is treated with cyclophosphamide.

Limited Scleroderma ("CREST" Syndrome)

Limited scleroderma presents with the following:

- **C**alcinosis of the fingers
- **R**aynaud
- **E**sophageal dysmotility
- **S**clerodactyly
- **T**elangiectasia

It does not present with the following:

- Joint pain
- Heart involvement
- Lung involvement (except for pulmonary hypertension)
- Kidney involvement

CREST syndrome frequently has anti-centromere antibodies and less often has anti-Scl70.

> CREST does present with primary pulmonary hypertension.

> CREST is characterized by anticentromere antibodies.

Eosinophilic Fasciitis

Eosinophilic fasciitis (rare condition) presents with thickened skin that looks like scleroderma.

Symptoms include:

- Marked eosinophilia
- Appearance of an "orange peel" (peau d'orange) on skin
- Symptoms worse with exercise

Symptoms do not include the following:

- Hand involvement
- Raynaud
- Heart, lung, or kidney involvement

Treatment is corticosteroids. If no response, try methotrexate.

Myositis

Polymyositis (PM) and Dermatomyositis (DM)

In both PM and DM, the patient cannot get up from a seated position without using the arms. There can also be muscle pain and tenderness.

For polymyositis, look for the following:

- Proximal muscle weakness
- Signs of muscle inflammation on blood tests, electromyography, and biopsy

For dermatomyositis, you find the same thing and various rashes.

- Gottron papules: over metacarpophalangeal joint surfaces
- Heliotrope rash: periorbital and purplish lesion around the eyes
- Shawl sign: shoulder and neck erythema

Diagnostic testing includes the following:

- Elevated CPK and aldolase
- Abnormal electromyogram
- For CCS, order all the liver function tests as well as ANA
- Biopsy (**most accurate test**)

> - Weakness + ↑ CPK + ↑ Aldolase + Biopsy = Polymyositis
> - Weakness + ↑ CPK + ↑ Aldolase + Biopsy + Skin rash = Dermatomyositis

A 50-year-old woman presents with muscle weakness of the girdle with increased CPK and aldolase. Her anti-Jo-1 antibody is positive. Which of the following is most likely to happen to her?

a. Stroke
b. Myocardial infarction
c. Septic arthritis
d. DVT
e. Interstitial lung disease

Answer: **E.** PM/DM presents with weakness and increased markers of muscle inflammation. The presence of **anti-Jo-1** indicates a markedly increased risk of interstitial lung disease.

What is the most common serious complication of PM/DM?

a. Rhabdomyolysis
b. Hyperkalemia
c. Metabolic acidosis
d. Malignancy

Answer: **D.** For unclear reasons, the most common serious threat to life from PM/DM is malignancy. DM has a greater risk than PM. Cancer hits the cervix, lungs, pancreas, breasts, and ovaries.

> LDH, AST, and ALT can all be elevated in PM and DM.

Treatment is glucocorticoids. If there is no response to steroids, use azathioprine or methotrexate. For treatment resistance, use rituximab/IVIG. For skin, use hydroxychloroquine.

Inclusion Body Myositis

- Slowly progressive weakness of both distal and proximal muscles
- Distal upper extremity flexors are particularly affected
- Ability to engage quadriceps and make a fist at same time is weak
- Elevated CK
- Muscle biopsy (**most accurate diagnostic test**)

There is no effective treatment.

Mixed Connective Tissue Disease

Mixed connective tissue disease (MCTD) is the overlap between SLE, scleroderma, and polymyositis.

Symptoms include:

- Hand edema
- Synovitis
- Possible myositis and pulmonary hypertension
- Sclerodactyly, calcinosis, malar rash, and Gottron rash
- Kidney involvement (25% of cases)
- Serositis and sicca symptoms (50% of cases)

The **most specific diagnostic test** is anti-U1 ribonucleoprotein (RNP). If anti-Smith or DS-DNA is positive, it is more likely just SLE.

Treatment is steroids, azathioprine, or methotrexate. Cyclophosphamide is for interstitial lung disease.

Fibromyalgia

Fibromyalgia is a chronic pain disorder common among women (females:males 10:1). This is a pain syndrome with tender trigger points.

- Muscle aches and stiffness
- Trigger points on palpation
- Nonrefreshing sleep
- Exercise intolerance
- Depression and anxiety (common); cognitive fatigue

Diagnostic tests are CBC (all blood tests are normal). There is no objective evidence of disease.

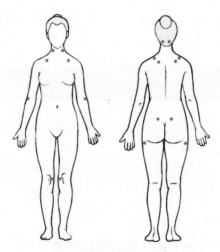

Fibromyalgia Trigger Points

Treatment is as follows:

- Aerobic exercise, cognitive behavioral therapy
- Milnacipran, duloxetine, pregabalin, or gabapentin
- Tricyclic antidepressants such as amitriptyline are effective but have more adverse effects.

NSAIDs are **not** first line for fibromyalgia.

Polymyalgia Rheumatica

Polymyalgia rheumatica is an inflammatory disorder seen age >50.

- Profound pain and stiffness of the proximal muscles, such as shoulders and pelvic girdle
- Stiffness worse in morning than in evening
- Stiffness localized to the muscles, not the joints
- Refreshing (normal) sleep
- Elevated ESR

In polymyalgia rheumatica, pain is much more prominent than weakness.

Nonspecific features include the following:

- Fever, weight loss, and malaise
- Normocytic anemia
- Normal CPK, electromyogram, aldolase, and muscle biopsy
- No muscle atrophy

Treatment is steroids, which have a very positive response.

Age >50 + proximal muscle pain + ↑ ESR = PMR

Note the differences between chronic fatigue syndrome, fibromyalgia, and polymyalgia rheumatica below.

	Chronic Fatigue Syndrome	Fibromyalgia	Polymyalgia Rheumatica
Fatigue/malaise	+++++ >6 months	++	++
Nonrefreshing sleep	+++++	++	No
Trigger points	No	Yes	No
Blood tests	All normal	All normal	↑ ESR
Treatment	None	Pain relief	Prednisone

Complex Regional Pain Syndrome (Reflex Sympathetic Dystrophy)

- Severe, excruciating pain in a limb (arms, legs) with allodynia (pain elicited by normal stimuli)
- Look for vasomotor symptoms with intermittent edema and skin color changes.
- Previous history of trauma damaging myelin of peripheral nerves
- Cause unknown and no precise test, but nuclear bone scan/MRI is abnormal.

Treatment is the same as peripheral neuropathy: NSAIDs, TCAs, gabapentin, and pregabalin

Vasculitis

All forms of vasculitis have some features in common:
- On presentation, they can all have:
  - Fatigue, malaise, weight loss
  - Fever: may present as a fever of unknown origin (FUO)
  - Skin lesions: palpable purpura, rash
  - Joint pain
  - Neuropathy: mononeuritis multiplex
- Common laboratory features:
  - Normocytic anemia
  - Elevated ESR
  - Thrombocytosis

Biopsy is the **most accurate diagnostic test** for vasculitis.

Methotrexate causes liver and lung fibrosis.

Treatment is prednisone and glucocorticoids. If no response, consider cyclophosphamide or rituximab. If no response, try azathioprine/6-mercaptopurine and methotrexate.

Polyarteritis Nodosa (PAN)

PAN has all of the features of vasculitis described, plus the following unique features:

- Abdominal pain (65%)
- Renal involvement (65%)
- Testicular involvement (35%)
- Pericarditis (35%)
- Hypertension (50%)

The lungs are not affected.

Diagnostic testing is angiogram of abdominal vessels (**best initial diagnostic test**) and biopsy (of skin, muscle, or sural nerve) (**most accurate test**).

> **Hepatitis B surface antigen** is found in 30% of patients with PAN.

CCS Tip: There is no good blood test for PAN.

Treatment is prednisone and cyclophosphamide or rituximab. Acute, life-threatening disease may respond to plasma exchange.

Granulomatosis with Polyangiitis

Granulomatosis with polyangiitis (formerly, Wegener) can affect the majority of the body, as PAN can. However, there are added upper and lower respiratory findings and c-ANCA (anti-proteinase 3).

> Upper and lower respiratory findings + c-ANCA = Wegener

Biopsy is the **most accurate test**.

Treatment is prednisone and cyclophosphamide.

Eosinophilic Granulomatosis with Polyangiitis

Although eosinophilic granulomatosis with polyangiitis (or Churg-Strauss Syndrome) can affect any organ in the body, it involves vasculitis, eosinophilia, and asthma.

Although the p-ANCA (anti-myeloperoxidase) can be positive, too, these findings are not as uniquely suggestive as the presence of eosinophilia and asthma.

> Vasculitis + Eosinophilia + Asthma = Churg-Strauss

Biopsy is the **most accurate test**.

Treatment is as follows:

- Steroids, which give an excellent response, plus an immunosuppressive agent (often cyclophosphamide but also azathioprine, methotrexate) to help reduce steroid dose
- Inhibitors of interleukin-5 (IL-5) such as mepolizumab or reslizumab (can induce remission in about 50% of cases)

Step 3 will ask you about leukotriene modifiers as a cause of Churg-Strauss syndrome. Look for zafirlukast, montelukast, or zileuton in the history.

Temporal Arteritis

Temporal arteritis is a type of giant cell arteritis (GCA). It is related to polymyalgia rheumatica. Fever, weight loss, malaise, and fatigue can be present, as they are in all forms of vasculitis.

Biopsy is the **most accurate test**.

> A patient presents with headache, jaw claudication, visual disturbance, and tenderness of the scalp. ESR is elevated. What is the next best step in management?
>
> Answer: Treatment with steroids is more important than getting a specific diagnostic test in temporal arteritis.

Tocilizumab is an inhibitor of interleukin 6 (IL-6) that controls giant cell arteritis (GCA) and gets patients off steroids.

Takayasu Arteritis

Half of patients with Takayasu arteritis have the usual vasculitis findings present before the loss or decrease of pulse:

Young Asian woman +
diminished pulses =
Takayasu arteritis

- Fatigue, malaise, weight loss, arthralgia
- Anemia, increased ESR

Symptoms of this vasculitis that are distinctive are TIA and stroke from vascular occlusion.

Diagnostic testing is distinctive in that the **most accurate test** is aortic arteriography or MRA, not biopsy.

Treatment is steroids. As with many autoimmune diseases, use azathioprine or methotrexate to get off steroids.

Cryoglobulinemia

Cryoglobulinemia has all the usual features of vasculitis, such as fatigue, malaise, skin lesions, and joint pain. There is an association with hepatitis C and renal involvement. Cryoglobulins and rheumatoid factor are very similar.

Treatment is as follows:

- For hepatitis C, standard treatment: sofosbuvir/ledipasvir, elbasvir/grazoprevir, daclatasvir/sofosbuvir, ombitasvir/paritaprevir/dasabuvir, or velpatasvir
- For the cryoglobulinemia and its vasculitis if severe (skin ulcers, renal failure, or stroke): rituximab
- For the vasculitis associated with cryoglobulinemia: cyclophosphamide is an alternative

Behcet Disease

This condition presents in patients of Middle Eastern or Asian ancestry.

Symptoms include:

- Oral and genital ulcers
- Ocular involvement (uveitis, optic neuritis): can lead to blindness
- Skin lesions: "pathergy," which is hyperreactivity to needle sticks, resulting in sterile skin abscesses
- CNS disease: 10% can have serious brain or spinal cord involvement
- Pulmonary artery aneurysm

There is no specific diagnostic test for Behcet disease. Use the features described.

Treatment is prednisone and colchicine. For severe disease, add cyclophosphamide.

Familial Mediterranean Fever (FMF)

Look for a patient with:

- Recurrent episodes of abdominal pain, tenderness, and fever (95%)
- Episodic chest and joint pain (50%)
- Multiple negative abdominal US and CT scans, negative stool studies, and normal colonoscopy
- Elevated ESR, CRP, WBC, fibrinogen

Treatment is colchicine. A long-term complication of FMF is amyloidosis.

> MEFV gene supports diagnosis of FMF.

Inflamed Joints

To diagnose inflamed joints, you need to look at the fluid. Inflamed joints will generally have effusions.

- Septic arthritis: cell count (**best initial test**); note that infectious septic arthritis could be present with as few as 20,000 white cells, although most cases have >50,000–100,000
- Gout, pseudogout, and septic arthritis: joint aspiration (**most accurate test**)
- Gram stain lacks sensitivity and, even in bacterial septic arthritis, detects only 50–60% of infections

The table compares synovial fluid cell count values.

Normal	Inflammatory (Gout/Pseudogout)	Infectious
<2,000 WBCs	2,000–50,000 WBCs	>50,000 WBCs

Pegloticase breaks down uric acid to allantoin. Use if allopurinol and febuxostat are not enough.

- Gout = negative birefringence
- Pseudogout = positive birefringence

Of all gout patients, 30% can have at least one normal uric acid level, especially during the attack, because the uric acid is being deposited into the joints from the blood.

Elevated uric acid level alone is not an indication for treatment in an asymptomatic patient. You must tap the joint.

Gout

Look for a man with a sudden onset of severe pain in the toe at night. The toe will be red, swollen, and tender, and it can look very similar to a toe with an infection.

The following can precipitate acute gouty attacks:

- Binge drinking of alcohol
- Thiazides
- Nicotinic acid

Diagnostic testing includes:

- Arthrocentesis (aspiration of joint fluid) (**best initial test**)
- Polarized light examination of the fluid will show negatively birefringent needles (**most accurate test**)

For CCS, also do the following:

- Joint fluid examination for cell count, culture, and protein level
- Serum uric acid level (however, do not rely on this to make an accurate diagnosis; 25% have normal uric acid during an acute event; don't treat asymptomatic hyperuricemia)
- X-ray of the toe: may show "punched-out" lesions
- Extremity examination for tophi

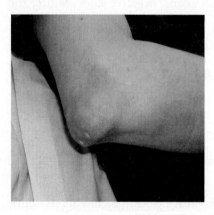

Tophus on elbow

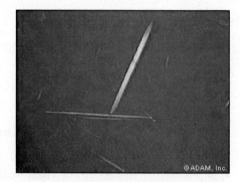

Negatively birefringent crystals of gout

Treatment for acute gouty attack is as follows:

- NSAIDs (**best initial therapy**); never use allopurinol
- Steroids if NSAIDs cannot be used; use injection for single joint and IV/oral for multiple joints
- Colchicine only under the following conditions:
  - First 24 hrs of an acute attack
  - If NSAIDs are contraindicated (e.g., renal insufficiency)
  - If steroids cannot be used
  - If part of preventive therapy to reduce the risk of a gouty attack (side effects of colchicine include nausea, diarrhea, bone marrow suppression)

- Anakinra: interleukin antagonist
- Prevention
  - Weight loss and avoiding alcohol
  - Uric level control
    - Allopurinol lowers uric acid (side effects include rash, allergic interstitial nephritis, hemolysis).
    - If allopurinol cannot be tolerated, use febuxostat (a xanthine oxidase inhibitor that markedly lowers uric acid).
    - If still not controlled, use uricase (pegloticase), a benign drug that breaks down uric acid.
    - Probenecid (rarely used for gout) increases urinary excretion of uric acid, which is contraindicated in those with renal insufficiency; it blocks absorption of uric acid at the kidney tubules; administer with xanthine oxidase inhibitors
  - Colchicine: prophylaxis, as described above
  - BP control: an ARB, e.g., losartan

> Steroids are much more the standard of care than colchicine in acute gout and pseudogout. Use colchicine for gout only if NSAIDs and steroids cannot be used.

> Do not start allopurinol during an acute attack of gout.

Pseudogout

In pseudogout (or calcium pyrophosphate deposition disease), the knee and wrist are involved but not the toes. It has a much slower onset than gout, and the patient will not wake up with severe pain.

Diagnostic testing involves tapping the joint and looking for positively birefringent rhomboid-shaped crystals.

Treatment is NSAIDs. Colchicine is an option but it is less effective. For acute disease, consider steroids.

CCS Tip: With pseudogout, expect hemochromatosis, hyperparathyroidism, acromegaly, or hypothyroidism in the history.

Baker Cyst

A Baker cyst is a posterior herniation of the synovium of the knee. Look for a patient with osteoarthritis or rheumatoid arthritis who has a swollen calf.

A ruptured Baker cyst is a "pseudo-phlebitis." An unruptured cyst can be palpated.

Diagnostic testing is ultrasound to exclude a DVT.

Treatment is NSAIDs and an occasional steroid injection.

Morton Neuroma

This condition presents with the following:

- Painful burning sensation in the interdigital web space between the 3rd and 4th toes
- Tenderness when pressure is applied between the heads of the 3rd and 4th metatarsals
- Sharp, intermittent pain radiating into the toes that feels better when shoes are taken off

Plantar Fasciitis and Tarsal Tunnel Syndrome

The table compares these 2 conditions.

Plantar Fasciitis	Tarsal Tunnel Syndrome
Pain on bottom of foot	Pain on bottom of foot
Very severe in the morning, better with walking a few steps	More painful with more use; like carpal tunnel of the foot; may have numbness of the sole, too
Stretch the foot and calf	Avoid boots and high heels; may need steroid injection
Resolves spontaneously over time	May need surgical release

> Do not order a foot x-ray for plantar fasciitis or tarsal tunnel syndrome. Heel spurs make no difference.

Septic Arthritis

The more abnormal the joint, the more likely a patient is to have septic arthritis. Any arthritic joint or prosthetic joint is a risk factor for septic arthritis.

prosthetic joint > rheumatoid arthritis > osteoarthritis > normal joint

Septic arthritis presents with a swollen, red, immobile, tender joint.

The etiology is as follows:

- *Staphylococcus aureus* (40%)
- *Streptococcus* (30%)
- Gram-negative bacilli (20%)

CCS Tip: In a CCS case, call an orthopedic surgery consult when you suspect a septic joint. The consultation won't offer much but it needs to be done.

Diagnostic testing includes:

- Tap the joint/arthrocentesis (**best initial test**): >50,000 white cells is consistent with infection
- Gram stain is 50–60% sensitive
- Culture is 90% sensitive (**most accurate test**) but is never available when you must make an acute treatment decision

> Disseminated gonorrhea is diagnosed by culture of:
> - Joint fluid (50% positive)
> - Pharynx (10–20% positive)
> - Rectum (10–20% positive)
> - Urethra (10–20% positive)
> - Cervix (20–30% positive)

Empiric treatment with IV ceftriaxone and vancomycin is effective. This is the choice for CCS when you have to write in one answer.

Other medications, seen below, are used in combination: one for *Staphylococcus/Streptococcus* and one for gram-negative bacilli.

Staph and Strep Drug	Gram-Negative Bacilli Drug
• Oxacillin • Nafcillin • Cefazolin	• Ceftriaxone • Ceftazidime • Gentamicin
• Penicillin allergy: anaphylaxis • Vancomycin • Linezolid • Daptomycin • Clindamycin	Penicillin allergy: anaphylaxis • Aztreonam • Fluoroquinolone

Three years after a hip replacement, a 64-year-old woman is seen for dental work that will cause bleeding. For the earlier surgery, the patient had a rash after the use of penicillin. What is the next step in management?

a. Administer clindamycin 1 hour before procedure

b. Administer cephalexin 1 hour before procedure

c. Desensitize the patient to penicillin, then give amoxicillin

d. Nothing

Answer: **D.** Prosthetic joint replacements do not need treatment with antibiotics before procedures. Even dental work that involves bleeding does not increase the risk of septic arthritis.

> Bisphosphonates can cause fever and flu-like symptoms in new users.

Upper Extremity Disorders

Diagnosis	Presentation	Testing & Treatment
Adhesive capsulitis	• Diabetic with shoulder pain & immobility • Loss of both active & passive ROM • Loss of abduction & external rotation	• No imaging needed • Physical therapy, stretching, and steroid injections
Medial epicondylitis (Golfer's elbow)	• Pain, inside of elbow	• NSAIDs, ice, stretching • Refractory cases need steroid injection
Lateral epicondylitis	• Pain, outside of elbow	• Same as medial epicondylitis
Rotator cuff tear	• Pain, lateral deltoid • Worse with overhead activity • Weak external rotation	• MRI confirms • Physical therapy, exercise and some need surgery

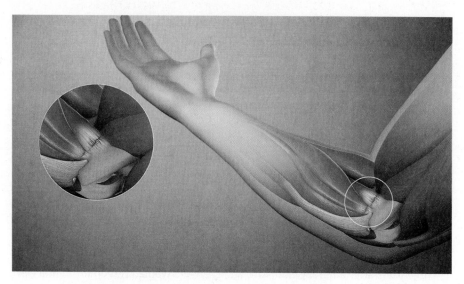

Medial Epicondylitis © Kaplan

Bone Disorders

Osteoporosis

The most common site of symptomatic osteoporosis is in the vertebral bodies, leading to crush fractures, kyphosis, and decreased height. The next most common sites are the hip and wrist.

The most common risk factor is positive family history in a thin, white woman. Other risk factors are steroid use, low calcium intake, sedentary lifestyle, smoking, and alcohol.

- Screen every woman with bone densitometry at least by age 65; screen after age 50 if risk factors are present.
- Prevent with calcium and vitamin D, weight-bearing exercise, and elimination of cigarettes and alcohol.

Diagnostic testing is as follows:

- DEXA scan (dual-energy x-ray absorptiometry) to assess bone density; results are reported as a T-score
  - T-score –2.5 or more indicates the presence of osteoporosis
- A 24-hour urine hydroxyproline or NTX (N-telopeptide, a bone breakdown product) to assess calcium loss

First-line treatment is bisphosphonates or denosumab.

- Bisphosphonates (e.g., alendronate, risedronate, ibandronate, zoledronic acid) inhibit osteoclastic activity.
  - If patient has osteopenia plus a fracture, add bisphosphonate.
- Denosumab (alternative first-line agent) is a RANKL inhibitor.
- Calcium and vitamin D (for everyone)

> DEXA scan results:
> - T-score –1.5 to –2.5 = osteopenia
> - T-score ≥–2.5 = osteoporosis

Estrogen is never first-line treatment for osteoporosis because of associated risks of clots and endometrial cancer.

Repeat the bone densitometry at 2 years. If there is continued bone loss, move to **second-line agents**.

- Selective estrogen receptor modulators (SERMs) increase bone density.
  - Protect the heart and bones but do not help vasomotor symptoms of menopause
  - Tamoxifen has endometrial and bone agonist effects but breast antagonist effects
  - Raloxifene has bone agonist effects but endometrial antagonist effects
- PTH analogs: teriparatide and abaloparatide

Third-line agent is calcitonin.

Paget Disease of Bone

Paget disease of bone is often asymptomatic. It may lead to pain, stiffness, aching, and fractures.

Soft bones lead to bowing of the tibias. Sarcoma arises in 1% of patients.

Diagnostic testing is as follows:

- Alkaline phosphatase level (**best initial test**) will be elevated
- Nuclear bone scan (**most accurate test**)
- For CCS, also order the following:
  - Urinary hydroxyproline
  - Serum calcium level (it will be normal)
  - Serum phosphate level (it will be normal)
  - Bone scan

Treatment is bisphosphonates. If the patient cannot tolerate bisphosphonates, use calcitonin. Bisphosphonates can cause flulike symptoms and jaw necrosis.

Stop bisphosphonates 6 weeks before dental surgery.

Denosumab is a RANKL inhibitor that inhibits osteoclast function.

Romosozumab, a sclerostin-inhibitor, can be tried as an alternative to bisphosphonates.

In cases of Paget, osteolytic lesions will be found initially. These may be replaced with osteoblastic lesions. So on Step 3,
- If osteolytic, then think Paget or osteoporosis; but
- If osteoblastic, think about metastatic prostate cancer in the differential diagnosis.

Anemia

All forms of anemia lead to fatigue and a subjective sense of loss of energy.

- Generalized anemia: fatigue, malaise, loss of energy
- More severe anemia: short of breath, lightheadedness, confusion (but other diseases can also present with fatigue or shortness of breath)

Symptoms include pallor, flow murmur described as I/VI or II/VI systolic murmur, and pale conjunctiva. Hemolysis will also give jaundice and scleral icterus (yellow eyes).

CCS Tip: There are no unique physical findings in anemia to allow you a specific diagnosis. For CCS cases, you find one anyway. For single best answer questions, go straight for the CBC. For physical exams, choose the following: general appearance, CV, chest, extremities, and HEENT.

Diagnostic testing includes:

- CBC with peripheral smear (**best initial test**): pay special attention to the mean corpuscular volume (MCV) and mean corpuscular hemoglobin concentration (MCHC)
  - MCV may clarify whether the anemia is microcytic, macrocytic, or normocytic
  - MCHC may reveal whether there is a problem with the synthesis of hemoglobin; based on this measurement, anemia can be further categorized as hypochromic, hyperchromic, or normochromic
- Reticulocyte count, haptoglobin, LDH, total and direct bilirubin, TSH with T4, B12/folate, iron
- Urinalysis with microscopic analysis
- Chest exam (if there is shortness of breath) to exclude other causes of shortness of breath, even though there are no positive findings in anemia
- ECG (for severe anemia) to exclude ischemia; anemia kills through myocardial ischemia

> If the question describes a craving for ice or dirt (i.e., forms of pica), think anemia. Step 3 loves to use pica as a lead-in to anemia.

> Hypoxia, carbon monoxide poisoning, methemoglobinemia, and ischemic heart disease have similar presentations to anemia.

> ### Basic Science Correlate
>
> Dyspnea occurs in anemia when there is no oxygen delivery to tissues. If there is low hemoglobin, there is no way to transport oxygen to the tissues.
>
> Anemia is perceived the same way as hypoxia. Carbon monoxide poisoning does not release the oxygen from hemoglobin. All of these cause light-headedness and ultimately, myocardial ischemia. Anemia kills via left ventricular ischemia and infarction.

Microcytic Anemia

Specific Diagnostic Tests and Treatments				
When this is in the history/physical...	Blood loss Elevated platelet count	Rheumatoid arthritis End-stage renal disease or Any chronic infectious, inflammatory, or connective tissue disease	Very small MCV with few or no symptoms Target cells	Alcoholic Isoniazid Lead exposure
...this is the diagnosis.	Iron deficiency	Anemia of chronic disease	Thalassemia	Sideroblastic anemia
What is the best initial diagnostic test?	Iron studies: • Low ferritin • High TIBC • Low Fe • Low Fe sat • Elevated RDW	Iron studies: • High ferritin • Low TIBC • Low Fe • Normal or low Fe sat	Iron studies: • Normal	Iron studies: • High Fe
What is the most accurate diagnostic test?	Bone marrow biopsy (do not do this on CCS)	No specific diagnostic test	Hemoglobin Electrophoresis Beta: Elevated HgA2,HgF Alpha: Normal	Prussian blue stain
What is the best initial therapy?	Prescribe ferrous sulfate orally	Correct the underlying disease EPO only with renal failure	No treatment for trait	Major: Remove the toxin exposure Minor: Prescribe pyridoxine replacement

A 62-year-old-man with a history of anemia from a bleeding peptic ulcer comes for evaluation. He is constipated and has black stool. His medications are omeprazole, oral ferrous sulfate, and occasional liquid antacids. What is the next step?

a. EGD

b. Colonoscopy

c. Guaiac testing/hemoccult

d. Discontinue omeprazole

e. Increased dose of ferrous sulfate

Answer: **C.** Oral ferrous sulfate can turn the stool black, but elemental iron such as this does not make the stool guaiac positive. Only the iron in hemoglobin or myoglobin can make the stool guaiac card positive.

> Alpha thalassemia is most accurately diagnosed by DNA sequencing.

Diagnostic testing is as follows:

- Iron studies/profile (Fe level, Fe saturation, ferritin, TIBC) (**most important test**)
- Bone marrow biopsy (**most accurate test**)

Only iron deficiency is associated with elevated red cell distribution of width (RDW). That is because the newer cells are progressively smaller and smaller, so the red cell width changes over time. Prussian blue is an iron stain. Sideroblastic anemia is associated with iron building up inside the mitochondria of the red cell.

Patients with severe thalassemia need regular transfusion to maintain circulating hemoglobin levels. The same is true for myelofibrosis, but the risk of hemochromatosis is less because these patients are typically older.

- For hemochromatosis due to overabsorption of iron in the duodenum, treatment is phlebotomy. Phlebotomy removes much more iron than chelating agents such as deferasirox, deferiprone, or deferoxamine.
- For iron overload from transfusion, treatment is deferasirox or deferiprone to remove iron. Phlebotomy cannot be used because you need the blood.

> HgH has beta-4 tetrads with 3-gene deleted alpha thalassemia.

A 68-year-old woman is found on routine CBC to have a hematocrit 32% (normal 37–42) and MCV 70 (normal 80–100). Stool is heme negative. What is the next step?

a. Colonoscopy
b. Sigmoidoscopy
c. Barium enema
d. Upper endoscopy
e. Two more stool tests now
f. Repeat stool test in a year
g. Capsule endoscopy

Answer: **A.** Colonoscopy is indicated as routine screening for everyone age >50, so this patient needs it anyway, regardless of the stool test results. Another reason to go straight to colonoscopy is the presence of microcytic anemia. Unexplained microcytic anemia age >50 is most likely caused by colon cancer. Sigmoidoscopy will do nothing to evaluate the right side of the colon and would miss nearly 40% of cancers. No matter what a sigmoidoscopy showed, you would need to inspect the right side of the colon. Capsule endoscopy is done to evaluate bleeding when the upper and lower endoscopy are normal and the source of bleeding is likely to be in the small bowel.

A patient comes with end stage renal disease for evaluation of shortness of breath. After dialysis, he is found to have a hematocrit of 28 with MCV 68. Iron studies are performed. What do you expect to find?

	Iron	Total Iron Binding Capacity	Ferritin	RDW
a.	Low	High	Low	High
b.	Low	Low	Normal	Normal
c.	Normal	Normal	Normal	Normal
d.	High	High	Normal	Normal

Answer: **B.** The anemia of chronic disease, such as that found in patients with end stage renal disease, is associated with normal or increased amounts of iron in storage (ferritin/TIBC) but the inability to process the iron into usable cells and hemoglobin. The only form of anemia of chronic disease that reliably responds to erythropoietin is caused by end stage renal disease.

> The only microcytic anemia with a high reticulocyte count is HgH.

Macrocytic Anemia

"Extravascular" hemolysis occurs in spleen and liver, so you cannot see it on the smear.

All anemia presents with fatigue, including macrocytic anemia, which is caused by vitamin B12 (folate) deficiency.

- B12 deficiency presents with neurological findings as well.
  - The most common is peripheral neuropathy, but any form of neurological abnormality can develop at any part of the peripheral or central nervous system.
  - The least common neurological problem is dementia.
  - Neurological problems resolve with treatment if they have been present for a short period of time.
- B12 deficiency also causes a smooth tongue (glossitis) and diarrhea.
- Folate deficiency: This does not present with neurological problems.

> Metformin blocks B12 absorption.

  - Drugs that cause megaloblastic anemia are the purine and pyrimidine modulators: azathioprine, mycophenolate, fludarabine, hydroxyurea, methotrexate, and trimethoprim.
  - Drugs that block GI absorption of folate are alcohol, nitrofurantoin, estrogens, and phenytoin.

Diagnostic testing is as follows:

- CBC with peripheral blood smear (**best initial test**): look for hypersegmented neutrophils and oval cells
  - Average number of lobes in normal white cell is 3.5
  - If the average number of lobes >4 or if more than 5% of the cells have >6 lobes, the patient has megaloblastic anemia and macrocytosis (megaloblastic anemia means the presence of hypersegmented neutrophils and macrocytosis means "big cells," i.e., large MCV)

- For CCS cases, also order a bilirubin level and LDH, which are commonly elevated.
- Reticulocyte count will be decreased
- Oval cells will be visible on the peripheral smear
- The 3 images that follow show hypersegmented neutrophils (megaloblastic anemia).

> Reticulocytes are low in B12 deficiency.

> RBC **bigger** than lymph = **Macro**
>
> RBC **smaller** than lymph = **Micro**

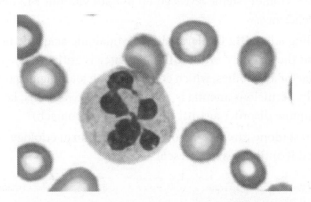

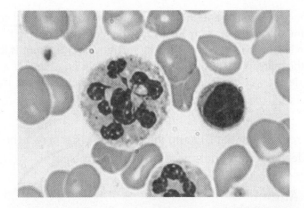

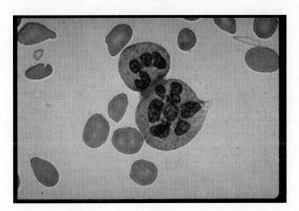

- Low B12 (for B12 deficiency) and folate (for folate deficiency) (**most accurate tests**)
  - Up to 30% of patients with B12 deficiency can have a normal B12, because transcobalamin is an acute phase reactant and any form of stress can cause its elevation.
  - If you suspect B12 deficiency but B12 is normal, order a methylmalonic acid level. Homocysteine levels go up in both vitamin B12 deficiency and folate deficiency.
- After finding a low B12 or elevated methylmalonic acid, the **next best test to confirm the etiology of the B12 deficiency** is antiparietal cell and anti-intrinsic factor antibodies, which confirm pernicious anemia as the etiology (essentially, pernicious anemia is an allergy to parietal cells, i.e., it is a kind of autoimmune disorder against this part of the stomach).
- Schilling test (done rarely) is an older way to confirm etiology and not usually needed if antibodies are present

> After B12 replacement therapy:
> - Reticulocytes will improve first (in iron deficiency)
> - Neurological abnormalities will improve last

Basic Science Correlate

B12 deficiency raises LDH and indirect bilirubin by destroying red cells early, as they come out of the bone marrow. This phenomenon is called "ineffective erythropoiesis," and it is why the reticulocyte count is low. Although the marrow itself is hypercellular, B12 deficiency creates a molecular defect that breaks down the cells just as they leave the marrow.

Treatment is replacement of B12 and folate. Folate will correct the blood problems in B12 deficiency, but not the neurological problems.

Hemolytic Anemia

All forms of hemolytic anemia present with the sudden onset of weakness and fatigue associated with anemia. The first thing to improve is the reticulocyte count and LDH.

Hemolysis shows the following:

- Elevated indirect bilirubin level
- Elevated reticulocyte count
- Elevated LDH level
- Decreased haptoglobin level
- Spherocytes on smear

> Autoimmune hemolysis also gives spherocytes.

Basic Science Correlate

Mechanism of Lab Abnormalities in Hemolysis

When cells are destroyed, they release indirect (lipid-soluble) bilirubin. The
liver has limited capacity to glucuronidate it into direct (water-soluble)
bilirubin. Indirect bilirubin never goes into the urine, because it is attached
to albumin and cannot be filtered. Haptoglobin is a transport protein for
newly released indirect bilirubin and is rapidly used up during hemolysis.
LDH increases from any form of tissue breakdown and is extremely
nonspecific.

CCS Tip: In a case of hemolysis, order a peripheral smear, LDH, bilirubin level,
reticulocyte count, and haptoglobin level on the first CCS screen.

Intravascular hemolysis also shows the following:

- Abnormal peripheral smear (schistocytes, helmet cells, fragmented cells)
- Hemoglobinuria

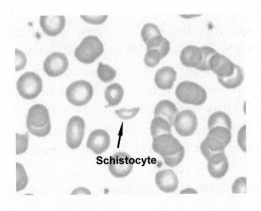

Schistocyte

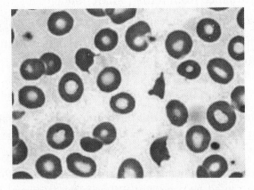

Microangiopathic Intravascular Hemolysis

Sickle Cell Anemia

Sickle cell anemia is seen frequently on the Step 3 exam. The case will describe severe pain in the chest, back, and thighs.

Diagnostic testing is as follows:

- Oxygen, fluids, analgesics, and antibiotics
- Complete physical examination if there is a fever; findings may include:
  - HEENT: retinal infarction
  - CV: flow murmur from anemia
  - Abdomen: splenomegaly in children; absence of spleen in adults
  - Chest: rales or consolidation from infection or infarction
  - Extremities: skin ulcers (unclear etiology in sickle cell) and aseptic necrosis of hip; aseptic necrosis found on MRI
  - Neurological: stroke, current or previous

Treatment is as follows:

- **Next best step**: oxygen, hydration with normal saline continuously, and pain medication
- If fever is present, give ceftriaxone, levofloxacin, or moxifloxacin with the first screen (fever in a patient with sickle cell disease is an **emergency** because there is no spleen).
  - So when fever is present, the most urgent next step is antibiotics. This is more important than waiting for results of testing.
  - If it is a CCS question, answer blood cultures, urinalysis, reticulocyte count, CBC, and chest x-ray with the first screen as well, but if fever is present, do not wait for results.

When do you answer "exchange transfusion" in sickle cell disease?

- **Eye:** visual disturbance from retinal infarction
- **Lung:** pulmonary infarction leading to pleuritic pain and abnormal x-ray
- **Penis:** priapism from infarction of prostatic plexus of veins if local drainage does not work
- **Brain:** stroke

> The goal of exchange transfusion is to decrease hemoglobin S to 30–40%.

> For priapism, aspirate first. If ineffective, exchange transfusion.

A patient admitted for sickle cell crisis has a drop from her usual hematocrit of 34 to 26 over 2 days in the hospital. Reticulocyte count is 2%. What is the diagnosis? What is the most accurate test? What is the treatment?

Answer: Sudden drops in the hematocrit in sickle cell patients or those with hemoglobinopathy can be caused by parvovirus B19 or folate deficiency. Sickle cell patients should universally be on folate replacement. A normal reticulocyte in sickle cell is a dangerous sign. Reticulocyte count should be 10–20%, so if it is 1–2% it means there is a very serious disorder in marrow production.

If the patient is on replacement therapy, then the diagnosis shifts to parvovirus B19, an infection that invades the marrow and stops production of cells at the level of the pronormoblast. The **most accurate diagnostic test** is PCR for DNA of the parvovirus. This is more accurate than IgM or IgG antibody testing or bone marrow.

Treatment is transfusions and IV immunoglobulins. When the patient is ready for discharge, prescribe folate replacement; pneumococcal vaccination; and hydroxyurea to prevent further crises if they happen >3× per year.

> For hydroxyurea dosing, increase until fetal Hg is 15% and crises stop or WBC count starts to drop.

Basic Science Correlate

Mechanism of Hydroxyurea in Sickle Cell Disease

Hydroxyurea increases the percentage of hemoglobin that is hemoglobin F, or fetal hemoglobin. Increased fetal hemoglobin dilutes the sickle hemoglobin and decreases the frequency of painful crises.

Hemoglobin Sickle Cell (SC) Disease

This condition is like a mild version of sickle cell disease with fewer crises. Visual disturbance is frequent. Painful crises do not occur. Renal problems are the only significant manifestation, including hematuria, isosthenuria (inability to concentrate or dilute the urine), and UTIs.

There is no specific treatment for hemoglobin SC disease.

> Sickle cell trait is not a disease, but rather an indication that someone has inherited the sickle cell gene from a parent. The only findings are hematuria and a concentrating defect. With hypoxia (as in scuba diving), splenic vein thrombosis can occur.

Autoimmune Hemolysis

Look for other autoimmune diseases in the history, such as SLE or rheumatoid arthritis. Other clues are a history of chronic lymphocytic leukemia (CLL), lymphoma, or medications such as penicillin, alpha-methyldopa, quinine, or sulfa drugs.

Diagnostic testing includes:

- LDH, indirect bilirubin level, and reticulocyte count (all will be elevated)
- Haptoglobin level can be decreased in both intravascular and extravascular forms of hemolysis
- Peripheral smear may show spherocytes
- Coombs test (**most accurate test**)

Basic Science Correlate

Mechanism of Spherocytes in Autoimmune Hemolysis

A normal RBC is a biconcave disc. When antibodies attack the RBC membrane, they pull out pieces of it. Removing membrane decreases the surface area, which turns the RBC into a sphere. It takes more surface area to maintain biconcave disc than a sphere.

Treatment is steroids such as prednisone. If that is not effective, do splenectomy. Rituximab works on both IgG and IgM.

The antibodies found in Coombs test are also called "warm antibodies," which are IgG. Only IgG antibodies respond to steroids and splenectomy.

A response to IVIG predicts a response to splenectomy.

CCS Tip: If the case describes severe hemolysis not responsive to prednisone or repeated blood transfusion, use IV immunoglobulins as the best therapy to stop acute episodes of hemolysis.

Cold-Induced Hemolysis (Cold Agglutinins)

Look for the following:

- Mycoplasma or Epstein-Barr virus in the history
- Standard Coombs test is negative
- Complement test is positive
- Treatment is rituximab. Steroids, splenectomy, and IV immunoglobulins have no role.

CCS Tip: CCS does not require you to know dosing, and in fact, there is no way even to order dosage on CCS.

> **Basic Science Correlate**
>
> Rituximab is an antibody against the CD20 receptor on lymphocytes. The CD20 positive cells are the ones that make antibodies, such as the IgM against red cells known as the "cold agglutinin." Rituximab's effect in both this disease and rheumatoid arthritis is to remove antibody-producing cells.

Glucose-6-Phosphate Dehydrogenase (G6PD) Deficiency

Sudden onset of hemolysis, which can be quite severe, is seen. As an X-linked disorder, hemolysis from G6PD deficiency is much more often described in males.

The most common form of oxidant stress to cause acute hemolysis with G6PD deficiency is an infection. Oxidizing drugs, such as sulfa medication, primaquine, or dapsone, are frequently in the history. Fava bean ingestion may also be in the history.

The **best initial diagnostic test** is Heinz body test, leading to characteristic bite cells. The **most accurate test** is G6PD level, but only after 2 months have passed (a normal level taken immediately after an episode of hemolysis does not exclude G6PD deficiency). On the day of the hemolysis, the most deficient cells have been destroyed, and the level of G6PD is normal.

Basic Science Correlate

Heinz bodies are collections of oxidized, precipitated hemoglobin embedded in the red cell membrane. **Bite cells** appear when pieces of the red cell membrane have been removed by the spleen.

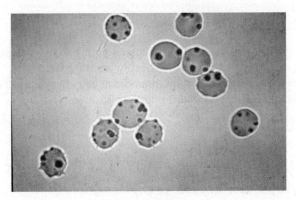

Heinz bodies

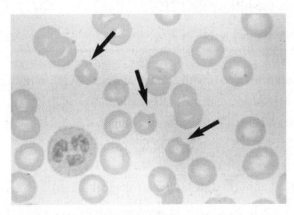

Bite cells

There is no specific treatment for G6PD deficiency. Avoid oxidant stress and give folic acid.

Test for G6PD before using dapsone and rasburicase.

Pyruvate Kinase Deficiency

Presents the same way as G6PD deficiency in terms of hemolysis. However, pyruvate kinase deficiency is not provoked by medications or fava beans; what precipitates the hemolysis with pyruvate kinase deficiency is not clear.

Hereditary Spherocytosis

This condition presents with:

- Recurrent episodes of hemolysis
- Splenomegaly
- Bilirubin gallstones
- Elevated mean corpuscular hemoglobin concentration (MCHC)

The **most accurate diagnostic test** is an eosin-5-maleimide (EMA), which is more accurate than osmotic fragility. The other alternative is the acidified glycerol lysis test.

Treatment is splenectomy, which will prevent hemolysis since the cells are destroyed in the spleen. Splenectomy helps in these patients.

> **Basic Science Correlate**
>
> Hereditary spherocytosis is the genetic loss of both ankyrin and spectrin in the red cell membrane. Ankyrin and spectrin are the basis of the cytoskeleton that maintains the RBC membrane in its biconcave disc. Without this cytoskeleton, the RBC pops into a sphere.

Hemolytic Uremic Syndrome (HUS) and Thrombotic Thrombocytopenic Purpura (TTP)

Look for *E. coli* 0157:H7 in the history for HUS. Look for medication use such as ticlopidine in the history for TTP.

Diagnosis is based on:

- HUS triad: **ART**
  - Intravascular hemolysis with abnormal smear (**A**: autoimmune hemolysis)
  - Elevated BUN and creatinine (**R**: renal failure)
  - Thrombocytopenia (**T**: thrombocytopenia)
- TTP pentad (**FAT RN**) also has the following:
  - Fever (**F**: fever)
  - Neurological abnormalities (**N**: neurological issues)

ADAMTS-13 level is decreased in TTP. PT/aPTT are normal in HUS and TTP.

Treatment is as follows:

- Some cases resolve on their own
- Plasmapheresis for severe cases of TTP and HUS
- Steroids are of no help
- Antibiotics for HUS from *E. coli* may make it worse
- Platelet transfusion for either condition will definitely make it worse
- HUS not from infection is treated with eculizumab, an antibody against complement C5
- Eculizumab stops complement mediated RBC destruction

Never use platelets in HUS or TTP.

Get an ADAMTS-13 level in TTP/HUS.

Vaccinate for meningococcus before using eculizumab. Complement deficiency predisposes to meningococcal infection.

> ### Basic Science Correlate
>
> **Mechanism of HUS/TTP**
>
> ADAMTS-13 is the metalloproteinase that breaks down von Willebrand factor (VWF) to release platelets from one another. When VWF is not dissolved, the platelets form abnormally prolonged strands that serve as a barrier to RBCs. RBCs that run into these strands break down and are destroyed. The purpose of plasmapheresis in the treatment of severe TTP is to replace the ADAMTS-13. This is why giving platelets only makes matters worse: It increases the size of the abnormal platelet strands.

Paroxysmal Nocturnal Hemoglobinuria

Paroxysmal nocturnal hemoglobinuria (PNH) presents with pancytopenia and recurrent episodes of dark urine, particularly in the morning. The most common cause of death is large vessel venous thrombosis, such as portal vein thrombosis.

The **most accurate diagnostic test** is CD 55 and CD 59 antibody (also known as decay accelerating factor).

Treatment is as follows:

- Glucocorticoids e.g., prednisone
- Eculizumab for transfusion-dependent patients with severe illness; before administering eculizumab, give the meningococcal vaccine

PNH can develop into aplastic anemia or acute myelogenous leukemia (AML).

> Eculizumab inhibits C-5 and prevents complement activation. PNH is treated with eculizumab.

A pregnant woman comes with weakness and elevated liver function tests. She is in her 35th week of pregnancy. Prothrombin time is normal. The smear of blood shows fragmented red cells. Platelet count is low. What is the treatment?

a. Transfuse platelets
b. Plasmapheresis
c. Fresh frozen plasma
d. Deliver the baby
e. Prednisone

Answer: **D.** Deliver the baby with the HELLP syndrome. HELLP syndrome stands for hemolysis, elevated liver function tests, and low platelets. This disorder is idiopathic and can be distinguished from DIC by the normal coagulation studies, such as the prothrombin time and aPTT.

Methemoglobinemia

Methemoglobinemia is blood locked in an oxidized state that cannot pick up oxygen. Symptoms include with shortness of breath for no clear reason, with clear lungs on exam and normal chest x-ray.

Look for an exposure to drugs such as nitroglycerin, amyl nitrate, nitroprusside, dapsone, or any of the anesthetic drugs that end in -caine (e.g., lidocaine, bupivacaine, tetracaine). Methemoglobinemia can occur with as little exposure as to a topical anesthetic administered to a mucous membrane. Look for brown blood in the case description.

Treatment is methylene blue.

Transfusion Reactions

Match the most likely diagnoses with each of the following cases:

a. ABO incompatibility

b. Transfusion-related acute lung injury (TRALI) or "leukoagglutination reaction"

c. Urticarial reaction

d. IgA deficiency

e. Febrile nonhemolytic reaction

f. Minor blood group incompatibility

Case 1: Twenty minutes after a patient receives a blood transfusion, the patient becomes short of breath. There are transient infiltrates on the chest x-ray. All symptoms resolve spontaneously.

Case 2: As soon as a patient receives a transfusion, he becomes hypotensive, short of breath, and tachycardic. LDH and bilirubin levels are normal.

Case 3: During a transfusion, a patient becomes hypotensive and tachycardic. She has back and chest pain, and there is dark urine. LDH and bilirubin are elevated, and the haptoglobin level is low.

Case 4: A few days after a transfusion, a patient becomes jaundiced. The hematocrit does not rise with transfusion, and he is generally without symptoms.

Case 5: A few hours after a transfusion, a patient becomes febrile with a rise in temperature of about 1 degree. There is no evidence of hemolysis.

Answers:

Case 1: B. TRALI presents with acute shortness of breath from antibodies in the donor blood against recipient white cells. There is no treatment, and it resolves spontaneously.

Case 2: D. IgA deficiency presents with anaphylaxis. In the future, use blood donations from an IgA deficient donor or washed red cells.

Case 3: A. ABO incompatibility presents with acute symptoms of hemolysis while the transfusion is occurring.

Case 4: F. Minor blood group incompatibility to Kell, Duffy, Lewis, or Kidd antigens or Rh incompatibility presents with delayed jaundice. There is no specific therapy.

Case 5: E. Febrile nonhemolytic reactions result in a small rise in temperature and need no therapy. These reactions are against donor white cell antigens. They are prevented by using filtered blood transfusions in the future to remove the white cell antigens.

Leukemia

Acute Leukemia

Presents with signs of pancytopenia, such as fatigue, bleeding, and infections from white cells that don't work. Patients have a functional immunodeficiency.

The **best initial test** is a peripheral smear showing blasts.

Treatment is as follows:

- For acute myelogenous leukemia: chemotherapy with idarubicin (or daunorubicin) and cytosine arabinoside (best initial therapy)
- For M3 (acute promyelocytic) leukemia, add all trans retinoic acid (ATRA) (arsenic trioxide is extremely effective for M3 when combined with ATRA)
- For acute lymphocytic leukemia (ALL), add intrathecal methotrexate

The most important prognostic finding in acute leukemia is cytogenetic abnormalities, such as specific karyotypic abnormalities. Cytogenetics tell who will relapse. If the patient is at high risk for relapse after chemotherapy, bone marrow transplantation should be performed as soon as chemotherapy induces remission.

> A patient presents with shortness of breath, confusion, and blurry vision. His white cell count is over 100,000. What is the best initial therapy?
>
> Answer: Acute leukemia can sometimes present with an extremely high white cell count. When >100,000, these cells result in sludging of the blood vessels of the brain, eyes, and lungs. Chronic lymphocytic leukemia rarely does this, because lymphocytes are much smaller and do not occlude vessels. Leukostasis is treated with leukapheresis, which removes white cells via centrifugation of blood. Hydroxyurea is also added to lower the white cell count.

Myelodysplasia

This condition presents in elderly patients with pancytopenia, elevated MCV, low reticulocyte count, and macroovalocytes. There is a special neutrophil with two lobes called a "Pelger-Huet cell." Look for a normal B12 level. There will be a small number of blasts (<20%) but not enough to be considered acute leukemia. Myelodysplasia is like a mild, slowly progressive preleukemia syndrome. Just as cervical dysplasia may sometimes progress to cervical cancer, myelodysplasia may progress to acute leukemia. The most common cause of death is not leukemia; most patients die of infection or bleeding.

Auer rods are associated with acute myeloid leukemia (AML).

M3, acute promyelocytic leukemia, is associated with disseminated intravascular coagulation. This is a common Step 3 question about acute leukemia.

Arsenic trioxide treats M3 (acute promyelocytic) leukemia.

Lenalidomide has tremendous efficacy in decreasing transfusion dependence in MDS.

Treatment is largely supportive with transfusions as needed. Azacitidine, decitabine, and lenalidomide are specific therapies for myelodysplasia (MDS). Those with the 5q minus syndrome are treated with lenalidomide. Only azacitidine increases survival.

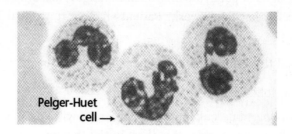

Pelger-Huet cell →

Myeloproliferative Disorders

Chronic Myelogenous Leukemia (CML)

Look for an elevated white cell count that is predominantly neutrophils. Splenomegaly is frequent.

> **Basic Science Correlate**
>
> **Mechanism of Early Satiety in CML and CLL**
> The spleen is anatomically right on top of the stomach. When the spleen is enlarged, it presses on the stomach and compresses it. This stomach compression makes a person feel full right after eating.

> Untreated CML has the highest risk of transformation into acute leukemia of all forms of myeloproliferative disorders.

Diagnostic testing is as follows:

- Elevated neutrophil count with a low LAP score is CML. Reactive high white blood cell counts from infection give an elevated LAP score. LAP is up in normal cells, not CML.
- Philadelphia chromosome by PCR of blood or BCR/ABL by FISH (**most accurate test**)

Treatment is imatinib, which leads to 90% hematologic remission with no major adverse effects; if that is not effective, try dasatinib and nilotinib, tyrosine kinase inhibitors. The only curative treatment is bone marrow transplantation.

Following are wrong answers for CML treatment:

- Interferon: much less effective; causes uncomfortable, flulike symptoms
- Hydroxyurea: never makes the Philadelphia chromosome negative
- Busulfan: never right for anything, unless the exam asks what causes pulmonary fibrosis

> Q: Interferon for CML?
> A: Only in **pregnant patients**.

Chronic Lymphocytic Leukemia (CLL)

CLL presents exclusively age >50 with elevated white cell count that is described as "normal appearing lymphocytes." CLL is often asymptomatic and found on "routine" testing.

Diagnostic testing is as follows:

- Peripheral blood smear shows "smudge" cells, which are ruptured nuclei of lymphocytes (similar to squished jelly donuts) (**best initial diagnostic test**)
  - Stage 0: elevated white cell count alone
  - Stage 1: enlarged lymph nodes
  - Stage 2: enlarged spleen
  - Stage 3: anemia
  - Stage 4: low platelets

Basic Science Correlate

Mechanism of Infection and Hemolysis in CLL

The lymphocytes in CLL produce abnormal or insufficient immunoglobulins.

- When IgG produced is abnormal, it is inappropriately directed against RBCs or platelets, causing immune thrombocytopenia or hemolysis.
- When IgG supply is insufficient, it leads to infection.

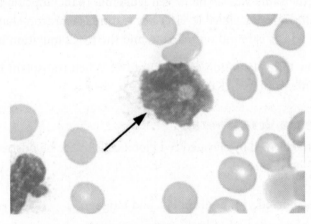

Smudge cell (found in CLL)

Treatment for CLL is based entirely on the stage of the disease.

Use bendamustine in elderly patients with CLL and relapsed lymphoma.

- Early stages (stages 0 and 1): no therapy required
- More advanced stages: fludarabine + rituximab (an antibody against CD20) to extend survival; chlorambucil is less effective
  - Although fludarabine + rituximab are used for most symptomatic CLL patients age <70, there is **no clear first-line therapy** between the agents discussed here.
  - You will not be asked to choose between them.

- Alemtuzumab (an anti-CD52 agent) is better than chlorambucil; use it with ibrutinib (an inhibitor of Bruton tyrosine kinase) when fludarabine fails
- Fludarabine can be combined with cyclophosphamide as well; adding cyclophosphamide increases both efficacy and toxicity
- The 3-drug combination is better for younger, more functional patients

Venetoclax increases apoptosis in CLL when there is 17p deletion.

When is **venetoclax** the answer?

- When there is CLL which fails initial therapy and there is a 17p deletion

Hairy Cell Leukemia

This condition presents with the following:

- Pancytopenia
- Massive splenomegaly
- Middle-aged patient (50s)

Smear showing hairy cells and immunophenotyping (or flow cytometry) is the **most accurate test**.

Treatment is cladribine (2-CDA).

Myelofibrosis

Presents in the same way as hairy cell leukemia (pancytopenia and spleno-megaly) with a normal TRAP level. A key feature is teardrop-shaped cells on the smear. Fibrosis is found on marrow, and the JAK2 mutation is found.

Bone marrow transplantation can be curative. When transplant is not possible, ruxolitinib inhibits JAK2.

Polycythemia Vera (Pvera)

Pvera is characterized by elevated red blood cells in the bloodstream.

Symptoms include:

- Headache, blurred vision, dizziness, and fatigue
- Pruritus, often after a hot bath or shower, due to the release of histamine from basophils
- Splenomegaly (common)

Most accurate diagnostic test is CBC, showing a markedly high hematocrit in the absence of hypoxia with a low MCV.

- Low erythropoietin level
- Possible elevated white cell count and platelet count
- Elevated B12 and LAP

- The high hematocrit can lead to thrombosis; once it has been revealed by CBC, order an arterial blood gas to exclude hypoxia as a cause of erythrocytosis
- If the case is a CCS, order an erythropoietin level, which should be low, and hematology consultation. The test for the JAK2 mutation is 97% sensitive.

Treatment is phlebotomy, hydroxyurea to lower the cell count, and daily aspirin. If hydroxyurea fails, use anagrelide or ruxolitinib (a JAK2 inhibitor).

> JAK2 mutation is found in Pvera and ET.

Essential Thrombocythemia

Essential thrombocythemia is a rare disorder often found in asymptomatic patients on routine CBC.

Symptoms include:

- Markedly elevated platelets (**key feature**)
- Headache, visual disturbance, and pain in the hands ("erythromelalgia")
- Thrombosis and bleeding (most common causes of death)
- It is hard to distinguish a reactive elevation in platelets from ET; CALR is a mutation found in ET that helps.

Treatment is hydroxyurea to lower the platelet count. (Anagrelide is an agent specific to the treatment of ET but it is not as strong as hydroxyurea.) Daily aspirin should also be given if patient is thrombosing.

> In Pvera on a CCS, order a B12 and LAP in addition to the CBC. If you are asked the "single best test," question, however, these tests would not be the most accurate tests.

Plasma Cell Disorders

Multiple Myeloma

The most frequent presentation of multiple myeloma (MM) is bone pain caused by a fracture occurring under normal use. The most common causes of death are infection (those with MM are effectively immunodeficient) and renal failure.

Initial diagnostic testing is as follows:

- Skeletal survey to detect punched out osteolytic lesions (which would suggest metastatic prostate cancer)
- Serum protein electrophoresis (SPEP): look for elevated monoclonal antibodies (usually IgG); 20% are IgA
- Urine protein electrophoresis (UPEP): detects Bence-Jones protein
- Peripheral smear: shows "rouleaux" formation of blood cells; mean platelet volume (MPV) is elevated because the cells stick together
- Elevated calcium level: makes sense with the osteolytic lesions
- Beta 2 microglobulin level: a prognostic indicator
- BUN and creatinine: to detect the frequent occurrence of renal insufficiency; bortezomib reverses renal dysfunction

> If plasma cells >60% in marrow or FLC ratio >100, treatment is needed.

Other testing includes serum free light chain (FLC) (ratio of 100:1 is highly consistent with myeloma) and low anion gap for myeloma (IgG is cation and raises the chloride level, narrowing the gap).

Basic Science Correlate

Mechanism of Renal Failure in Myeloma
- Hypercalcemia leads to nephrocalcinosis.
- Hyperuricemia is directly toxic to kidney tubules.
- Bence-Jones protein clogs up glomeruli and is toxic to kidney tubules.
- Amyloid occurs in myeloma.

The **most specific test** is the bone marrow biopsy, which detects high numbers of plasma cells (10–60%).

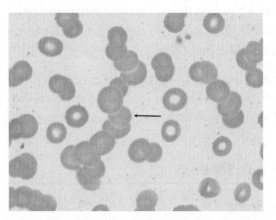

"Rouleaux" formation of blood cells

In Pvera, the B12 and LAP levels are elevated.

There is no single, clear treatment for MM. Any of the following medications can be used (on the exam, you will not be asked to choose between them).

- Melphalan and steroids
- Consider adding thalidomide, lenalidomide, or bortezomib (thalidomide is an inhibitor of TNF that has the same efficacy as chemotherapy)
  - Thalidomide and lenalidomide have a high risk of clotting; give prophylaxis against clotting when using these agents.
  - Bortezomib has a high risk of neurological complications.
- Autologous stem cell bone marrow transplantation (**most effective therapy**) is reserved for those relatively young (age <70) with advanced disease

Also remember to treat the hypercalcemia (hydration), bone fractures (bisphosphonates), renal failure (hydration), and anemia (erythropoietin) and to prophylax against infections with vaccinations (e.g., flu, Pneumovax, tetanus, etc.).

Smoldering Myeloma

In this disorder, 10–60% of bone marrow is plasma cells, and there is a high M-spike on serum protein electrophoresis (SPEP). Urine monoclonal protein level is elevated, and the FLC ratio is increased. There is no "CRAB" organ damage (i.e., no hyper**c**alcemia, **r**enal failure, **a**nemia, or **b**one lesions).

There is no specific therapy. The physician should undertake close follow-up.

Monoclonal Gammopathy of Unknown Significance (MGUS)

MGUS presents with an asymptomatic elevation of IgG on an SPEP. The SPEP is done because of an elevated total protein level found in an elderly patient, typically age >70.

There are 10% plasma cells.

There is no treatment for MGUS.

Waldenstrom Macroglobulinemia

This presents with hyperviscosity from IgM overproduction. The question will describe blurry vision, confusion, and headache. Enlarged nodes and spleen can be found.

There are no specific findings on CBC. The best initial test is a serum viscosity level, which will be markedly increased, and an SPEP, which will show an elevated IgM level.

Treatment is plasmapheresis, if symptomatic. For further treatment, use the agents you would use for CLL, such as fludarabine, chlorambucil, or rituximab.

Aplastic Anemia

This condition presents with pancytopenia with no identified etiology.

- When patient is young (age <50) and has a match, the best treatment is bone marrow transplantation.
- When bone marrow transplantation is not possible (age >50 and/or no match), use antithymocyte globulin and cyclosporine.

Aplastic anemia never has cytogenetic abnormalities. Most cases are idiopathic. Chronic hepatitis B and C can cause it.

Lymphoma

Lymphoma presents with enlarged lymph nodes, most commonly in the cervical area.

- **Hodgkin disease (HD)** spreads centrifugally away from the center, starting at the neck.
- **Non-Hodgkin lymphoma (NHL)** more often presents as widespread disease.

The major difference between HD and NHL is that **HD has Reed-Sternberg cells**.

Diagnostic testing is as follows:

- **Best initial test for both HD and NHL** is excisional lymph node biopsy.
- After the initial excisional biopsy shows the abnormal architecture of the cells, further tests determine the stage of the lymphoma. Staging is critical to guide therapy.
  - Stage I: single lymph node group
  - Stage II: two lymph node groups on one side of the diaphragm
  - Stage III: lymph node involvement on both sides of the diaphragm
  - Stage IV: widespread disease
- **80–90% of HD** cases present with stages I and II, while **80–90% of NHL** cases present with stages III and IV
- Staging involves chest x-ray; CT scan with contrast (chest, abdomen, pelvis, head); and bone marrow biopsy

Treatment is as follows:

- Localized disease (stages I and II) without "B" symptoms: radiation and low-dose chemotherapy
- More advanced stage disease (stages III and IV): chemotherapy exclusively
  - HD: ABVD (adriamycin [doxorubicin], bleomycin, vinblastine, dacarbazine)
  - NHL: CHOP (cyclophosphamide, hydroxydaunorubicin, Oncovin [vincristine], prednisone); also test for anti-CD20 antigen and if present, add rituximab, which adds efficacy to CHOP (rituximab can reactivate hepatitis)

Chemotherapy-Induced Nausea

There are 3 classes of medication for chemotherapy-induced nausea. In severe cases they can be combined:

- 5-hydroxytryptamine (5HT) inhibitors: ondansetron, granisetron, palonosetron, dolasetron (**best initial treatment**)
  - Do not give with QT prolongation on EKG—this is a good Step 3 question.
- Glucocorticoids: dexamethasone used first
  - Have a major anti-nausea effect
  - Are permissive on 5HT drugs, adding to their effect

The "B" symptoms of lymphoma, which imply more widespread disease, are the following:
- Fever
- Weight loss
- Night sweats

Wrong answers for diagnostic testing of lymphoma include:
- Needle biopsy (useful for infections such as TB, but is not sufficient for lymphoma because the visual appearance of lymphoma cells is normal, i.e., not grossly abnormal)
- Lymphangiogram or exploratory laparotomy of the abdomen

Test for hepatitis B before initiating rituximab.

- Neurokinin-1 (NK) receptor antagonists: aprepitant, rolapitant, netupitant (use these if 5HT inhibitors do not work or cannot be given because of QT prolongation on EKG)

Other antiemetic medications include the dopamine antagonists:

- Phenothiazines
- Metoclopramide (for the nausea of diabetic gastroparesis)

These medications have no utility in combination since they are all dopamine-receptor antagonists. Look for a question describing worsening Parkinson disease after the patient starts an antiemetic—one of these dopamine antagonists is the answer.

Coagulation Disorders

Von Willebrand Disease (VWD)

VWD presents with bleeding from platelet dysfunction—superficial bleeding from the skin and mucosal surfaces, such as the gingiva, gums, and vagina.

- Epistaxis (consistent with platelet dysfunction) (the exam question may say the bleeding is worse with aspirin use)
- Normal platelet count
- Elevated aPTT (in up to 50% of patients) because VWF deficiency destabilizes factor VIII

The **most accurate test** is ristocetin cofactor assay and von Willebrand factor (VWF) level. VWF carries factor VIII in the blood. If the VWF level is normal, ristocetin testing will tell if it is working properly.

Treatment is as follows:

- Desmopressin or DDAVP (first-line) will release subendothelial stores of VWF and factor VIII, which will stop the bleeding
- If that is not effective, use factor VIII replacement, which has both VWF and factor VIII.
- If DDAVP and factor VIII are not effective, use recombinant VWF.

> Prochlorperazine and chlorpromazine are antiemetics, but note the following:
> - Much less effective than 5HT and NK antagonists. They are never the correct answer.
> - Have an anticholinergic effect as well, but look for worsening dementia after their use.

> A case of VWD is likely to present with epistaxis and/or petechiae.

Basic Science Correlate
Mechanism of Ristocetin Testing Ristocetin acts as an artificial endothelial lining. If VWF is present, platelets will stick to it. Ristocetin is a functional test of VWF activity.

| Distinguishing Types of Bleeding ||
Platelet-Type Bleeding	**Factor-Type Bleeding**
• Petechiae • Epistaxis • Purpura • Gingiva • Vaginal	• Hemarthrosis • Hematoma

Immune Thrombocytopenic Purpura (ITP)

ITP presents with platelet-type bleeding if platelet count $<10,000$–$30,000/mm^3$.

Diagnostic testing is as follows:

- Peripheral smear shows large platelets.
- Sonogram to assess for normal spleen size found in ITP
- Bone marrow to find increased numbers of megakaryocytes

Antibody testing does not help in ITP.

> A generally healthy patient comes with epistaxis and petechiae. No spleen is felt on examination. Platelet count is $24,000/mm^3$. What is the next step in management?
>
> a. Prednisone
> b. Bone marrow biopsy
> c. Antiplatelet antibodies
> d. Sonogram
> e. Hematology consultation
>
> Answer: **A.** Prednisone is the most important thing to do first in mild ITP. Since ITP is a diagnosis of exclusion, the main point of most exam questions is that initiating therapy is more important than determining a specific diagnosis. All the answers listed would be given on a CCS case at the same time. In a single best answer case, however, the most important thing is to start therapy.

> A patient comes in with ITP and a platelet count of $5,000/mm^3$. The patient has epistaxis and petechiae as well as an intracranial hemorrhage and melena. What is the best initial step?
>
> Answer: **IVIG administration.** The fastest way to raise the platelet count with ITP is to use intravenous immunoglobulins (IVIG) or RhoGAM. IVIG is the answer when the platelet count is low ($< 20,000/mm^3$) and the case describes life-threatening bleeding, such as that into the bowel or brain.

Romiplostim and eltrombopag treat chronic ITP. They directly stimulate megakaryocytes.

> Romiplostim and eltrombopag are thrombopoietin analogs.

Treatment is as follows:

Case presents with...	Treatment
Platelet count >50,000/mm3	No treatment
Count <50,000 with minor bleeding	Prednisone
Count <10,000–20,000 with serious bleeding	IVIG or RhoGAM (Rho[D] immune globulin)
Recurrent episodes	Splenectomy, rituximab
No response to splenectomy	Romiplostim, eltrombopag

Basic Science Correlate

Mechanism of IVIG Effect in ITP

IVIG has no direct activity against platelets. It is administered in order to prevent the action of macrophages against platelets: By stopping up all the FC receptors on the macrophages, IVIG leaves no room for the antibodies on the platelets. Thus it shuts off platelet destruction.

> Rituximab, an anti-CD20 antibody, removes B cells that make antibodies against platelets.

Platelet Function Disorders

Uremia-Induced Platelet Dysfunction

Uremia by itself prevents platelets from working properly; they do not degranulate. Look for a normal platelet count with platelet-type bleeding in a patient with renal failure. The ristocetin test and VWF level will be normal.

Treatment is desmopressin (DDAVP), dialysis, and estrogen.

CCS Tip: Mixing study is the first test to determine the difference between a clotting factor deficiency and a factor inhibitor antibody. The aPTT will correct to normal with a clotting factor deficiency.

Glanzmann Thrombasthenia and Bernard-Soulier Syndrome

These disorders present with platelet-type bleeding (epistaxis, petechiae) despite normal platelet count and normal vWF level. Both are diagnosed with platelet studies, which in Bernard-Soulier reveals giant platelets. Glanzmann is like being on abciximab permanently.

Treatment is as follows:

- Desmopressin releases subendothelial stores of vWF and factor VIIIa.
- Tranexamic and epsilon amino caproic acid inhibit fibrinolysis and plasminogen.
- Recombinant factor VIIa
- Estrogen upregulates VWF

Clotting Factor Deficiencies

Deficiency	Factor VIII	Factor IX	Factor XI	Factor XII
Presentation	Joint bleeding or hematoma in a male child	Joint bleeding or hematoma; Less common than factor VIII deficiency	Rare bleeding with trauma or surgery	No bleeding
Diagnostic Test	Mixing study first, then specific factor level	Same	Same	Same
Treatment	Severe deficiency: (<1% activity): Factor VIII replacement Minor deficiency: DDAVP	Factor IX replacement	Fresh frozen plasma (FFP) with bleeding episodes	No treatment necessary

A woman presents with bleeding into her thigh after minor trauma. The aPTT is prolonged, and prothrombin time is normal. Mixing study does not correct the aPTT to normal. What is the diagnosis?

Answer: **Factor VIII antibody** is the most common cause of a prolonged aPTT and bleeding that does not correct with a mixing study. Treat severe bleeding from factor VIII antibodies with factor VII replacement. This therapy bypasses usual pathway to activate factor X directly. Antibodies attack recombinant factor VIII, not porcine factor VIII.

Treatment is as follows:

- Recombinant versions of factor VII, VIII, IX, and X are available for those with deficiencies.
- DDAVP will only work for factor VIII deficiency and Von Willebrand disease (VWD).
- Recombinant VWF is available to treat VWD. Prothrombin complex concentrate (PCC) reverses warfarin toxicity. PCC has all the vitamin K–dependent factors: factors II, VII, IX, and X and protein C and S.
- PCC works faster than vitamin K or fresh frozen plasma (FFP).

> Bleeding from factor VIII antibodies is treated with factor VII replacement, directly stimulating factor X.

Heparin-Induced Thrombocytopenia

Heparin-induced thrombocytopenia (HIT)

- Reduced platelets (at least 50% of cases) a few days after the start of heparin (the amount of heparin does not matter, because HIT is an allergic reaction)
- Thrombosis (**most common symptom**); venous thromboses are 3× more common than arterial thromboses
- Although low molecular weight heparin is less likely to cause HIT, both types of heparin can do so

> HIT can start after heparin is stopped.

The best initial diagnostic test is platelet factor 4 antibodies or heparin-induced, antiplatelet antibodies.

Treatment is to stop the heparin and use fondaparinux or a NOAC.

> Fondaparinux is safe in HIT.

If HIT happens with IV unfractionated heparin, do not answer "switch to low molecular weight heparin."

- If fondaparinux is not among the answer options, look for bivalirudin or argatroban.
- If both fondaparinux and argatroban are in the options, choose fondaparinux (argatroban needs aPTT testing every 2 hours and causes more bleeding).

Thrombophilia/Hypercoagulable States

Cause	Antiphospholipid Syndromes (Lupus Anticoagulant or Anticardiolipin Antibodies)	Protein C Deficiency	Factor V Leiden Mutation	Antithrombin Deficiency
Presentation	Venous or arterial thrombosis Elevated aPTT with a normal PT Spontaneous abortion False positive VDRL	Skin necrosis with the use of warfarin Venous thrombosis	Most common cause of thrombophilia Venous thrombosis	No change in the aPTT with a bolus of IV heparin Venous thrombosis
Diagnostic Test	Mixing study first Russel viper venom test is most accurate for lupus anticoagulant	Protein C level	Factor V mutation test	Level of antithrombin III
Treatment	Heparin followed by warfarin	Heparin followed by warfarin	Heparin followed by warfarin	Large amounts of heparin or direct thrombin inhibitor followed by warfarin

Basic Science Correlate

Protein C inactivates factor V, but only in its normal form. If factor V has a mutation, protein C will not inhibit it. Factor V mutation functions like protein C deficiency.

Anti-beta-2 glycoprotein is an anti-phospholipid.

Gastroenterology 10

Esophageal Disorders

In general, esophageal disorders with any degree of anatomic damage that leads to narrowing will result in dysphagia. All forms of dysphagia can lead to weight loss.

- If dysphagia is present and you do not know the diagnosis, do a barium study first (in the stomach, do endoscopy first).
- Endoscopy is indispensable for diagnosing cancer and the precancerous histologic change called "Barrett esophagus." Biopsy is necessary to diagnose both of these.

> Dysphagia (difficulty swallowing) is different from odynophagia (painful swallowing). Odynophagia suggests an infectious process, i.e., HIV, HSV, *Candida,* or CMV.

Dysphagia

Achalasia

Achalasia presents in a young nonsmoker who has dysphagia to both solids and liquids at the same time. There may also be regurgitation of food particles and aspiration of previously eaten material that is regurgitated and falls into the lungs. This can be a progressive form of dysphagia in which the symptoms get worse over time.

The **best initial test** is a barium swallow or chest x-ray. The **most accurate test** is esophageal manometry.

Other tests include:

- Endoscopy to exclude malignancy (it is not necessary to diagnose achalasia)
- Manometry to show an absence of normal esophageal peristalsis. (Achalasia presents with abnormally high pressure at the lower esophageal sphincter, since it involves a failure of the gastroesophageal sphincter to relax. There is no mucosal abnormality.)

Treatment is surgical myotomy; if not successful, do pneumatic dilation. If the patient refuses surgery or pneumatic dilation, use a botulinum toxin injection.

Basic Science Correlate

Mechanism of Botulinum Toxin

Botulinum toxin inhibits the release of acetylcholine at the neuromuscular junction. This inhibits nicotinic receptors and relaxes all skeletal muscle.

Esophageal Cancer

Esophageal cancer presents with the following:

- Dysphagia: solids first, liquids later
- Possible heme-positive stool or anemia
- Often found in patients age >50 who smoke and drink alcohol

- Dysphagia + Weight Loss = Esophageal pathology
- Dysphagia + Weight Loss + Heme-positive stool/Anemia = Cancer

The **best initial test** is endoscopy; if that is not one of the answer choices, do a barium swallow. Manometry will not be useful since cancer can only be diagnosed with biopsy.

CCS Tip: Just order the procedures you think you need on the CCS. Do not wait for a consult. If you need a consult for a procedure, the computer will tell you.

Treatment is surgical resection (as long as there are no local or distant metastases), followed by 5-fluorouracil chemotherapy. Use palliative stenting for obstruction.

Rings and Webs

Rings and webs (or "peptic strictures") can be caused by the repetitive exposure of the esophagus to acid, resulting in scarring and stricture formation. Previous use of sclerosing agents for variceal bleeding can also cause strictures, and this is why variceal banding is a superior procedure.

Eosinophilic esophagitis:
- Dysphagia
- History of allergies
- Scope + biopsy
- Treat with PPIs and budesonide

The **best initial test** is a barium study.

Treatment depends on the kind of stricture that presents:

- Plummer-Vinson syndrome, a proximal stricture associated with iron deficiency anemia and squamous cell esophageal cancer; it is common in middle-aged women: treat with iron replacement
- Schatzki ring (peptic stricture), a distal ring of the esophagus that presents with intermittent symptoms of dysphagia: treat with pneumatic dilation
- Peptic stricture from acid reflux: treat with pneumatic dilation

Zenker Diverticulum

Look for a patient with dysphagia with horrible bad breath. There is rotting food in the back of the esophagus from dilation of the posterior pharyngeal constrictor muscles.

To avoid perforation, do not do endoscopy or place a nasogastric tube with Zenker diverticulum.

The **best initial test** is barium study.

Treatment is surgical resection.

Spastic Disorders

Diffuse esophageal spasm and "nutcracker esophagus" are essentially the same disease.

Look for a case of severe chest pain, often without risk factors for ischemic heart disease. Pain may occur after drinking a cold beverage.

- There is always pain but there is not always dysphagia.
- EKG, stress test, and possibly the coronary angiography will be normal.

The **most accurate diagnostic test** is manometry. Barium study may show a corkscrew pattern but only during an episode of spasm.

Treatment is CCBs and nitrates (as you would treat Prinzmetal angina). If CCBs cannot be used, try TCAs.

Scleroderma (Progressive Systemic Sclerosis)

Scleroderma presents as symptoms of reflux.

Treatment is PPIs.

> Esophageal disorders can mimic Prinzmetal variant angina, because the pain is sudden, severe, and not related to exercise. However, Prinzmetal will give you ST segment elevation and an abnormality on stimulation of the coronary arteries, while esophageal spasm will not.

> An HIV-positive man comes in with progressive dysphagia and odynophagia. He has 75 CD4 cells but no history of opportunistic infections. What is the next best step in management?
>
> a. Fluconazole
> b. Amphotericin
> c. Barium swallow
> d. Endoscopy
> e. Antiretroviral therapy
>
> Answer: **A.** Odynophagia is pain on swallowing, while dysphagia is simply difficulty swallowing (i.e., food getting "stuck" in the esophagus). When odynophagia occurs in an HIV-positive patient (particularly when <100 CD4 cells), the diagnosis is most likely esophageal candidiasis, and giving empiric fluconazole is both therapeutic as well as diagnostic. Amphotericin is not necessary.

Esophagitis

Esophagitis presents with pain on swallowing (odynophagia) as the food rubs against the esophagus.

In HIV-positive patients, Candida esophagitis causes >90% of esophagitis. Other causes are pills such as doxycycline or a bisphosphonate such as alendronate. (If caused by pills, the patient should sit up and drink more water when taking pills and remain upright for at least 30 minutes afterward.)

Eosinophilic esophagitis presents with swallowing difficulty, food impaction, and heartburn. Look for a patient with a history of asthma and allergic diseases and findings of multiple concentric rings on endoscopy.

Diagnostic testing includes biopsy finding eosinophils (**most accurate test**).

Treatment starts with PPIs and eliminating allergenic foods. Swallowing steroid inhalers is the **most effective treatment**.

- In **HIV-positive** patients with <100 CD4 cells, give fluconazole; if there is no response, do endoscopy.
- In **HIV-negative** patients, do endoscopy first.

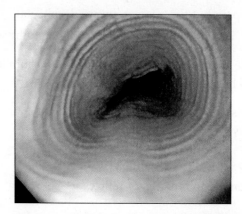

Eosinophilic Esophagitis (source: WikiCommons)

Mallory-Weiss Tear

This is not a cause of dysphagia, although Mallory-Weiss tear is clearly an esophageal disorder. It presents as sudden upper GI bleeding with violent retching and vomiting of any cause. There may be hematemesis or black stool.

Diagnose with endoscopy.

Most cases resolve spontaneously. If bleeding persists, treat with an injection of epinephrine to stop the bleeding.

CCS Tip: How do I know I am doing the right thing on CCS?

- You may get spontaneous nurse's notes telling you whether the patient is doing well or not. You get these automatically as you move the clock forward.
- You can get an "interval history" as a choice under physical exam. This is a 2-minute advance of the clock that will "check in" with the patient. This often tells you how the patient is doing and, consequently, how you are doing in management.

Gastroesophageal Reflux Disease (GERD)

In addition to the epigastric pain and substernal chest pain of GERD, several other symptoms are clearly associated with acid reflux:

- Sore throat
- Metallic or bitter taste
- Hoarseness
- Chronic cough (20–25% of those with chronic cough also have GERD)
- Wheezing

> 25% of chronic cough is caused by GERD.

PPI administration is both diagnostic and therapeutic. If there is no response to PPIs and the diagnosis is not clear, do a 24-hour pH monitor.

Basic Science Correlate

Mechanism of Bad Taste in GERD

Sweet taste receptors are on the anterior 2/3 of the tongue, and sweet taste is controlled by CN VII. The bitter taste receptors are on the back of the tongue, and bitter taste is controlled by CN IX and X.

Treatment is lifestyle medication for mild disease.

- Losing weight
- Not eating within 3 hours of going to sleep
- Elevating the head of the bed
- Quitting smoking and limiting alcohol, caffeine, chocolate, and mint ingestion

If that does not work:

- PPIs (control nearly 95% of cases); all PPIs are equal in efficacy
- H2 blockers, e.g., ranitidine, famotidine, nizatidine (70% success rate)
- Promotility agents, e.g., metoclopramide, are equal to H2 blockers but much less effective than PPIs, so not routinely used
- If disease is still not controlled, consider a surgical or endoscopic procedure to narrow the distal esophagus and reconstrict the lower esophageal sphincter (e.g., Nissen fundoplication or endoscopically suturing the LES tighter); make sure esophageal motility is adequate before you tighten the sphincter surgically

A patient comes with epigastric pain that is associated with substernal chest pain and an unpleasant metallic taste in the mouth. What is the next best step in management?

a. Endoscopy
b. Barium studies
c. PPIs
d. H2 (histamine) blockers
e. 24-hour pH monitor

Answer: **C.** PPIs are preferred as the first line of therapy and also serve as a diagnostic test. Using them is far easier than other testing.

Treatment for *Helicobacter pylori* is not effective or necessary for GERD. Such treatment will not tighten the LES.

Basic Science Correlate

H2 blockers reduce only 70% of gastric acid production. Why?

Because histamine is only one of the 3 stimulants to acid production on the parietal cell, namely: gastrin, histamine, and acetylcholine via the vagus nerve.

Histamine potentiates the other 2, resulting in a 70% reduction in acid. By contrast, PPIs inhibit acid output of the cell no matter what the stimulant.

When is reflux alarming, and when is **endoscopy** used in GERD?

- When weight loss, anemia, blood in the stool, and dysphagia are present

Barrett Esophagus

Barrett esophagus is a precancerous lesion (0.5% cases per year will develop into esophageal cancer). That is why adenocarcinoma is an increasingly frequent histological type of esophageal cancer.

Testing is endoscopy, where you are able to visualize and biopsy the distal esophagus. With GERD, the timing of the initial endoscopy looking for Barrett esophagus is not clear.

- Perform endoscopy for all the symptoms described (weight loss, anemia, heme-positive stool).
- Perform endoscopy in anyone with symptoms of reflux disease for >5–10 years.

Barrett is a biopsy diagnosis. Although the color is different, the only way to be certain that the histology has changed from squamous epithelium to columnar epithelium ("Barrett esophagus") with metaplasia is by endoscopy.

Treatment is as follows:

- **Barrett esophagus**: PPI and repeat endoscopy every 2–3 years
- **Low-grade dysplasia**: PPI and repeat endoscopy in 3–6 months
- **High-grade dysplasia**: endoscopic mucosal resection, ablative removal, or distal esophagectomy

Epigastric Pain

A 58-year-old man seeks an evaluation of epigastric discomfort for the last several weeks. He is otherwise asymptomatic with no weight loss. His stool is heme-negative. What is the next best step in management?

a. Upper endoscopy
b. Serology for *Helicobacter pylori*
c. Urea breath testing for *Helicobacter pylori*
d. PPI, amoxicillin, and clarithromycin for 2 weeks
e. Ranitidine empirically

Answer: **A.** Upper endoscopy should be performed in any patient age >45 with persistent symptoms of epigastric discomfort. The purpose is to exclude the possibility of gastric cancer. There is no way to be certain of gastric cancer without performing an endoscopy. [There is no way to be certain of gastric cancer without performing an endoscopy.]

Nonulcer Dyspepsia

Nonulcer dyspepsia is the most common cause of epigastric discomfort.

This is a diagnosis of exclusion, i.e., it can be diagnosed only after endoscopy has excluded ulcer disease, gastric cancer, and gastritis.

Treatment is symptomatic therapy with H2 blockers, liquid antacids, or PPIs. *Helicobacter* is sometimes treated in refractory disease.

> There is no proven benefit to treating *Helicobacter* for non-ulcer dyspepsia.

Peptic Ulcer Disease

Peptic ulcer disease can be either duodenal ulcer (DU) or gastric ulcer (GU) disease. After *Helicobacter*, the most common causes of ulcer are NSAIDs, head trauma, burns, intubation, Crohn disease, and Zollinger-Ellison syndrome.

Gastric cancer occurs in 4% of those with GU.

There is no way to distinguish DU and GU by symptoms alone. The alteration of pain with food is only suggestive, not definitive. Food more often makes GU pain worse and DU pain better.

However, if the patient is age >45 and has epigastric pain, you must scope to exclude gastric cancer.

Gastritis

Gastritis can be associated with *Helicobacter pylori*. If it is present, treat with a PPI and 2 antibiotics.

Gastritis can also be atrophic, caused by pernicious anemia and associated with vitamin B12 deficiency. This type of gastritis will not improve with treatment for *H. pylori*.

Diagnostic testing is as follows:

- **Most accurate test**: endoscopy with biopsy; if this is done, no further testing is necessary for *Helicobacter*
- Serology: very sensitive but not specific; if serology is negative, this excludes *Helicobacter*
  - A positive test cannot distinguish between new and previous infection.
- Breath testing and stool antigen testing are 95% sensitive and specific. They are used after treatment to test for cure of the infection.
  - These can distinguish between new and previous disease.

Treatment is a PPI, clarithromycin, amoxicillin. Only treat *Helicobacter* if it is associated with gastritis or ulcer disease. There is no benefit in treating *Helicobacter* for GERD.

If treatment for *H. pylori* fails to control symptoms, proceed as follows:

- Repeat treatment with 2 new antibiotics and a PPI. Try metronidazole and tetracycline instead of clarithromycin and amoxicillin. Adding bismuth may help.
- If repeat treatment fails, then evaluate for Zollinger-Ellison syndrome (gastrinoma).

You should routinely test for the cure of *Helicobacter*.

Be aware of the adverse effects of PPIs. PPIs interfere with:

- Calcium absorption, possibly leading to fractures
- Magnesium absorption
- Vitamin B12 absorption (acid frees B12 from food)
- Iron absorption (low acid blocks iron absorption)
- Resistance to bacterial invasion (PPIs reduce the acid barrier, increasing the risk of pneumonia and *Clostridium difficile*)
- Kidney function, leading to interstitial nephritis (urinating eosinophils)

Stress Ulcer Prophylaxis

Routine prophylactic use of a PPI should be used only if one of the following is present (NSAID or steroid use alone is not an indication for routine stress ulcer prophylaxis):

- Head trauma
- Intubation and mechanical ventilation
- Burns
- Coagulopathy and steroid use in combination

H2 blockers and sucralfate have less efficacy in preventing stress ulcer prophylaxis than a PPI.

> The **only** time tetracycline is used is for *Helicobacter pylori*.

> USMLE Step 3 does not want routine "GI prophylaxis" on every patient. Do that only for those with:
> - Head trauma
> - Burns
> - Intubated
> - Sepsis with coagulopathy

A 52-year-old man has epigastric discomfort. He is seropositive for *Helicobacter pylori*. Upper endoscopy reveals no gastritis or ulcer disease. Biopsy of the stomach shows *Helicobacter*. What is the next step?

a. Breath testing
b. PPI alone as symptomatic therapy
c. Repeat endoscopy after 6 weeks of PPIs
d. PPI, amoxicillin, and clarithromycin

Answer: **B.** You do not need to treat *Helicobacter pylori* unless there is gastritis, mucosa-associated lymphoid tissue lymphoma (MALToma), or ulcer disease. This patient has epigastric pain and *Helicobacter* but no ulcer or gastritis. This is non-ulcer dyspepsia. Treat it symptomatically with a PPI. Enormous numbers of people are colonized with *H. pylori*; you do not need to eradicate it from the world without evidence of disease. *H. pylori* is not the cause of nonulcer dyspepsia.

A man is found to have ulcer disease. There are 3 ulcers in the distal esophagus 1–2 cm in size. The ulcers persist despite treatment for *Helicobacter*. What is the next step?

a. Switch antibiotics

b. Breath testing

c. Gastrin level and gastric acid output

d. CT scan of the abdomen

e. ERCP

Answer: **C.** Gastrin level and gastric acid output testing should be done when there is the possibility of Zollinger-Ellison syndrome. ERCP will only show the ducts of the pancreas and gallbladder; it will not reveal gastrinoma.

Zollinger-Ellison Syndrome

Zollinger-Ellison syndrome (ZES) (also called gastrinoma) is diagnosed with an elevated gastrin level and elevated gastric acid output.

Most ulcers have the following features:

- Small size (<1 cm)
- Single ulcer
- Proximal location near the pylorus
- Resolve easily with treatment

Therefore, when the following are present, test the gastrin level and gastric acid output:

- Large size (>1 cm)
- Multiple ulcers
- Distal location near the ligament of Treitz
- Recurrent or persistent despite *Helicobacter* treatment

If both are elevated, the next step is to localize the gastrinoma.

If hypercalcemia is present, that is a clue to the presence of a parathyroid problem with ZES and, therefore, is the clue to a multiple endocrine neoplasia (MEN) syndrome.

> Everyone on an H2 blocker or PPI has elevated gastrin.

Testing is as follows:

- Endoscopic ultrasound (similar to a transesophageal echocardiogram): much more sensitive than a surface ultrasound
- Nuclear somatostatin scan: very sensitive, because patients with ZES have an enormous increase in number of somatostatin receptors
- Secretin suppression (**most accurate test**)

Treatment is surgical resection for local disease, and lifelong PPIs for metastatic disease.

With an infusion of IV secretin, healthy people will show decreased gastrin level and decreased acid output. Those with ZES will show increased (or unchanged) gastrin level and no decrease in acid output.

Effect of Infusing IV Secretin		
	Normal	**ZES**
Gastrin secretion	Decreases	No change
Gastric acid output	Decreases	No change

Inflammatory Bowel Disease (IBD)

Both Crohn disease (CD) and ulcerative colitis (UC) can present with fever, weight loss, abdominal pain, diarrhea, and blood in the stool. (Abdominal pain and bloody diarrhea are more common in UC.)

The extraintestinal manifestations of IBD are as follows:

- Joint pain
- Eye findings (iritis, uveitis)
- Skin findings (pyoderma gangrenosum, erythema nodosum)
- Sclerosing cholangitis

Features more common to Crohn disease are the following:

- Masses
- Skip lesion
- Upper GI tract involvement
- Perianal disease
- Transmural granulomas
- Fistulae
- Hypocalcemia from fat malabsorption
- Obstruction
- Calcium oxalate kidney stones
- Cholesterol gallstones
- Vitamin B12 malabsorption from terminal ileum involvement

Endoscopy is diagnostic in both CD and UC, as is barium study.

If the diagnosis is still not clear, blood tests are helpful.

	CD	**UC**
ASCA	Positive	Negative
ANCA	Negative	Positive

Both CD that involves the colon and UC can lead to colon cancer. Screen with colonoscopy every 1–2 years after 8–10 years of colonic involvement.

Treatment for IBD is as follows:

- **Best initial therapy for both CD and UC**: mesalamine
- Sulfasalazine is not the best initial therapy for CD or UC because of side effects (rash, hemolytic anemia, and interstitial nephritis)
- Steroids: budesonide is a glucocorticoid that can be used to control acute exacerbations of IBD. It has extensive first-pass effect in the liver and, therefore, has limited systemic adverse effects
- Azathioprine and 6-mercaptopurine for severe disease with recurrent symptoms when steroids are stopped; these medications help wean patients off of steroids
- TNF inhibitors for CD associated with fistula formation. TNF is what maintains a granuloma in place. Plant a PPD and give isoniazid if the PPD is positive prior to the use of infliximab. TNF inhibitors can reactivate TB by releasing dormant TB from granulomas. There is no need to wait 9 months to start the TNF drug.
- Antibiotics metronidazole and ciprofloxacin for perianal involvement in CD
- Surgery can be curative in UC by removing the colon, although CD will recur at the site of surgery (occasionally, surgery must still be done in CD if there is a stricture and obstruction)
- Vedolizumab is an integrin receptor antagonist administered by IV for severe IBD not controlled with the other medications
  - Vedolizumab induces and maintains IBD remission
  - Natalizumab (an integrin antagonist) gives progressive multifocal leukoencephalopathy (PML), but vedolizumab does not

> TNF inhibitors for IBD include adalimumab, certolizumab, etanercept, golimumab, and infliximab.
> - If those are not effective, check TNF level and antibodies, and switch TNF drug.
> - If the level is good but there are no antibodies, switch drug class.

> TNF inhibitors reactivate TB. Screen with a PPD prior to its use in fistulizing CD.

Diarrhea

Infectious Diarrhea

The most important feature of infectious diarrhea on presentation is the presence of blood. Blood means the presence of an invasive bacterial pathogens:

- *Campylobacter* (most common cause of food poisoning): can be associated with Guillain-Barre and reactive arthritis
- *Salmonella*: transmitted by chickens and eggs
- *Vibrio parahaemolyticus*: associated with seafood
- *E. coli*: has several variants, some of which are associated with blood. *E. coli* 0157:H7 is most commonly associated with hemolytic uremic syndrome (via effects of verotoxin). Look for undercooked beef in the history. Do not give platelet transfusions or antibiotics, which can make it worse.

> Give eculizumab for HUS, not for infection.

- *Vibrio vulnificus:* look for shellfish (oysters, clams) in a person with liver disease and skin lesions
- *Shigella:* secretes Shiga toxin; associated with reactive arthritis
- *Yersinia:* transmitted by rodents via vegetables, milk-derived products, and meat (case may describe pork) that are contaminated with infected urine or feces
- Amebic: perform 3-stool ova and parasite exams or serologic testing; treat with metronidazole; may be associated with liver abscesses

The **best initial test** is fecal leukocytes. The **most accurate test** is stool culture.

If blood is not described in the case, test fecal leukocytes, which tell you that an invasive pathogen is present and will indicate the same diseases described that are associated with the presence of blood.

Treatment is as follows:

- **Mild disease**: hydration only; this will resolve on its own
- **Severe disease** (presence of blood, fever, abdominal pain, or hypotension/tachycardia): fluoroquinolones, e.g., ciprofloxacin

Nonbloody Diarrhea

All of the pathogens described can present without blood as well as with blood. The presence of blood does exclude the following pathogens, which never result in blood:

- **Viruses:** rotavirus, norovirus (also called "Norwalk virus")
- *Giardia:* look for camping/hiking and men who have sex with men
  - Stool ELISA antigen >90% sensitive and specific (and more accurate than 3-stool ova and parasite exams)
  - Look for bloating, flatus, and signs of steatorrhea
  - Treatment is metronidazole or tinidazole
- *Staphylococcus aureus:* presents with vomiting in addition to diarrhea; will resolve spontaneously
- *Bacillus cereus:* associated with refried Chinese rice and vomiting; will resolve spontaneously
- Cryptosporidiosis: look for an HIV-positive patient with <100 CD4; diagnose with a modified acid-fast stain; treatment is antiretrovirals to raise CD4, i.e., nitazoxanide and paromomycin (only partially effective)
- Scombroid (histamine fish poisoning): has fastest onset of diarrhea/wheezing, e.g., within 10 minutes of eating infected tuna, mackerel, or mahi-mahi; treatment is antihistamines, e.g., diphenhydramine

Antibiotic-Associated Diarrhea/*Clostridium difficile (C. diff)*

This develops several days to weeks after the use of antibiotics. Although clindamycin is the most common cause, it can be caused by any antibiotic. Recently, fluoroquinolones have also come to be associated with *C. diff.* There can be both blood and fecal leukocytes with *C. difficile* colitis.

Diagnostic testing is stool toxin assay (**best initial test**) and stool PCR (**most accurate test**).

Treatment is oral vancomycin, with oral fidaxomicin as an alternative. IV vancomycin is not useful.

- If diarrhea resolves with vancomycin and then recurs again later, retreat with vancomycin. Treat severe disease with combination metronidazole + vancomycin.
- Consider fidaxomicin, an alternative to vancomycin
- Stool transplant: multiple recurrences after vancomycin and fidaxomicin
- Surgery for severe disease (toxic megacolon, elevated lactate, leukocytosis, or elevated creatinine)
- Bezlotoxumab to prevent recurrence

> PPIs increase the risk of *C. diff* in hospitalized patients.

> When treating antibiotic-associated diarrhea, use oral vancomycin or fidaxomicin as initial therapy.

Chronic Diarrhea

- Lactose intolerance (most common cause of chronic diarrhea and flatulence)
  - Diagnose with a lactose-intolerance test
  - Stool osmolarity increased
  - Treatment is removal of all milk and milk-related products from the diet except yogurt
- Carcinoid syndrome (associated with flushing and episodes of hypotension)
  - Diagnose with urinary 5-HIAA level
  - Not premalignant; no extra screening needed
  - Treatment is octreotide (somatostatin-analog)
- IBD
  - Look for blood, fever, and weight loss

Malabsorption

This type of chronic diarrhea is always associated with weight loss. Fat malabsorption is associated with steatorrhea, which leads to oily, greasy stools that float on the water in the toilet. There is a particularly foul smell to the stool.

The causes of fat malabsorption are as follows:

- Celiac disease (gluten sensitive enteropathy), or nontropical sprue
- Tropical sprue
- Chronic pancreatitis
- Whipple disease

All forms of fat malabsorption are associated with the following:

- Hypocalcemia from vitamin D deficiency, which may lead to osteoporosis
- Oxalate overabsorption and oxalate kidney stones
- Easy bruising and elevated prothrombin time/INR from vitamin K malabsorption
- Vitamin B12 malabsorption from destruction of the terminal ileum or loss of the pancreatic enzymes necessary for B12 absorption

Diagnostic testing is as follows:

- Sudan black stain of stool to test for the presence of fat (**best initial test**)
- 72-hour fecal fat (**most sensitive test**)

Celiac Disease (Gluten-Sensitive Enteropathy)

Celiac disease can also present with malabsorption of iron and microcytic anemia. This does not happen with pancreatic insufficiency, since pancreatic enzymes are not necessary for iron absorption. Folate malabsorption also occurs from destruction of villi. Celiac disease is associated with a vesicular skin lesion not present on mucosal surfaces (called dermatitis herpetiformis).

Diagnostic testing is as follows:

> Celiac can cause LFT rise in 10%.

- Antigliadin, antiendomysial, and antitissue transglutaminase antibodies (**best initial test**)
- Small bowel biopsy (**most accurate test**)
- D-xylose testing is abnormal in celiac disease, Whipple disease, and tropical sprue, because the villous lining is destroyed and D-xylose cannot be absorbed. However, this test is rarely necessary, because the specific antibody tests eliminate the need for it.
- Bowel biopsy is always necessary for celiac disease, even if the diagnosis is confirmed with antibody testing, to exclude bowel wall lymphoma.

Treatment is elimination of wheat, oats, rye, and barley from the diet. It may take several weeks for symptoms to resolve. Beer, whiskey, and most vodkas are derived from wheat. Wine is okay.

Tropical Sprue

This presents in the same way as celiac disease. There will be a history of the patient being in the tropics.

Serologic tests, such as antitissue transglutaminase, will be negative.

The **most accurate test** is a small bowel biopsy showing microorganisms.

Treatment is doxycycline or TMP/SMX for 3–6 months.

Whipple Disease

Whipple disease has several additional findings on presentation, such as the following:

- Arthralgia
- Neurological abnormalities
- Ocular findings

Diagnostic testing is as follows:

- Small bowel biopsy showing PAS positive organisms (**most accurate test**)
- Alternate test: PCR of stool for *Tropheryma whippeli*

Treatment is TMP/SMX or tetracycline for 12 months.

Chronic Pancreatitis

Look for a history of alcoholism and multiple episodes of pancreatitis. Amylase and lipase levels will most likely be normal, since the fat malabsorption does not develop until the pancreas is burnt out and largely replaced by calcium and fibrosis.

Malabsorption of fat-soluble vitamins, such as vitamin K and vitamin D, is less common than with celiac disease.

- **Best initial tests**:
  - Abdominal x-ray (50–60% sensitive for detection of pancreatic calcifications)
  - Abdominal CT scan without contrast (60–80% sensitive)
- **Most accurate test**: secretin stimulation testing

Iron and folate levels will be normal, since pancreatic enzymes are not necessary to absorb these. D-xylose testing will be normal. B12 levels can be low.

> **Basic Science Correlate**
>
> A normal person should release a large volume of bicarbonate-rich pancreatic fluid in response to the intravenous injection of secretin.

Treatment is replacement of the pancreatic enzymes chronically by mouth. Amylase, lipase, and trypsin can be combined in one pill for chronic use.

Irritable Bowel Syndrome

> Irritable bowel syndrome presents with pain. There is no fever, no weight loss, and no blood in the stool.

Irritable bowel syndrome is a pain syndrome with altered bowel habits. This condition presents with the following symptoms:

- Abdominal pain relieved by a bowel movement
- Abdominal pain that is less at night
- Abdominal pain with diarrhea alternating with constipation

All diagnostic tests will be normal:

- Stool guaiac, stool white cells, culture, ova, and parasite exam
- Colonoscopy
- Abdominal CT scan

Treatment is fiber, because bulking up the stool helps relieve the pain. Fiber gives the guts a "stretch," like sending the colon to yoga class!

If there is no relief of pain with fiber, add antispasmodic/anticholinergic agents, such as dicyclomine or hyoscyamine, to "relax" the bowel.

If there is no response to the antispasmodic/anticholinergic agents, add a tricyclic antidepressant such as amitriptyline.

Additional principles for treating diarrhea-predominant IBS:

- Rifaximin: nonabsorbed antibiotic with modest effect in diarrhea-predominant IBS
- Alosetron: serotonin inhibitor with modest effect in IBS; needs special permission to use
- Eluxadoline: a mu-opioid receptor agonist for diarrhea IBS that relieves pain/slows the bowel
- Probiotics: unclear; do not use

Additional principles for treating constipation-predominant IBS:

- Start with fiber, always
- Then try polyethylene glycol, a nonabsorbed bowel "lubricant"
- If still no effect, consider a chloride-channel activator (lubiprostone) or guanylate cyclase agonist (linaclotide or plecanatide)

Basic Science Correlate

Tricyclic antidepressants help IBS because they are anticholinergic; relieve neuropathic pain; and are antidepressant.

Colon Cancer

Screening guidelines are the most important thing to know about colon cancer. Diagnostic testing is as follows:

- **General population**: begin screening at **age 50**
  - Colonoscopy every 10 years (**best test by far**)
  - If positive, fecal occult blood testing and scope yearly
  - Sigmoidoscopy every 5 years
  - Fecal immunochemistry test and stool DNA every 3 years
- **One family member with colon cancer**: colonoscopy starting at age 40 or 10 years before the age of the family member who had cancer
- **Three family members, two generations, one premature (age <50)**: colonoscopy starting at age 25, done every 1–2 years ("Lynch syndrome," or hereditary nonpolyposis colon cancer)
- **Familial adenomatous polyposis** (FAP): begin screening sigmoidoscopy at age 12 and perform a colectomy once polyps are found

> - Hamartomas and hyperplastic polyps: benign
> - Dysplastic polyps: malignant

Virtual colonoscopy lacks both sensitivity and specificity (you cannot biopsy and it misses small lesions), so it is used only when a real colonoscopy cannot be done.

Gardner Syndrome

Gardner syndrome is a subvariant of FAP and so gets the same level of screening. It presents with benign bone tumors known as osteomas, and other soft tissue tumors.

Gardner is similar to FAP in its long-term risk of colon cancer (remember it as FAP with cancers outside the colon). There is more cancer of the thyroid, pancreas, and small bowel in Gardner than in FAP.

Screen at the same starting age of 12 with sigmoidoscopy.

Peutz-Jeghers Syndrome

This presents with melanotic spots on the lips. There are hamartomatous polyps throughout the small bowel and colon. The risk of cancer is much higher than previously thought, and Peutz-Jeghers has been changed to the same category as FAP.

As with FAP, screening is with sigmoidoscopy starting at age 8.

Juvenile Polyposis

There are multiple extra hamartomas in the bowel. Screen both the upper and lower GI tracts. The risk of cancer is significant and premature.

Start screening at age 12.

Dysplastic Polyp Found

Repeat colonoscopy 3–5 years after the polyp was found.

> Carcinoembryonic antigen (CEA) is never a screening test. It is used to follow response to therapy.

Colon cancer screening recommendations are summarized below.

General Population	Single Family Member with Colon Cancer	Three Family Members, Two Generations, One Age <50	FAP, Gardner, Peutz-Jeghers, Turcot's	Juvenile Polyposis
• Start screening at age 50 • Colonoscopy every 10 years	• Start screening at age 40 or 10 years earlier than the age at which family member contracted cancer	• Start screening at age 25 • Colonoscopy every 1–2 years	• Start screening at age 12 • Sigmoidoscopy every 1–2 years (for Peutz-Jeghers start at age 8)	• Screen upper & lower tract starting at age 12

On routine x-ray, a man is found to have several osteomas. What is the next step?

Answer: Perform a colonoscopy to screen for cancer. This is Gardner syndrome.

Diverticular Disease

Diverticulosis (very common in older Americans) is caused by a low-fiber, high-fat, hamburger-filled, low-residue diet.

- Symptoms include left lower quadrant (LLQ) abdominal pain and lower GI bleed.
- Colonoscopy is the **most accurate test.**
- Treatment is a high-fiber diet.

Diverticulitis is a complication of diverticulosis. It presents with LLQ abdominal pain, tenderness, fever, and elevated white cells.

LLQ Pain + Tenderness + Fever + Leukocytosis = Diverticulitis

- Abdominal and pelvic CT is the **best diagnostic test**.
- Treatment is antibiotics. Combine agents against gram-negative bacilli (e.g., a quinolone or cephalosporin) with an agent against anaerobes (e.g., metronidazole). Ciprofloxacin and metronidazole are a standard combination.
- Colonoscopy and barium enema are contraindicated because of an increased risk of perforation.

Gastrointestinal (GI) Bleeding

GI bleeding presents in various ways:

- Red blood usually indicates lower GI bleeding. In 10% of cases, extremely brisk/rapid or high-volume upper GI bleeding leads to red blood from the rectum.
- Black stool: Indicates upper GI bleeding, which is usually defined as that occurring proximal to the ligament of Treitz (demarcation between the duodenum and the jejunum). Black stool usually results from at least 100 mL of blood loss.

- Heme-positive brown stool can occur from as little as 5–10 mL of blood loss.
- Coffee ground emesis needs very little gastric, esophageal, or duodenal blood loss—as little a 5–10 mL.

The most important thing to do in acute GI bleeding is to determine if there is hemodynamic instability. Orthostatic hypotension means a drop in blood pressure or rise in pulse when going from a lying to a standing or seated position.

CCS Tip: On CCS with large-volume GI bleeding, order the following:

- Bolus of normal saline or Ringer lactate
- CBC
- Prothrombin time/INR
- Type and cross
- Consultation with gastroenterology
- EKG

As you move the clock forward on CCS, the results of all tests will automatically pop up. You do not have to do anything for them to come. Test results on CCS are like your phone bill: you do not have to do anything for your bills to arrive; they automatically show up as time passes.

> A 74-year-old man with a history of aortic stenosis comes to the ED having had 5 red/black bowel movements over the last day. His pulse is 112 beats/min and blood pressure 96/64 mm Hg. What is the next best step in management?
>
> a. Colonoscopy
> b. Consult gastroenterology
> c. CBC
> d. Bolus of normal saline
> e. Transfer to ICU
>
> **Answer: D.** The most urgent step in severe GI bleeding is fluid resuscitation. When systolic blood pressure is low or pulse high, there has been at least a 30% volume loss. The Step 3 exam will not ask you to order specific doses, so all you can order is a "bolus." Colonoscopy is important, but not as important as fluid resuscitation at the moment.

Test	Route of Administration	Time Ordered	Report Available
CBC	Applies to medications ordered	09:00	09:15

When do I transfuse **packed red blood cells?**

- When hematocrit <30 in older patient or <20–25 in younger patient with no heart disease

When do I transfuse **fresh frozen plasma (FFP)?**

- When there is elevated prothrombin time/INR and vitamin K is too slow

---

Orthostasis is a drop in systolic pressure >20 mm Hg or rise in pulse >10 beats per minute. It presents with one of the following:

- Systolic blood pressure <100 mm Hg
- Heart rate >100 beats/min

Either of these implies >30% volume loss.

CT and US cannot detect the source of a GI bleed.

When do I transfuse **platelets**?

- When patient is bleeding or to undergo surgery; transfuse platelets when <50,000

What is the **most common cause of death** in GI bleeding?

- Myocardial ischemia, which is why an EKG should be done in older patients with severe GI bleeding.
- The myocytes of the left ventricle cannot distinguish between ischemia, anemia, carbon monoxide poisoning, and coronary artery stenosis. All of these lead to myocardial infarction.

When is **nasogastric (NG) tube** the answer?

- When you are unsure whether bleeding is from an upper or lower GI source; the NG tube has no therapeutic benefit, i.e., it will not stop bleeding
- Iced saline lavage is worthless and is always wrong.

Why not use the **NG tube to identify all bleeding**?

- If the NG tube shows bile, you can be sure the pyloric sphincter is open and there is no blood in the duodenum. But if the pyloric sphincter is closed, no blood will be detectable in the NG tube even if it is present in the duodenum.
- Also, if you are going to scope the patient anyway, it does not matter what the NG tube shows.

Treatment of GI bleed of large volume is fluid resuscitation, first. Fluid resuscitation is more important than determining the specific etiology of the source of the bleed. With adequate fluid resuscitation, 80% of GI bleeding stops, even without endoscopy.

> Fluid resuscitation beats scoping!

> Fix the coagulopathy with GI bleed before worrying about a scope or NG tube.

- The most important measures of severity are the pulse and blood pressure. If pulse is elevated or blood pressure is decreased, you can always give more fluid.
- If you must give so much fluid to maintain blood pressure that the patient becomes hypoxic, then give the fluid and increase oxygenation, even if it means intubating the patient.
- Hypotension supersedes all other therapeutic priorities. Start PPIs in upper GI bleeding.
- Correcting anemia, thrombocytopenia, or coagulopathy is more important than endoscopy.
- If platelets are low, then giving platelets is more important than consulting gastroenterology or moving the patient to the ICU.
- If you scope the patient but do not correct anemia, thrombocytopenia, or elevated prothrombin time/INR, the bleeding will not stop.
- If PT or INR is increased, give FFP.
- If warfarin caused the increase of the INR, give PCC (II, VII, IX, X concentrate).

Ulcer Disease

Add a PPI to the initial resuscitation of fluids, blood, platelets, and plasma. Note, however, that unnecessary stress ulcer prophylaxis with PPIs increases the risk of pneumonia and *Clostridium difficile* colitis.

Variceal Bleeding

Look for an alcoholic with hematemesis and/or liver disease (cirrhosis). The other clues to the presence of esophageal varices are the presence of spleno-megaly, low platelets, and spider angiomata or gynecomastia.

Varices produce the highest mortality of any GI bleed.

Treatment is as follows:

- Add octreotide to the initial orders. This is a somatostatin analog and it decreases portal hypertension. Add ceftriaxone if ascites is present with variceal bleeding to prevent SBP.
- Do prompt upper endoscopy to band the varices
- If the bleeding persists with moving the clock forward, perform a TIPS procedure (using a catheter to place a shunt between the portal and hepatic veins) which will replace the need for surgical shunt placement. The most common complication of a TIPS procedure is hepatic encephalopathy.
- Blakemore gastric tamponade balloon (rarely performed) will temporarily stop bleeding from varices; it is only a temporary measure to stop bleeding to allow a shunt to be placed

Propranolol prevents future episodes of variceal bleeding.

Sources of Bleeding

Bleeding in the upper GI can have the following causes:

- Ulcer disease
- Esophagitis, gastritis, duodenitis
- Varices
- Cancer

Goal INR is <1.4 with variceal bleeding

Bleeding in the lower GI can have the following causes:

- Angiodysplasia
- Diverticular disease
- Polyps
- Ischemic colitis
- Inflammatory bowel disease
- Cancer

Diagnostic testing is as follows:

- Technetium bleeding scan ("tagged red cell scan") to detect the site of bleeding if endoscopy does not reveal the source; it will identify the location but not the precise cause

- Angiography to identify the vessel that is bleeding (can be done preoperatively in massive GI bleeding to let you know which part of the colon to resect)
- Capsule endoscopy (swallowing a capsule that contains a camera) to detect the location of GI bleeding from the small bowel, if not revealed by upper and lower endoscopy; it takes a large number of pictures but does not allow a biopsy or therapeutic intervention

Acute Mesenteric Ischemia

This is an embolus from the heart resulting in an infarction of the bowel. There is a sudden onset of extremely severe abdominal pain and possible bleeding as well. Physical examination shows a relatively benign abdomen. Look for an older patient with a history of valvular heart disease and the very sudden onset of pain.

Diagnostic testing includes:

> Abdominal pain out of proportion to physical exam = Mesenteric ischemia

- Elevated lactic acid (look for metabolic acidosis)
- Elevated amylase
- Angiography (**most accurate test**)

Treatment is surgical resection of the bowel, if it is dead. Very ill patients should go straight to the operating room for surgical resection. This is a **surgical emergency**. If left undetected and untreated, the patient will die quickly.

In ischemia that is not caused by emboli, treatment is for the underlying low flow state.

Constipation

The vast majority of constipation cases have no clear etiology. Although Step 3 seldom asks specifically for the diagnosis, it does ask for the management.

With constipation, treatment means correcting the underlying cause, so knowing the etiology is key. Following are possible causes of constipation:

- Dehydration: look for decreased skin turgor in an elderly patient with increased BUN-to-creatinine ratio (>20:1)
- CCBs
- Narcotic medication use
- Hypothyroidism
- Diabetes: loss of sensation in bowels leads to decreased detection of stretch in the bowel (a main stimulant of GI motility)
- Ferrous sulfate iron replacement
  - Stool is black and can look as though there is upper GI bleeding

- Blood is cathartic and will usually produce rapid bowel movement
- Ferrous sulfate is constipating and is also heme-negative when one tests for occult blood
- Anticholinergic medication, including tricyclic antidepressants

Treatment is hydration and increased fiber, first. Consider a bowel regimen with laxatives.

- Polyethylene glycol increases stool liquidity
- Lubiprostone, linaclotide, and plecanatide increase stool volume and lubrication
- Milk of magnesia increases osmotic draw into the bowel

Dumping Syndrome

Dumping syndrome (relatively rare) is related to prior gastric surgery, usually done for ulcer disease. Treatment and eradication of *H. pylori* have made surgery for ulcer disease rare.

The patient presents with shaking, sweating, and weakness.

Basic Science Correlate

Dumping syndrome may involve hypotension. There are 2 causes.
- Rapid release of the gastric contents into the duodenum, which causes an osmotic draw into the bowel
- Rapid rise in blood glucose resulting in a reactive hypoglycemia

---

Treatment is a change to frequent, small meals.

Diabetic Gastroparesis

Longstanding diabetes impairs the neural supply of the bowel. There is impairment of normal motility.

Symptoms include bloating and constipation, as well as diarrhea.

Basic Science Correlate

Mechanism of Gastroparesis

The main stimulant to gastric motility is distension. Diabetes damages sensory nerves of all kinds, including those in the bowel. Vascular damage to the nerves of the digestive tract impairs a person's ability to detect stretching or distention of the stomach. With longstanding diabetes, the result is bloating and constipation.

Treatment is erythromycin or metoclopramide. Erythromycin increases motilin in the gut, a hormone that stimulates gastric motility.

Acute Pancreatitis

This condition presents as severe midepigastric abdominal pain and tenderness in an alcoholic or someone with gallstones. Other causes are the following:

- Hypertriglyceridemia
- Trauma
- Infection
- ERCP
- Medications such as thiazides, didanosine, stavudine, or azathioprine

Other symptoms include vomiting without blood; anorexia; and tenderness in the epigastric area.

In severe cases, symptoms include:

- Hypotension
- Metabolic acidosis
- Leukocytosis
- Hemoconcentration
- Hyperglycemia
- Hypocalcemia caused by fat malabsorption
- Hypoxia

Diagnostic testing is as follows:

Acute pancreatitis:
- Diagnose with ultrasound, CT, and MRCP.
- Treat with ERCP.

- Amylase and lipase (lipase has higher specificity): **best initial test**
- Abdominal CT, which can detect dilated common bile ducts and even comment on intrahepatic ducts: **most accurate test**
- Magnetic resonance cholangiopancreatography (MRCP) detects causes of biliary and pancreatic duct obstruction not found on CT
- If there is dilation of the common bile duct without a pancreatic head mass, consider endoscopic retrograde cholangiopancreatography (ERCP); can detect the presence of stones or strictures in the pancreatic duct system (and can remove them); ERCP is predominantly a therapeutic tool

There are no medications that reverse pancreatitis.

Treatment is bowel rest (no feeding); hydration; and pain medication.

Necrotic Pancreatitis

In the past, Ranson criteria were the major method of determining the severity of pancreatitis. Ranson criteria are operative criteria to see who needs pancreatic debridement.

Today, the CT scan effectively replaces Ranson criteria as the most precise way to determine severity.

Treatment is as follows:

- If CT shows >30% necrosis of the pancreas: antibiotic such as imipenem and CT-guided biopsy
- If biopsy shows infected, necrotic pancreatitis: surgical debridement of the pancreas

Hepatitis

Patients with acute hepatitis will present is a very similar way.

- Jaundice
- Fatigue
- Weight loss
- Dark urine (bilirubin in urine)
- Serum sickness-phenomena, i.e., joint pain, urticaria, and fever (hepatitis B and C)
- Polyarteritis nodosa (30% of cases) (hepatitis B)
- Cryoglobulinemia (hepatitis C)

In pregnancy, hepatitis E is the most severe and can be fatal.

The etiology of acute hepatitis cannot be determined from history and presentation alone.

Diagnostic testing includes:

- Acute hepatitis: elevated conjugated (direct) bilirubin (all patients)
  - Will cause bilirubin in the urine (urobilinogen)
  - Unconjugated bilirubin, e.g., that associated with hemolysis, is not water soluble and will not pass into the urine; unconjugated bilirubin is attached to albumin
- Viral hepatitis: elevated ALT
- Drug-induced hepatitis: elevated AST
- Hepatitis A, C, D, and E: serology for antibodies (**most accurate test**)
- Hepatitis B: surface antigen, core antibody, e-antigen, or surface antibodies (**most accurate test**); note these are not present in hepatitis A, C, D, E

> - Viral: ↑ ALT
> - Drugs: ↑ AST

Acute Hepatitis B

The first test to become abnormal in acute hepatitis B infection is the surface antigen. Elevation in ALT, e-antigen, and symptoms all occur afterward.

Chronic hepatitis B gives the same serologic pattern, but the surface antigen persists beyond 6 months.

The table below shows the appearance of the antigens and antibodies through the course of the disease.

	Surface Antigen	e-Antigen	Core Antibody	Surface Antibody
Acute disease (hepatitis B)	+	+	+	−
Window period (recovering)	−	−	+	−
Vaccinated	−	−	−	+
Healed/recovered	−	−	+	+

These 3 tests are essentially equal in meaning. They all indicate active viral replication:

Hepatitis B DNA polymerase = e-Antigen = hepatitis B PCR for DNA

No treatment is available for acute hepatitis B.

Acute Hepatitis C

Acute hepatitis C is the only acute hepatitis that can be treated.

- Hepatitis C antibody (**best initial test**)
  - Cannot, however, tell activity level of the virus (PCR-RNA level tell if there is active disease)
  - Stays positive even after treatment
- Hepatitis C PCR for RNA (**most accurate test to tell activity level of the virus and degree of viral replication**); also the most accurate way to determine response to therapy
- Liver biopsy (**most accurate way to determine seriousness of the disease**)
  - Patient can have 10 years of active viral replication with relatively little liver damage
  - Use the biopsy to determine extent of damage to the liver, but biopsy is not needed to determine the need for treatment

Genotype can help in the selection of therapy.

Chronic Hepatitis B

The patient with surface antigen, e-antigen, and DNA polymerase or PCR for DNA is the patient who is most likely to benefit from antiviral therapy. Look for >6 months of positive serology.

Treatment is one of the following single agents:

- Lamivudine
- Adefovir
- Entecavir
- Telbivudine
- Tenofovir (side effects include bone demineralization and RTA)

> HIV is associated with a false-negative hepatitis C antibody.

> Tenofovir affects the proximal convoluted tubule.

- Interferon (seldom needed): use only when patient has hepatitis D co-infection; has the most side effects
  - Flu-like symptoms
  - Arthralgia, myalgia
  - Fatigue, depression
  - Thrombocytopenia

Chronic Hepatitis C

Everyone age 18 and over should be tested for hepatitis C.

To become infected, one does not need to have risk factors such as injection drug use, transfusion before 1989, or extensive unprotected sex.

Treatment depends on the genotype of the infecting organism.

All genotypes	Some genotypes
Sofosbuvir/velpatasvir	Sofosbuvir/ledipasvir
Glecaprevir/pibrentasvir	Sofosbuvir/daclatasvir
	Elbasvir/grazoprevir
	Ombitasvir/paritaprevir/ritonavir/dasabuvir

These agents all have nearly equal efficacy. Ribavirin is sometimes used in combination with them.

- In advance of therapy, the genotype of the virus is ascertained to determine which combination is ideal (you will not be asked which drug goes with which specific genotype).
- Treatment is oral therapy for 12 weeks (>95% cure rate)
- Cure is assessed by finding a suppressed PCR-RNA viral load 12 and 24 weeks after therapy stops

What predicts the response to therapy?

Answer: Genotype

What tells if there has been a response?

Answer: PCR-RNA viral load. Look for sustained viral response.

What tells the extent of liver damage?

Answer: Liver biopsy, but rarely needed

What is the most common *wrong* answer?

Answer: Liver function tests (AST/ALT). The correlation between disease activity and level is poor.

Vaccination

Vaccination for both hepatitis A and B is now done universally in childhood. Specific indications are as follows:

- Hepatitis A vaccine: travelers and homeless
- Hepatitis B vaccine: health care workers, patients on dialysis, diabetes

For adults, the strongest indications for vaccination for both hepatitis A and B are the following:

- Chronic liver disease: Someone with cirrhosis or another cause of liver disease who develops hepatitis A or B is at much greater risk of fulminant hepatitis.
- Household contacts of those with hepatitis A or B
- Men who have sex with men
- Chronic recipients of blood products
- Injection drug users

Hepatitis E

- Fecal-oral transmission; greater incidence in poor countries
- Worse in pregnant women (acute liver failure)
- Generally no treatment; resolves spontaneously
- Can progress to chronic disease in immunosuppressed patients; treat with ribavirin/interferon

Postexposure Prophylaxis

If there is exposure to hepatitis A, hepatitis A vaccine for postexposure prophylaxis is enough.

- Age >12 months: give a single dose of the vaccine
- Age <12 months: give immune globulin
- If exposed patient is immunocompromised or has chronic liver disease: give immune globulin

Meaningful exposures to hepatitis A are household and sexual contacts. Unvaccinated persons in daycare centers or changing diapers should get a single dose of vaccine.

> There is no vaccine and no postexposure prophylaxis for hepatitis C.

A health care worker gets stuck with a needle contaminated with blood from a person with chronic hepatitis B. The health care worker has never been vaccinated. What is the most appropriate action?

Answer: Give hepatitis B immune globulin and hepatitis B vaccine. The same recommendation would be made for a child born to a mother with chronic hepatitis B. If the person had already been vaccinated, then you would check for levels of protective surface antibody. If hepatitis B surface antibody were already present, then no further treatment would be necessary.

Cirrhosis

No matter what the cause of the cirrhosis, it will have a number of features:

- Edema from low oncotic pressure: treat with spironolactone and diuretics
- Gynecomastia
- Palmar erythema
- Splenomegaly
- Thrombocytopenia caused by splenic sequestration
- Encephalopathy: treat with lactulose or rifaximin
- Ascites: treat with spironolactone
- Esophageal varices: propranolol will prevent bleeding; if they do bleed, perform banding of the varices

Everyone with cirrhosis should get an ultrasound every 6 months to screen for cancer. Ultrasound is 95% sensitive at detecting cancer.

> **Basic Science Correlate**
>
> Propranolol is a nonspecific beta blocker. This agent decreases pulse pressure in the esophageal varices, which is thought to be the reason it decreases the risk of variceal bleeding. Propranolol has no effect during an acute episode of bleeding. This is why all patients with cirrhosis should undergo endoscopy. Prophylactic beta blockers are very useful.

Ascites

Perform a paracentesis for all patients with ascites if any of the following are present:

- New ascites
- Pain, fever, or tenderness

Diagnostic testing includes ascitic fluid albumin level. If the level is low, the difference between the ascites and the serum level of albumin will be very great (this is a serum-to-ascites albumin gradient [SAAG]). If SAAG >1.1, portal hypertension from cirrhosis or congestive failure is present.

- If SAAG <1.1, then portal hypertension is not present.
- If SAAG >1.1, then portal hypertension is present.

Spontaneous bacterial peritonitis (SBP) is diagnosed with a cell count >250 neutrophils.

Treatment is cefotaxime or ceftriaxone. Anyone with SBP needs lifelong prophylaxis.

Chronic Liver Disease (Causes of Cirrhosis)

Alcoholic cirrhosis is a diagnosis of exclusion. Exclude all the other causes of cirrhosis and look for a history of longstanding alcohol abuse. Treat as described for cirrhosis.

Obeticholic acid decreases alkaline phosphatase levels in PBC.

Primary biliary cholangitis (PBC) presents in middle-aged women complaining of itching. PBC increases the risk of osteoporosis. Xanthelasmas (cholesterol deposits) may be found on examination. Also look for a history of other autoimmune disorders.

- **Best initial tests**: elevated alkaline phosphatase with a normal bilirubin; elevated IgM
- **Most accurate tests**: antimitochondrial antibody (AMA), liver biopsy

Treatment is ursodeoxycholic acid. If no response, add obeticholic acid, a farnesoid X receptor agonist that suppresses bile acid synthesis and promotes bile acid transport out of hepatocytes. The most common side effect is intense pruritus (add antihistamine).

Primary Sclerosing Cholangitis

Inflammatory bowel disease (IBD) accounts for 80% of primary biliary cholangitis. It also presents with itching but is much more likely to give an elevated bilirubin. Alkaline phosphatase level is elevated.

Most accurate tests: ERCP (shows "beading" of the biliary system); anti-smooth muscle antibody (ASMA); and ANCA (positive)

Treatment is ursodeoxycholic acid.

Wilson Disease

Penicillamine can't be used if allergic to penicillin.

Wilson disease involves cirrhosis and liver disease in a person with a choreiform movement disorder and neuropsychiatric abnormalities. This condition also presents with hemolysis.

Diagnostic testing includes:

- **Best initial test:** Slit lamp looking for Kayser-Fleischer rings is more sensitive and specific than a low ceruloplasmin level. On CCS, order both.
- **Most accurate test:** liver biopsy (more accurate than a urinary copper level)

Treatment is penicillamine or trientine, possibly in combination with zinc.

Hemochromatosis

The most common cause of death from hemochromatosis is cirrhosis. Cardiac disease occurs in only 15% of cases.

Most often, hemochromatosis is caused by a genetic disorder resulting in the overabsorption of iron. The iron deposits throughout the body, most commonly in the liver. Other manifestations include:

- Restrictive cardiomyopathy
- Skin darkening
- Joint pain caused by pseudogout or calcium pyrophosphate deposition disease
- Damage to the pancreas leading to diabetes, referred to as "bronze diabetes"
- Pituitary accumulation with panhypopituitarism
- Infertility
- Hepatoma

Hemochromatosis gives high risk of liver cancer from any type of chronic liver disease.

Diagnostic testing is as follows:

- **Best initial test**: elevated serum iron and ferritin with a low iron-binding capacity; the iron saturation is enormously elevated (>45%)
- **Most accurate test**: liver biopsy. However, an MRI of the liver and the specific genetic test, the HFe gene mutation, in combination are sufficiently diagnostic to spare the patient a liver biopsy.

Treatment is phlebotomy. Iron chelators such as deferasirox or deferiprone are used only from overtransfusion, not the genetic overabsorption of iron.

Autoimmune Hepatitis

Look for a young woman with other autoimmune diseases, such as Coombs positive hemolytic anemia, thyroiditis, and ITP.

- **Best initial tests**: ANA (positive), antismooth muscle antibody, and serum protein electrophoresis (SPEP) (shows hypergammaglobulinemia)
- **Most accurate test**: liver biopsy

Treatment is prednisone. Other immunosuppressive agents, such as azathioprine, may be needed if one is attempting to wean the patient off steroids.

Nonalcoholic Fatty Liver Disease (NAFLD)

There are 2 degrees of NAFLD:

- Nonalcoholic fatty liver (NAFL)
- Nonalcoholic steatohepatitis (NASH)

NAFL is milder and does not cause cirrhosis. NASH is more severe. It leads to cirrhosis and, in some, to cancer. NASH can also result in the need for liver transplant. When cirrhosis develops, screen with US every 6 months.

NASH is strongly associated with obesity, diabetes, and hyperlipidemia. Hepatomegaly is often present.

- **Best initial test**: ALT > AST
- **Most accurate test**: liver biopsy showing fatty infiltration (looks just like alcoholic liver disease)

Treatment is only to control the underlying causes with weight loss, diabetes control, and management of the hyperlipidemia. Moderate-intensity exercise will help reduce fatty liver.

Nephrology 11

Acute Renal Failure

The first step with renal failure is to evaluate whether it is prerenal (perfusion), renal (parenchymal), or postrenal (drainage).

Acute renal failure will have the following:

- Normal kidney size
- Normal hematocrit
- Normal calcium level

Chronic renal failure (>2 weeks) will have the following:

- Reduced kidney size
- Reduced hematocrit due to loss of erythropoietin production
- Reduced calcium level due to loss of vitamin D hydroxylation (i.e., activation)

Prerenal Azotemia

Any cause of hypoperfusion will lead to renal failure:

- Hypotension (generally, systolic pressure <90 mm Hg)
- Hypovolemia from dehydration or blood loss
- Low oncotic pressure (low albumin)
- Congestive heart failure (you can't perfuse the kidney if pump does not work)
- Constrictive pericarditis (you can't perfuse the kidney if heart cannot fill)
- Renal artery stenosis (although the systemic pressure may be high, the kidney thinks the body is hypotensive because of the blockage [which must be bilateral])

Diagnostic testing is as follows:

- BUN to creatinine ratio >15:1 and often >20:1
- Low urinary sodium <20
- Fractional excretion of sodium <1% (largely the same thing as a low urine sodium): do not spend time learning to do the calculation
- Urine osmolality >500
- Possible hyaline casts on urinalysis

Basic Science Correlate

Mechanism of Elevation of BUN in Prerenal Azotemia
Low volume status increases ADH. ADH increases urea absorption at the collecting duct. There is a urea transporter that brings urea in. ADH increases the activity of the urea transporter.

Treatment is based on the underlying cause.

CCS Tip: On CCS, all renal cases should have the following tests performed:

- Urinalysis, urine sodium, potassium
- Chemistries
- Renal ultrasound

Postrenal Azotemia (Obstructive Uropathy)

Any cause of obstruction of the kidney will lead to renal failure:

- Stone in the bladder or ureters
- Bilateral strictures
- Cancer of the bladder, prostate, or cervix
- Neurogenic bladder (atonic or noncontracting, such as from MS or diabetes)
- Prostate hypertrophy/BPH

Diagnostic testing is as follows:

- BUN to creatinine ratio >15:1
- Distended bladder on exam
- Large volume diuresis after passing a urinary catheter
- Bilateral hydronephrosis on ultrasound

> The obstruction must be bilateral to cause renal failure. Unilateral obstruction cannot cause renal failure.

Intrarenal Causes of Renal Failure

Intrarenal causes of renal failure result in the following:

- BUN-to-creatinine ratio 10:1
- Urinary sodium >40
- Urine osmolality <350

Acute tubular necrosis (ATN) can be caused by hypoperfusion to the point of death of the tubular cells or by various toxic injuries to the kidney. It is often caused by a combination of both.

In cases of toxin-induced renal insufficiency, there is no single test to prove that a particular toxin caused the renal failure. Common causes are:

- Aminoglycosides, such as gentamicin, tobramycin, or amikacin (hypomagnesemia is suggestive of aminoglycoside-induced renal failure but it is not conclusive; it usually takes 4–5 days of use to effect damage)

- Amphotericin
- Contrast agents: low urine sodium <20; can happen 12 hours later
- Chemotherapy, such as cisplatin (presents the same as aminoglycosides)

Urinalysis may show "muddy brown" or granular casts.

There is no specific treatment to reverse toxin-induced renal failure.

> Contrast is extremely rapid in onset.

Basic Science Correlate

Contrast agents are directly toxic to kidney tubules, as are aminoglycosides. Contrast also causes an intense vasoconstriction of the afferent arteriole. This combination of direct toxicity and decreased perfusion explains why there is such a rapid rise in creatinine during contrast-induced renal failure. It is also why contrast-induced renal failure causes a low urine sodium, as in prerenal azotemia.

A man is admitted for pneumonia from a nursing home. He is placed on piperacillin-tazobactam, and he becomes afebrile. Two days later, his BUN and creatinine start to rise. He develops a new fever and a rash. What is the most likely diagnosis, and what is the most accurate diagnostic test?

Answer: Allergic interstitial nephritis is a hypersensitivity reaction to medications such as penicillin or sulfa drugs. Other common culprits are phenytoin, allopurinol, cyclosporine, quinidine, quinolones, or rifampin. The clue to diagnosis is the fever and rash. The best initial test is urinalysis (UA) that shows white cells. However, the UA is not capable of distinguishing between neutrophils and eosinophils. The most accurate test is a Wright stain or Hansel stain of the urine that will show eosinophils. This is more sensitive than either the blood eosinophil level or elevated IgE level. There is no specific therapy generally given for allergic interstitial nephritis; it resolves on its own.

> Cyclophosphamide causes hemorrhagic cystitis, not renal failure.

> If AIN does not improve in 48 hours, give steroids.

Rhabdomyolysis

In cases of rhabdomyolysis, large-volume muscular necrosis is associated with renal failure from the direct toxic effect of myoglobin on the kidney tubule. Look for the following in presentation:

- Crush injury
- Seizure or cocaine toxicity
- Prolonged immobility in an intoxicated patient
- Hypokalemia resulting in muscle necrosis
- A patient recently started on a "statin" medication for hyperlipidemia

> Low serum phosphate causes rhabdomyolysis.

Diagnostic testing includes:

- Urinalysis (**best initial test**) showing dipstick positive for large amounts of blood with no cells seen on microscopic examination
- CPK level: elevated

- Urine myoglobin (**most accurate test**)
- On a CCS, also order the following:
  - Potassium level (hyperkalemia): potassium elevates with any cellular destruction, i.e., tumor lysis, rhabdomyolysis
  - Calcium level (hypocalcemia): damaged muscle binds increased amounts of calcium; hyperphosphatemia may lead to binding of calcium with the phosphate
  - Chemistries especially for detecting a decreased serum bicarbonate

---

Basic Science Correlate

Mechanism of Low Calcium in Rhabdomyolysis
Damaged muscle binds calcium. Each skeletal muscle cell contains sarcoplasmic endoplasmic reticulum for calcium (SERCA). SERCA is the normal mechanism for ending contraction, which it achieves by pulling all the cell calcium out of the cytosol. When the outside covering, or sarcolemma, is damaged, the SERCA can suck up calcium and lower the blood level.

Treatment is as follows:

- Bolus of normal saline
- Mannitol diuresis to decrease the contact time of myoglobin with the tubule
- Alkalinization of the urine to decrease precipitation of myoglobin at the tubule

A patient is brought to the ED after a seizure leading to prolonged immobility on a sidewalk. He has dark urine and myalgias. What is the most urgent step in management?

a. Urinalysis
b. Urine myoglobin level
c. EKG
d. CPK level
e. Phosphate level
f. Creatinine

Answer: **C.** EKG is the most urgent step in an acute case of rhabdomyolysis. This case tests your knowledge of how people die with rhabdomyolysis. Severe muscle necrosis leads to hyperkalemia, which leads to arrhythmia. If this is a CCS case, then all of the tests should be done simultaneously. A specific diagnosis with urinalysis or urine myoglobin is not as important as detecting and treating potentially life-threatening conditions, such as hyperkalemia with peaked T-waves. This condition would be treated with immediate IV calcium gluconate, insulin, and glucose.

Crystal-Induced Renal Failure

This condition can result from oxalate crystals or uric acid crystals.

- Oxalate crystals: look for suicide by antifreeze ingestion (ethylene glycol); patient will be intoxicated with metabolic acidosis with elevated anion gap.
  - Urinalysis shows envelope-shaped oxalate crystals (**best initial test**)
  - Treatment is ethanol or fomepizole with immediate dialysis
- Uric acid crystals: look for tumor lysis syndrome, often after chemotherapy for lymphoma.
  - Treatment is hydration, allopurinol, and rasburicase
- Cholesterol embolism gives livedo reticularis, low C3 and C4, and increased eosinophils.

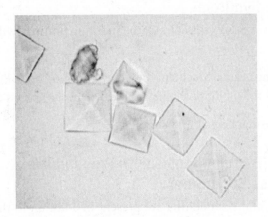

Oxalate crystals

Contrast-Induced Renal Failure

Regarding how to prevent contrast-induced renal failure, the exam may describe a patient who must have a radiologic procedure with contrast and common reasons for renal insufficiency, i.e., elderly patient with hypertension and diabetes. There will be no attempt to hide the etiology. Mild renal insufficiency with creatinine just above normal at 1.5–2.5 will be shown.

> **What is the best method to prevent contrast induced renal failure?**
>
> **Answer:** Give hydration with normal saline. Giving N-acetylcysteine or bicarbonate is not more effective than saline hydration alone.

The Step 3 exam wants you to know that even a very slight elevation in creatinine means the loss of 60–70% of renal function at a minimum. Preserve what is left!

Kidney Damage Caused by NSAIDs

NSAIDs can cause the following:

- Direct toxicity and papillary necrosis
- Allergic interstitial nephritis with WBCs and eosinophils in the urine
- Nephrotic syndrome
- Afferent arteriolar vasoconstriction and decreased perfusion of the glomerulus, worsening renal function

> Rasburicase breaks down uric acid.

Think: What are the few extra words to remember about each disease in order to answer the diagnostic and treatment questions? Step 3 does not generally emphasize the "most likely diagnosis" question.

Glomerulonephritis

All forms of glomerulonephritis (GN) can have the following characteristics:

- Red blood cells in urine
- Red cell casts in urine
- Mild degrees of proteinuria (<2 g per 24 hours)
- Edema
- May lead to nephrotic syndrome
- Are most accurately diagnosed with kidney biopsy, although this is not always necessary

Goodpasture Syndrome

Cough, hemoptysis, shortness of breath, and lung findings will be present in the case.

Diagnostic testing is anti–basement membrane antibodies, MPO-ANCA (**best initial test**), and renal biopsy showing "linear deposits" (**most accurate test**).

Treatment is plasmapheresis and steroids.

Eosinophilic Granulomatosis with Polyangiitis (Churg-Strauss Syndrome)

Asthma, cough, and eosinophilia are present in addition to the renal abnormalities.

The **best initial test** is CBC for eosinophil count. The **most accurate test** is biopsy.

Treatment is glucocorticoids (e.g., prednisone). If no response, add cyclophosphamide.

- Steroids must often be combined with an immunosuppressive agent, most commonly cyclophosphamide but also azathioprine, methotrexate, leflunomide, or mycophenolate.
- Inhibitors of interleukin-5 (IL-5) such as mepolizumab or benralizumab can induce remission in about 50% of cases.

Granulomatosis with Polyangiitis (Wegener)

Upper respiratory problems such as sinusitis and otitis are the key to diagnosis. Lung problems (cough, hemoptysis, abnormal chest x-ray) are present as well.

Wegener is a systemic vasculitis, so joint, skin, eye, brain, and GI problems are also present, but the key is both upper and lower respiratory involvement in addition to renal involvement. Often the case will be misdiagnosed as pneumonia.

The **best initial test** is c-ANCA (antineutrophil cytoplasmic antibodies) or antiproteinase 3-ANCA. The **most accurate test** is kidney biopsy (but lung biopsy is safer).

Treatment is cyclophosphamide (or rituximab) and steroids.

Microscopic Polyangiitis

- Lung and renal and systemic vasculitis
- No granulomas on biopsy
- No eosinophils or asthma
- MPO-ANCA present
- Treat with steroids and cyclophosphamide or rituximab.

Polyarteritis Nodosa (PAN)

Polyarteritis nodosa is a systemic vasculitis with involvement of every organ except the lung. Symptoms include:

- Renal
- Myalgias
- GI bleeding and abdominal pain
- Purpuric skin lesion
- Stroke
- Uveitis
- Neuropathy

The very nonspecific findings of fever, weight loss, and fatigue will also be present. Multiple motor and sensory neuropathy with pain are key to diagnosis.

Diagnostic testing is as follows:

- ESR and markers of inflammation (**best initial test**)
- Biopsy of sural nerve or the kidney (**most accurate test**)
- Test for hepatitis B and C (associated with 30% of PAN)
- Angiography showing "beading" can spare the need for biopsy
- Treatment is cyclophosphamide and steroids.

IgA Nephropathy (Berger Disease)

This condition presents with painless recurrent hematuria, particularly in an Asian patient after a very recent viral respiratory tract infection. Proteinuria and red cells and red cell casts can be present in all forms of glomerular disease. There is no specific physical finding that clearly defines the disease.

Diagnostic testing is as follows:

- No specific blood test; IgA is sometimes elevated
- Renal biopsy (**most accurate test** and essential for diagnosis), because there is no blood test or specific physical findings
- Complement levels are normal

There is no proven effective treatment to reverse IgA nephropathy.

- Steroids are used in boluses when there is a sudden worsening of proteinuria.
- ACE inhibitors are used as they are for all patients with proteinuria.
- Fish oil may have some effect on delaying progression.

Henoch-Schönlein Purpura

This presents in an adolescent or child with the following symptoms:

- Raised, nontender, purpuric skin lesions, particularly on the buttocks
- Abdominal pain
- Possible bleeding
- Joint pain
- Renal involvement

Diagnosis is made with a combined presentation of GI, joint, skin, and renal involvement. Biopsy showing deposition of IgA is the **most accurate test** but usually not necessary.

Treatment is not typically needed because Henoch-Schönlein purpura resolves spontaneously over time. If proteinuria worsens with ACE inhibitors, give steroids.

> Steroids are the answer for IgA nephropathy + HSP only when there is worsening proteinuria after ACE inhibitors.

Post-Streptococcal Glomerulonephritis (PSGN)

PSGN results in dark urine, described as "tea-" or "cola-colored." Periorbital edema and hypertension also occur. Many other infections can lead to glomerulonephritis; both throat and skin infections can lead to PSGN.

The **best initial test** is antistreptolysin O (ASLO), anti-DNase, antihyaluronidase in blood. Complement levels are low.

The **most accurate test** is biopsy, although it is not done routinely since blood tests are usually sufficient. Biopsy shows subepithelial deposits of IgG and C3.

Treatment is antibiotics (penicillin) for the infection, although they do not reverse the disease. Control the hypertension and fluid overload with diuretics.

Cryoglobulinemia

This presents in a patient with a history of hepatitis C with renal involvement. The patient may have joint pain and purpuric skin lesions.

The **best initial test** is serum cryoglobulin component levels (immunoglobulins and light chains, IgM). Complement levels (especially C4) are low.

The **most accurate test** is biopsy.

Treat the hepatitis C as described in the gastroenterology chapter. Rituximab helps with severe disease. Steroids do not help in IgM-related disease.

Lupus (SLE) Nephritis

The patient presents with a history of SLE. Note that drug-induced lupus spares the kidney and brain.

Diagnostic testing is as follows:

- ANA and anti-double-stranded DNA **(best initial test)**
- Renal biopsy **(most accurate test)**
  - The biopsy in the case of lupus nephritis is very important.
  - It is not to diagnose the presence of renal involvement but to determine the extent of disease to guide therapy.

Treatment is as follows:

- Sclerosis only: no treatment (this is a "scar" of the kidney)
- Mild, early stage, nonproliferative disease: steroids
- Severe, advanced, proliferative disease: mycophenolate mofetil (equal to cyclophosphamide) and steroids

Alport Syndrome

Alport syndrome is a congenital problem with eye and ear problems, such as deafness. Renal failure occurs in decades 2 or 3 of life.

There is no specific treatment.

Nephrotic Syndrome

Nephrotic syndrome is often a term of severity of renal disease. Any of the glomerular diseases just described can lead to nephrotic syndrome if they are severe.

Nephrotic syndrome is defined as follows:

- Hyperproteinuria
- Hypoproteinemia
- Hyperlipidemia
- Edema

Hypertension is common.

- When damage becomes severe enough, there is loss >3.5 g per day of protein in the urine; when that happens, albumin level in the blood falls and there is edema
- Hyperlipidemia is a part of nephrotic syndrome
- Thrombosis can occur because of loss of antithrombin III, protein C, and protein S in the urine

> **Basic Science Correlate**
>
> LDL and VLDL are removed from serum by lipoprotein signals. If the lipoprotein is lost in the urine with nephrotic syndrome, then the lipid levels in the blood rise.

Diagnostic testing is as follows:

- Urinalysis shows markedly elevated protein (**best initial test**)
- **Next best test**:
  - 24-hour urine protein collection shows >3.5 g of protein
  - Spot urine for protein-to-creatinine ratio >3.5:1 (equal in accuracy to 24-hour urine collection)
- Renal biopsy (**most accurate test**)

> Urine protein:creatinine ratio is same as 24-hour urine.

Other Primary Renal Disorders

In addition to the glomerular diseases previously described with systemic manifestations and specific blood tests, there are several primary renal disorders with no specific physical findings to make a precise diagnosis. There are features in the history that are suggestive.

Children	Adults, Cancer Such as Lymphoma	Hepatitis C	HIV, Heroin Use	Unclear
Minimal change disease	Membranous	Membranoproliferative	Focal segmental	Mesangial

Diagnostic testing is as follows:

- Urinalysis, followed by spot protein-to-creatinine ratio or 24-hour urine (**best initial test**)
- Renal biopsy (**most accurate test**)

Treatment is steroids. If there is no response, i.e., a decrease in urine protein excretion after 12 weeks, use cyclophosphamide. Biopsy findings will drive the choice of treatment.

Proteinuria

At any given time, 2–10% of the population has mild proteinuria (protein in urine). The first step in evaluation is to repeat the urinalysis. Oftentimes, the proteinuria will disappear on repeat testing.

- If proteinuria persists, see if the patient has a reason for transient mild proteinuria, such as CHF, fever, exercise, or infection.
- If not, consider orthostatic proteinuria. Look for a history of a job requiring one to stand all day (teaching, hair styling).

Diagnostic testing for proteinuria is as follows:

- Split the urine; do a morning urine for protein and then one in the afternoon; if protein is present in the afternoon but not in the morning, the patient likely has orthostatic proteinuria
- Orthostatic proteinuria needs no treatment
- If proteinuria is persistent and not orthostatic, do a 24-hour urine or spot protein/creatinine ratio. If elevated, do a renal biopsy.

End-Stage Renal Disease (ESRD)

When is **dialysis** indicated?

- When there is renal failure in hyperkalemia; metabolic acidosis; uremia with encephalopathy; fluid overload; and uremia with pericarditis
- When there is no renal failure but patient has toxicity with dialyzable drug (lithium, ethylene glycol, aspirin) and with uremia-induced malnutrition

The table summarizes other manifestations of uremia and their treatment.

> **Phosphate binders:**
> - Sevelamer
> - Lanthanum
> - Calcium acetate
> - Calcium carbonate

Hyperphosphatemia	Calcium acetate, calcium carbonate phosphate binders
Hypermagnesemia	Dietary magnesium restriction
Anemia	Erythropoietin replacement
Hypocalcemia	Vitamin D replacement

Complications of ESRD include:

- **Nephrogenic systemic fibrosis** (caused by MRI contrast agent gadolinium in patients with ESRD or severely low glomerular filtration rate (<30 mL)
  - Proliferation of dermal fibrocytes, leading to hardened areas of fibrotic nodules on the skin and in some cases, joint and skin contractures
  - No specific treatment
- **Calciphylaxis** (type of extraskeletal calcification)
  - Calcification of blood vessels with skin vessel clotting and necrosis
  - Caused by ESRD but also caused by hypercalcemia with milk-alkali syndrome or hyperparathyroidism
  - No diagnostic test
  - No specific treatment; manage by normalizing calcium level and increasing amount of dialysis

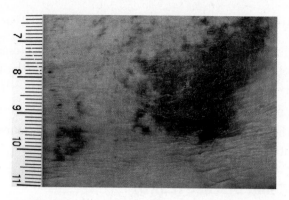

Calciphylaxis (© Niels Olson, MD. Used with permission.)

Potassium Disorders

Hyperkalemia

Hyperkalemia is predominantly caused by increased potassium release from tissues (muscles) or red blood cells (in rhabdomyolysis or hemolysis).

Other causes of hyperkalemia are the following:

- Metabolic acidosis from transcellular shift out of the cells
- Adrenal aldosterone deficiency, such as from Addison disease
- Beta blockers
- Digoxin toxicity
- Insulin deficiency, such as from diabetic ketoacidosis (DKA)
- Diuretics, such as spironolactone
- ACE inhibitors and angiotensin receptor blockers, which inhibit aldosterone
- Prolonged immobility, seizures, rhabdomyolysis, or crush injury
- Type IV RTA, resulting from decreased aldosterone effect
- Renal failure, preventing potassium excretion

> **Hyperkalemia can be caused by increased dietary potassium only if it is associated with renal insufficiency.**
>
> - If kidney function is normal, it is almost impossible to ingest potassium faster than the kidney can excrete it.
> - Also, the GI tract cannot absorb potassium faster than the kidney can excrete it. Since aldosterone functions to excrete potassium from the body, a deficiency or blockade of it will cause potassium levels will rise.

> **Basic Science Correlate**
>
> **Mechanism of Hyperkalemia with Beta Blocker Use**
> Normal Na/K ATPase activity lowers blood potassium. Beta blockers decrease the activity of the sodium/potassium ATPase. When you inhibit Na/K ATPase with a beta blocker, potassium levels can go up.

Pseudohyperkalemia is an artifact caused by the hemolysis of red cells in the laboratory or prolonged tourniquet placement during phlebotomy. No treatment is required, you need only repeat the test.

Hyperkalemia can lead to cardiac arrhythmia. Potassium disorders are not associated with seizures or neurological disorders.

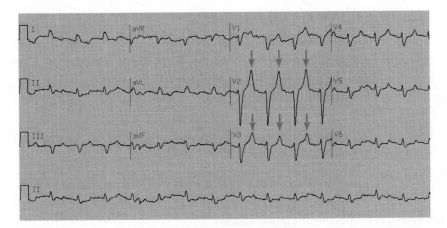

First the peaked T-waves occur, then the loss of the P-wave, and then the widened QRS complex.

Hyperkalemia Peaked T-Waves

Treatment is as follows:

- **Severe hyperkalemia** (EKG abnormalities, i.e., peaked T-waves): IV calcium gluconate to protect the heart, followed by IV insulin and glucose; conclude with sodium polystyrene sulfonate

- **Moderate hyperkalemia** (no EKG abnormalities): IV insulin and glucose; bicarbonate to shift potassium into the cell when the hyperkalemia is caused by acidosis or there is rhabdomyolysis, hemolysis, or other reason to alkalinize the urine; oral sodium polystyrene sulfonate (potassium-binding resin) to remove potassium from the body (takes several hours); patiromer and zirconium (oral binders of potassium in the bowel) to allow long-term use of ACEs, ARBs, and MRAs

  - Patiromer exchanges calcium and potassium, and allows continued use of medications which protect the kidneys but also cause hyperkalemia; can be used for chronic disease

  - Zirconium: oral binder of potassium in bowel, allowing use of ACE and ARBs

Basic Science Correlate

Mechanism of How Bicarbonate Lowers Potassium
When alkalosis pulls hydrogen cations out of cells, another cation must go in to maintain electrical neutrality. As hydrogen ions come out of cells, potassium goes in.

Hypokalemia

Dietary insufficiency can lead to hypokalemia. Other causes are:

- Increased urinary loss caused by diuretics
- High-aldosterone states, e.g., Conn syndrome
- Vomiting leads to metabolic alkalosis, which shifts potassium intracellularly, and volume depletion, which leads to increased aldosterone

- Proximal and distal RTA
- Amphotericin from the RTA it causes
- Bartter syndrome is the inability of the loop of Henle to absorb sodium and chloride. It causes secondary hyperaldosteronism and renal potassium wasting.

Signs include the following:

- Cardiac rhythm disturbance; EKG will show "U-waves" (have an extra wave after T-wave, indicating Purkinje fiber repolarization)
- Muscular weakness (due to contraction inhibition); can be severe and even cause rhabdomyolysis

Treatment is IV potassium replacement.

- Do not administer too rapidly so as to prevent possible arrhythmia.
- There is no maximum rate; the bowel will regulate the rate of absorption.

Also, avoid glucose-containing fluids, which would increase insulin release and worsen the hypokalemia.

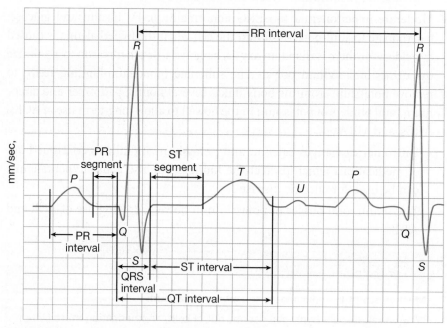

mm/mV   1 square = 0.04 sec/0.1mV

EKG-Normal Intervals

Sodium Disorders

Hypernatremia

Elevated serum sodium always implies a free water deficit. Dehydration is treated with normal saline replacement at first.

Besides simple dehydration, which can occur from poor oral intake, fever, pneumonia, or other types of increased insensible losses, the other main cause is diabetes insipidus (DI). DI can be caused by one of the following:

- Failure to produce antidiuretic hormone (ADH) in the brain (central)
- Insensitivity of the kidney (nephrogenic). Nephrogenic DI can result from hypokalemia, hypercalcemia, or lithium toxicity.

Hypernatremia leads to neurological abnormalities, such as confusion, disorientation, or seizures. The worst manifestation is a coma.

Sodium disorders do not cause cardiac rhythm disturbance.

Both central and nephrogenic DI produce the following:

- Low urine osmolality
- Low urine sodium
- Increased urine volume
- No change in urine osmolality with water deprivation

See below the management for central and nephrogenic DI.

> The Step 3 exam will not require knowledge of specific dosing. However, fluids should be first ordered as a bolus, then given continuously.

	Central DI	Nephrogenic DI
Urine volume	Prompt **decrease** in urine volume with administration of vasopressin (DDAVP)	**No change** in urine volume with DDAVP
Urine osmolality	Prompt **increase** in urine osmolality with DDAVP	**No change** in urine osmolality with DDAVP
Treatment	Treat with **DDAVP** or **vasopressin**	**Correct underlying cause**, such as hypokalemia or hypercalcemia. **Thiazide diuretics** are used in other cases.

Hyponatremia

Hyponatremia presents with neurological abnormalities, such as confusion, disorientation, seizures, or coma. There is no edema or dehydration.

The first step in management is to assess volume status to determine the cause.

- **Hypervolemic causes**: CHF; nephrotic syndrome; cirrhosis
- **Hypovolemic causes**: diuretics (urine sodium elevated); GI loss of fluids, i.e., vomiting, diarrhea (urine sodium low); skin loss of fluids, i.e., burns, sweating (urine sodium low)
  - The diuretics and sweating make the patient lose water and a little salt, but only free water is patient replaced
  - Over time, sodium level drops
- Correct underlying cause and replace with normal (isotonic) saline; check serum sodium frequently

Euvolemic (Normal) Volume Status

This can be caused by the following:

- Syndrome of inappropriate ADH release (SIADH)
- Hypothyroidism
- Psychogenic polydipsia
- Hyperglycemia (causes an artificial drop in sodium by 1.6 points of sodium for each 100 points of glucose)

Addison Disease

Addison disease also causes hyponatremia from insufficient aldosterone production. The key to this diagnosis is the presence of hyponatremia with hyperkalemia and mild metabolic acidosis. Treat with aldosterone replacement, such as fludrocortisone.

SIADH

Syndrome of inappropriate antidiuretic hormone secretion (SIADH) can be caused by any CNS abnormality; lung disease; cancer; or medication (e.g., sulfonylurea, SSRI, or carbamazepine).

It is associated with the following:

- Inappropriately high urine sodium (>20 mEq/L)
- Inappropriately high urine osmolality (>100 mOsm/kg)
- Low serum osmolality (<290 mOsm/kg)
- Low serum uric acid
- Normal BUN, creatinine, and bicarbonate

Treatment of hyponatremia is as follows:

- Mild hyponatremia (no symptoms): fluid restriction
- Moderate to severe hyponatremia (confused, seizures): saline infusion with loop diuretics; hypertonic (3%) saline; ADH blockers (conivaptan, tolvaptan); check serum sodium frequently (do not correct >10–12 mEq/L in first 24 hrs or >18 mEq/L in first 48 hrs; otherwise, possible central pontine myelinolysis)
- Chronic SIADH (i.e., from malignancy): demeclocycline to block the effect of ADH at the kidney; conivaptan and tolvaptan to inhibit ADH at the V2 receptor of the collecting duct

> Hyperglycemia causes an artificial drop in sodium by 1.6 points of sodium for each 100 points of glucose.

> Conivaptan raises sodium as an ADH blocker.

Magnesium Disorders

Hypermagnesemia

Hypermagnesemia is caused by the overuse of magnesium-containing laxatives or from iatrogenic administration, such as during premature labor when it is administered as a tocolytic. It is rare to have hypermagnesemia without renal insufficiency. Hypermagnesemia leads to muscular weakness and loss of deep tendon reflexes.

Treat hypermagnesemia as follows:

- Restricting intake
- Saline administration to provoke diuresis
- Occasionally dialysis

Hypomagnesemia

Hypomagnesemia is caused by the following:

- Loop diuretics
- Alcohol withdrawal, starvation
- Gentamicin, amphotericin, diuretics
- Cisplatin
- Parathyroid surgery
- Pancreatitis

Hypomagnesemia presents with hypocalcemia and cardiac arrhythmias.

Magnesium is required for parathyroid hormone release. This is particularly important in the management of torsade de pointes.

Acid-Base Disorders

Metabolic Acidosis

In metabolic acidosis, the blood's pH is low. Categories of this condition include increased or normal anion gap, according to whether unmeasured anions are present or absent in serum.

Metabolic Acidosis with Increased Anion Gap

- Lactic acidosis, caused by any form of hypoperfusion, e.g., hypotension, resulting in anaerobic metabolism. Anaerobic metabolism leads to glycolysis, which results in the accumulation of lactic acid. Treat the underlying cause of hypoperfusion.
- Aspirin overdose originally gives respiratory alkalosis from hyperventilation. Over a short period, metabolic acidosis develops from poisoning of mitochondria and the loss of aerobic metabolism. This gives lactic acidosis. Treat with bicarbonate, which corrects the acidosis and increases urinary excretion of aspirin.
- Methanol intoxication: this toxic alcohol leads to formic acid and formaldehyde production; look for an intoxicated patient with visual disturbance; get a methanol level and then give fomepizole or ethanol, which blocks the production of formic acid and allows time for dialysis to remove the methanol.
- Uremia: renal failure prevents the excretion of the 1 mEq/kg of organic acid that is formed each day; this is an indication for dialysis

- Diabetic ketoacidosis: acetone, acetoacetate, and beta hydroxybutyric acid lead to an increased anion gap; a low serum bicarbonate is the fastest test to tell if a patient's hyperglycemia is life-threatening. Treat with normal saline hydration and insulin. Place the patient in the ICU.

- Isoniazid toxicity: just stop the medication and move the clock forward on CCS

- Ethylene glycol: Look for an intoxicated patient with a renal abnormality, such as oxalate crystals in the urine. There is also renal failure and hypocalcemia, because the oxalate binds with calcium to form crystals. Suicide attempt with ethylene glycol is key. Treat the same as methanol intoxication with fomepizole or ethanol, which blocks the production of oxalic acid and allows time for dialysis to remove the ethylene glycol.

Metabolic Acidosis with Normal Anion Gap

This condition results from diarrhea or renal tubular acidosis (RTA).

- Diarrhea causes metabolic acidosis via increased bicarbonate loss from the colon. The colon secretes both bicarbonate and potassium, so potassium level will be low (hypokalemia) as well. Because there is increased chloride reabsorption, there is hyperchloremia, which is why there is a normal anion gap.

- RTA
  - **Distal RTA (type I):** An inability to excrete acid of hydrogen ions in the distal tubule leads to the accumulation of acid in the body. Urine pH rises because the body cannot excrete acid. In an alkaline environment, stones will form. Serum potassium is low (body excretes + ions in the form of K+ since it can't excrete H+) and serum bicarbonate is low.
    - Test by administering acid intravenously (ammonium chloride, which should lower urine pH secondary to increased H+ formation). In distal RTA the person cannot excrete the acid, and the urine pH stays abnormally basic.
    - Treat with bicarbonate. The proximal tubule is still working, so the patient will still absorb the bicarbonate.
  - **Proximal RTA (type II):** An inability to reabsorb bicarbonate in the proximal renal tubule leads to a drop in urine pH (after urine pH was initially elevated) after the body has lost substantial amounts of bicarbonate. Because urine pH is low, kidney stones do not often develop. A low serum bicarbonate leaches calcium out of the bones, and there is also osteomalacia.
    - Test by giving bicarbonate. A normal person with metabolic acidosis will absorb all of the bicarbonate, and there should still be a low urine pH. In proximal RTA, the patient cannot absorb the bicarbonate and the urine pH rises from the bicarbonate malabsorption.
    - Treat with a thiazide diuretic, which will produce a blood volume contraction and thus raise the concentration of serum bicarbonate. Give large quantities of serum bicarbonate (since bicarbonate is generally ineffective and so requires high amounts).

- **Hyporeninemic hypoaldosteronism (type IV):** Decreased aldosterone production or effect. Look for a diabetic patient with a normal anion gap metabolic acidosis.
  ○ This is the **only RTA with elevated potassium**.
  ○ Treat with aldosterone, in the form of fludrocortisone (steroid with the highest mineralocorticoid content).

The table compares Types I, II, and IV RTA.

	Distal RTA (Type I)	**Proximal RTA (Type II)**	**Type IV (Diabetes)**
Urine pH	High	Low	Low
Serum Potassium	Low	Low	High
Stones	Yes	No	No
Test	Give acid	Give bicarbonate	Urine sodium loss
Treatment	Bicarbonate	Thiazide diuretic **high dose** bicarbonate	Fludrocortisone

Urine Anion Gap (UAG)

The way to distinguish between diarrhea and RTA as the cause of the normal anion gap metabolic acidosis is with the urine anion gap (UAG):

$$UAG = urine\ Na^+ - urine\ Cl^-$$

When acid is excreted from the kidney, it goes out as NH_4Cl. Acid excretion from the kidney goes out with chloride.

- If you can excrete acid from the kidney, urine chloride goes up. If the urine chloride is up, this give a negative UAG number. Diarrhea causes a negative UAG, because the kidney can excrete acid and the net UAG is negative. In metabolic acidosis, a negative UAG means the kidney works.

- If you cannot excrete acid from the kidney, urine chloride goes down. This gives a positive UAG number. In RTA, you cannot excrete acid from the kidney. The urine chloride will be low, and the UAG will be positive.

Metabolic Alkalosis

In metabolic alkalosis, the blood's pH is elevated. This can be caused by various things:

- Volume contraction, because there is a secondary hyperaldosteronism that causes increased urinary loss of acid. Treat the underlying cause.

- Hyperaldosteronism resulting from primary hyperaldosteronism (Conn syndrome) or Cushing syndrome, which causes urinary acid loss. Also look for hypokalemia, which often accompanies the increased urinary acid loss. Treat by removing the adenoma surgically.

- Hypokalemia, because potassium ions shift out of the cell to correct the hypokalemia. This shifts hydrogen ions into the cell in exchange for the potassium ions leaving.

- Too much liquid antacid (milk-alkali syndrome)

- Vomiting, because it causes a loss of acid from the stomach. Also, the loss of fluids can lead to volume contraction and secondary hyperaldosteronism.

Cystic Disease

Cystic disease presents with recurrent hematuria, stones, and infections.

- Cysts throughout the body (e.g., in the liver, ovaries, and circle of Willis)
- Most common site of extrarenal cysts is the liver
- Mitral valve prolapse
- Diverticulosis

The most common cause of death is end-stage renal disease (not subarachnoid hemorrhage).

There is no specific treatment.

Incontinence

> Mirabegron relaxes the bladder by beta-3 stimulation.

The table summarizes the presentation, diagnosis, and treatment of incontinence.

	Urge Incontinence	Stress Incontinence
Presentation	Pain followed by urge to urinate	No pain
	No relationship to coughing, laughing, or straining	Brought on by coughing and laughing
Testing	Urodynamic pressure monitoring	Observe leakage with coughing

Treatment	• Behavior modification
	• Anticholinergic medications
	  - Tolterodine or fesoterodine
	  - Trospium
	  - Darifenacin
	  - Solifenacin
	  - Oxybutynin
	  - Mirabegron
		• Kegel exercises
		• Estrogen cream

Hypertension

The first step when a case of hypertension presents is to repeat the blood pressure measurement in 1–2 weeks. It may take 3–6 measurements to get an accurate assessment of blood pressure. BP >140/90 mm Hg is definitely defined as hypertension for all groups. Some consider >130/80 as hypertension. The exam will not ask questions about guidelines that differ between organizations.

CCS Tip: Routine tests for hypertension cases on CCS are:

- Urinalysis
- EKG
- Eye exam for retinopathy
- Cardiac exam for murmur and S4 gallop

Treatment is as follows:

- Lifestyle modification such as sodium restriction, weight loss, exercise, and relaxation techniques for 3–6 months
- If that has no effect, initiate medical therapy with a thiazide diuretic (hydrochlorothiazide or chlorthalidone plus a CCB or ACE inhibitor) (60–70% success rate)
- ACEI/ARB as first-line therapy for diabetics
- If blood pressure is still not controlled, add a second drug: ACE inhibitor, ARB, CCB, or beta blocker (metoprolol, carvedilol) (90–95% success rate)
- If blood pressure is still not controlled, add a third drug, and if there is still no success, investigate causes of secondary hypertension

Note: If any of the conditions below are present, do not start with a diuretic. Go straight to the specific medication.

> As a first drug, thiazides are not better than CCBs, ACEIs, or ARBs.

Condition	Medication
Coronary artery disease	Beta blocker
Congestive heart failure	Beta blocker, ACEI, or ARB
Migraine	Beta blocker, CCB
Hyperthyroidism	Beta blocker
Osteoporosis	Thiazide
Depression	No beta blockers
Asthma	No beta blockers
Pregnancy	Alpha methyldopa
BPH	Alpha blockers
Diabetes	ACEI/ARB

Thiazides are not better as a first choice than ACE inhibitors, ARBs, or CCBs.

- If baseline blood pressure >160/100 mm Hg, start with 2 medications.
- In those age >60, blood pressure need only be controlled to <150/90 mm Hg.
- Diabetes alone can be controlled to at least 140/90 mm Hg.

> For those age >60, BP target is 150/90 mm Hg.

Secondary Hypertension

Investigate for secondary hypertension if you see the following:

- Young (age <30) or old (age >60) patient
- Failure to control pressure with 3 medications
- Specific findings in the history or physical (see table)

> Weight loss is the most effective lifestyle modification for hypertension.

Specific Findings in the History or Physical	
Condition	**Finding**
Closure of renal artery (stenosis)	Bruit
Pheochromocytoma	Episodic hypertension
Conn syndrome	Hypokalemia
Cushing syndrome	Buffalo hump, truncal obesity, striae
Coarctation of the aorta	Upper extremity > lower extremity pressure
Congenital adrenal hyperplasia	Hirsutism
Sleep apnea	None

Renal Artery Stenosis

Look for an abnormal sound (bruit) auscultated in the flanks or abdomen. Hypokalemia may be present.

Diagnostic testing is renal ultrasound with Doppler (**best initial test**). Doppler is specific, but not sensitive.

If a small kidney is seen, do any of the following tests next:

- Magnetic resonance angiography (MRA) or CT angiogram confirms renal artery stenosis (**most accurate test**)
- Duplex ultrasonogram
- Nuclear renogram

Treatment is maximum medical control, including ACEs/ARBs. Renal artery angioplasty and stenting are not effective.

Basic Science Correlate

Diameter and Flow

Flow markedly increases as radius of a tube increases. The flow increases to the fourth power of the radius. For example, if the radius or diameter doubles in size, flow will go up 16 times, or $2 \times 2 \times 2 \times 2$.

For Step 3 in oncology, the most important thing to know is the screening tests.

Which of the following screening tests lowers mortality *the most*?

a. Mammography age >50

b. Mammography age >40

c. Colonoscopy

d. Pap smear

e. Prostate-specific antigen (PSA)

Answer: A. Mammography age >50 lowers mortality the most. Although screening should start at age 50, the mortality benefit is also greatest age >50 because the number of cases of cancer detected will be greater age >50.

The age cutoff for mammography is somewhat controversial. Step 3 will likely avoid the issue.

Breast Cancer

Screening mammography should begin at age 50. After age 75, it is not routinely indicated.

When an abnormality is found on mammogram, do the following:

- Do a breast biopsy, which will both show cancer (or not) and test for the presence of estrogen and progesterone receptors and HER2/neu overexpression.
- With a sentinel node biopsy, a dye or tracer is placed into the operative field. The first node it goes to is biopsied (called the "sentinel node").
  - If node is free of cancer, then an axillary node dissection is not necessary
  - If node does have cancer, then an axillary lymph node dissection is performed

Genetic testing for BRCA genes is not a routine screening test. All that can be said for certain about BRCA is that it is associated with an increased risk of familial breast cancer and of ovarian cancer.

> Use tamoxifen, raloxifene, or aromatase inhibitors if ≥2 first-degree relatives have breast cancer. Those agents decrease the risk of breast cancer.

Treatment is as follows:

- Lumpectomy with radiation to the site at the breast (equal to modified radical mastectomy)(**best initial treatment**)
- Hormonal inhibition therapy
  - Tamoxifen is used if either the estrogen or progesterone receptors are positive (the response is greater if both are positive); adverse side effects include DVT, hot flashes, and endometrial cancer.
  - Aromatase inhibitors (anastrozole, letrozole, exemestane) are pure estrogen antagonists. They do not have the selective estrogen receptor agonist (stimulatory) activity that tamoxifen has. Adverse side effects include osteoporosis (because they are antagonistic to estrogen receptors in the bone), but do not include DVT.
- Adjuvant chemotherapy only if cancer is in the axilla and cancer >1 cm in size. Adjuvant therapy is more effective when the patient is still menstruating. Breast cancer in menstruating women will not likely be controlled with estrogen antagonists, such as tamoxifen or aromatase inhibitors.
- Trastuzumab and pertuzumab (used in combination for metastatic disease): monoclonal antibodies against the breast cancer antigen HER2/neu; have modest efficacy and some cardiotoxicity (trastuzumab)
- Atezolizumab (PD inhibitor): only drug for triple receptor-negative breast cancer

For primary preventive therapy, tamoxifen is used for anyone with multiple first-degree relatives (mother, sister) who have had breast cancer; start treatments at age 40. Tamoxifen reduces the risk by 50%.

A 42-year-old woman has a 2-cm breast cancer tumor removed by lumpectomy and the breast is irradiated. The cancer is negative for estrogen receptors and positive for progesterone receptors. Three of 14 nodes removed from the axilla are positive for cancer. What is the next best step in management?

a. Adjuvant chemotherapy and radiation of the axilla
b. Tamoxifen for 5 years
c. Anastrozole (aromatase inhibitor) for 5 years
d. Tamoxifen and adjuvant chemotherapy
e. Oophorectomy and chemotherapy

Answer: **D.** Tamoxifen is used when there are positive estrogen- or progesterone-receptors. (If both receptors are positive, tamoxifen will be of greater benefit.) Adjuvant chemotherapy is used whenever the axillary nodes are positive or the size of the cancer >1 cm.

Colon Cancer

The table below shows the recommended screening for colon cancer.

General Population	Single Family Member with Colon Cancer	Three Family Members, Two Generations, One Age <50	FAP, Gardner, Peutz-Jeghers, Turcot's	Juvenile Polyposis
• Start screening at age 50 • Colonoscopy every 10 years	• Start screening at age 40 or 10 years earlier than the age at which family member contracted cancer	• Start screening at age 25 • Colonoscopy every 1–2 years	• Start screening at age 12 • Sigmoidoscopy every 1–2 years (for Peutz-Jeghers start at age 8)	• Screen upper & lower tract starting at age 12

Which of the following colon cancer screening methods lowers mortality the most?

a. Colonoscopy every 10 years
b. Sigmoidoscopy every 5 years
c. Fecal immunochemical test every year
d. Fecal occult blood test (FOBT) every year
e. CT colonography ("virtual colonoscopy")
f. Fecal immunochemical test (FIT) for DNA

Answer: **A.** Because 40% of colon cancer occurs proximal to the sigmoid colon, colonoscopy is the most accurate test for detection. If the question had said "Which of the following screening methods finds colon cancer and lowers mortality?", the answer would be "All of them." But this is not a very exam-like question: USMLE avoids both "All of the above" and "None of the above" as answer options.

Managing anticoagulation in colonoscopy is important.

• Stop novel oral anticoagulants (NOACs) only 1 day before the colonoscopy and restart the day after colonoscopy; so if colonoscopy is on Tuesday, skip Monday's dose and restart on Wednesday

• Stop warfarin 3–5 days before the colonoscopy; the length of time is based on the reason for the anticoagulation, i.e., those with metal heart valves should be off warfarin for the shortest period of time

Treatment of colon cancer is surgical resection and chemotherapy centered around a 5-fluorouracil regimen (for cancers which are high-risk stage 2 and greater).

Lung Cancer

Lung cancer screening (chest CT) should be performed annually in all smokers with >30 pack-years of smoking history age 55–75. (Start long-term smokers at age 55.)

> A 52-year-old smoker has a 1.5-cm calcified nodule found on chest x-ray done for other reasons. He has no symptoms. What is the next step?
>
> Answer: Excisional biopsy should be done on solitary lung nodules >1 cm in size in those who smoke. Age >50 lends additional urgency to the need for biopsy. Even though calcification goes against malignancy, the age of the patient, size of the nodule, and history of smoking are more important.

Treatment is based on whether the disease is localized enough to be surgically resectable. Lesion size alone is not enough to determine whether a cancer is resectable. If the lesion is large but peripheral, without metastases, it can be resected.

A cancer is not resectable if any of the following are present:

- Bilateral disease
- Metastases
- Malignant pleural effusion
- Involvement of the aorta, vena cava, or heart
- Lesions within 1–2 cm of the carina
- Laryngeal nerve involvement

Small-cell cancer is nonresectable because one of these features is present in >95% of cases.

When a cancer tests positive for the programmed death (PD) biomarker, give a PD inhibitor. Although pembrolizumab and nivolumab are the answer for lung cancer, it is the presence of the PD biomarker—not the specific histology—that makes them the right answer as targeted therapy.

PD inhibitors are more effective and better tolerated than platinum therapy for non–small cell lung cancer.

> Lung cancer screening (annual chest CT):
> - Age 55–80
> - 30 pack-years
> - Has not quit in past 15 years

Prostate Cancer

The area of prostate cancer screening is controversial. Prostate-specific antigen (PSA) and digital rectal exam are not proven to lower mortality from prostate cancer.

Besides the spread of the disease, the most important prognostic factor for prostate cancer is the Gleason score, a measure of the level of differentiation of the histology. The higher the score, the more aggressive the cancer.

> There is no proven screening method that lowers mortality for prostate cancer.

A 65-year-old man comes to you requesting screening for prostate cancer. What is the next step?

Answer: Patients requesting screening for prostate cancer should undergo PSA and digital rectal exam. Though seemingly self-contradictory, the recommendation is that the physician should not "routinely offer" screening but, if requested, should perform it if the patient is age <75.

Treatment is as follows.

- Localized prostate cancer: surgery plus either external radiation or implanted radioactive pellets (nearly equal in efficacy)
- Metastatic prostate cancer: androgen blockade
  - No particularly good chemotherapy
  - Hormonal treatments: flutamide (testosterone receptor blocker) and leuprolide or goserelin (gonadotropin-releasing hormone [GnRH] agonists)
  - Abiraterone, a 17 hydroxylase inhibitor which stops production of all androgens in the body including adrenal production, decreases risk of death by over 35%

Do not confuse treatment for prostate cancer with the 5 alpha-reductase inhibitor finasteride. Finasteride treats benign prostatic hypertrophy and male pattern hair loss—not prostate cancer.

> Abiraterone lowers mortality in metastatic prostate cancer.

What is the fastest way to lower androgen/testosterone levels?

Answer: Orchiectomy. We did not say to do it, but this is the fastest way.

A man with prostate cancer presents with severe, sudden back pain. MRI shows cord compression and he is started on steroids. What is the next best step in management?

a. Flutamide
b. Flutamide and leuprolide simultaneously
c. Leuprolide followed by flutamide
d. Ketoconazole

Answer: **A.** Flutamide should be started first to block the temporary flare up in androgen levels which accompany GnRH agonist treatments. When cord compression is described, GnRH agonists can worsen the compression if used too soon. Ketoconazole, at a high dose, blocks the production of androgens, but it is not as effective as the other therapies.

> Scalp hypothermia can improve the alopecia (hair loss) of chemotherapy.

Ovarian Cancer

There is no routine screening test for ovarian cancer. CA125 is a marker of progression and response to therapy for ovarian cancer, not a diagnostic test.

Look for a woman age >50 with increasing abdominal girth at the same time as weight loss.

Treatment is surgical debulking followed by chemotherapy, even in cases of extensive local metastatic disease.

Ovarian cancer is unique in that surgical resection is beneficial even when there is a large volume of tumor spread through the pelvis and abdomen. Removing all visible tumor still helps.

Testicular Cancer

Testicular cancer presents with a painless scrotal lump in a man <age 35.

For diagnostic testing, perform an inguinal orchiectomy of the affected testicle. Do not do a needle biopsy.

Of all testicular cancers, 95% are germ cell tumors (seminoma and nonseminoma). Alpha fetoprotein (AFP) is secreted only by nonseminomas.

Diagnostic testing is as follows:

- AFP, LDH, and beta-hCG levels
- CT scan of the abdomen and pelvis for staging purposes

> It is not diagnosed by biopsy of the testicle.

Testicular cancer is extremely curable with a 90–95% 5-year survival rate. Treatment is radiation for local disease and chemotherapy for widespread disease; even metastatic disease can be cured with chemotherapy.

PART 2

Preventive Medicine

Screening

"Screening" means a test done in an asymptomatic person to detect disease. There are some tests that provide no screening benefit to the patient:

- Carotid artery imaging (duplex)
- Annual chest x-ray
- Stress (exercise tolerance) testing
- CBC
- Carotid stenosis in asymptomatic persons
- Thyroid hormone level

The tests that do provide benefit to the patient are as follows:

Cancer Screening

The single most important oncology question on Step 3 is about **prevention**. While what you need to know in terms of volume is extremely small, it is very highly tested.

Breast Cancer

Mammography is the cancer screening test that lowers mortality most. It should be started in all women **age >50** (this age group sees the great benefit in mortality).

Mammography guidelines are controversial at this time.

Routine breast self-examination has no proven benefit.

Cervical Cancer

Cervical cancer screening with Pap smear also lowers mortality.

- Start Pap smear at **age 21**, regardless of the onset of sexual activity.
- Continue doing Pap smear at least **every 3 years** until age 29. From 30 to 65 Pap smear combined with HPV testing is done every 5 years until age 65 when it can be stopped.

> HPV testing is right for ASCUS. If ASCUS is HPV-positive, do colposcopy.

Colon Cancer

Colon cancer screening is started with a **colonoscopy at age 50** and is performed **every 10 years. No screening after age 85.**

- If a close family member has had the disease, begin screening at age 40 or 10 years earlier than the family member was diagnosed, whichever is earlier.
  - If the family member is age <60, do colonoscopy every 5 years. If the family member is age >60, do colonoscopy every 10 years.
- If family has hereditary nonpolyposis colon cancer syndrome (HNPCC) (formerly known as Lynch syndrome) defined as colon cancer in 3 family members spanning 2 generations, with 1 family member having it prematurely (age <50), begin screening at age 25 and perform every 1–2 years.

Other screening methods such as sigmoidoscopy and fecal occult blood testing are less effective at detecting cancer than colonoscopy. Virtual colonoscopy with CT scanning is not accurate, and barium enema is not effective.

- Sigmoidoscopy: every 5 years
- Fecal occult blood testing (FOBT): yearly
- Fecal immunochemical test (FIT) with DNA: every 3 years

Prostate Cancer

There is no clear recommendation to screen all patients routinely for prostate cancer with either a prostate-specific antigen (PSA) or a digital rectal exam.

There is specific evidence to recommend **against the PSA** for men age >75 on the basis that they will accrue the disadvantages of treatment, such as erectile dysfunction or incontinence, without any benefit.

Lung Cancer

Perform lung cancer screening yearly in long-term smokers age 55–80 with 30 pack-years. Use a low-dose chest CT to do the screening.

Stop if it has been >15 years since the patient quit smoking.

Osteoporosis

All women should be screened with bone densitometry at age 65.

Abdominal Aortic Aneurysm

All men age **65–75** who have ever smoked should be screened 1× with an ultrasound.

Diabetes

Diabetes screening is routine only in those with hypertension or who are obese.

HIV

Everyone age 15–65 should be tested for HIV regardless of risk factors.

The interval between tests is unclear. Check more frequently in those patients on pre-exposure prophylaxis (PreP).

Hepatitis C

Test everyone age 18 and over.

Screening is especially beneficial in those with a history of injection drug use, men who have sex with men, and those who have received blood products.

Vaccinations

Influenza and Pneumococcal Vaccine

The indications for influenza vaccination and pneumococcal pneumonia vaccination have a lot of overlap:

- Patients with chronic lung, heart, liver, kidney, and cancer conditions
- HIV-positive patients
- Patients on steroids
- Patients with diabetes

Influenza Vaccine

Influenza vaccine is recommended yearly in the general population. It has the greatest benefit in the following persons:

- Everyone age >50
- Pregnant women
- Health care workers

Use inactivated influenza vaccine in those age >50 or immunocompromised. The inhaled live attenuated vaccine is the least powerful form.

Egg allergy is not a contraindication to influenza vaccination.

Pneumococcal Vaccine

Pneumococcal vaccine is different from influenza vaccine in that:

- Everyone age >65
- Tobacco smokers

The pneumococcal vaccine is routinely 2 injections given one year apart.

- **First injection**: 13-polyvalent vaccine
- **Second injection one year later**: 23-polyvalent vaccine
  - If patient already received the 23-polyvalent, then give 13-polyvalent one year later.
  - If patient is immunocompromised, give the 23-polyvalent vaccine 8 weeks after the 13-polyvalent. If immunocompromised, do not wait for age 65.

> Flu vaccine is indicated for everyone yearly.

> Healthy: 13 now, 23 in a year
>
> Immunocompromised: 13 now, 23 in 8 weeks

> Group B meningococcal vaccine exists as a separate injection.

Meningococcal Vaccination

Meningococcal vaccination is routine at **age 11–18** for serogroups B, C, and Y.

Children at especially high risk, who should be vaccinated even earlier, are those with functional anatomic asplenia, HIV positive, or those with terminal complement deficiency. Group B vaccination is also given.

There is no clear association between meningococcal vaccine and Guillain-Barré syndrome. If the question says the patient is to receive the medication with ocrelizumab, choose the answer "Vaccinate against meningococcus."

HPV Vaccination

This is a quadrivalent vaccine that should be administered to **all females age 13–45.** Studies are looking at the benefits of administering the vaccine to women outside this age range, but currently the guideline is age 13–45.

HPV vaccine is acceptable in boys to age 21.

Varicella-Zoster Vaccination

> Zoster vaccine at age 50.

Vaccination against the reactivation of varicella-zoster (shingles) should be performed in everyone age >50. The vaccine is a higher-dose form of the varicella vaccine given to children.

Tetanus Vaccination

> Use yellow fever vaccine for travel to parts of Africa:
> - Vaccine = 100% effective
> - Infection = 50% fatal

A booster of tetanus vaccine should be given **1 × every 10 years**. At least one of these boosters should be **Tdap** (both the tetanus toxoid and vaccination for acellular pertussis).

- Tdap is safe in pregnancy; revaccination with Tdap should be done with every pregnancy.
- If a patient has a wound strongly contaminated with dirt that might have a high volume of tetanus spores, the patient is considered protected for only 5 years after the last injection; revaccination, or booster, should be with Tdap as well.
- Tetanus immune globulin is used only if the patient has never been vaccinated.

Issues Surrounding Vaccination

Vaccine hesitancy is a term used to describe refusal of vaccination or a delay in acceptance of vaccination. The Step 3 exam will expect you to know what type of hesitancy patients/parents have regarding vaccinations, so that you can provide proper education and reassurance.

- MMR vaccine does not cause autism.
- Meningococcal vaccine has not been proved to cause Guillain-Barré syndrome.
- HPV vaccine does not encourage sexual promiscuity.
- Egg allergy is not a contraindication for influenza vaccine.
- Hepatitis B vaccine does not cause demyelinating neurologic disorders.

Lifestyle Management

Smoking Cessation

All patients should be screened for tobacco use and advised against it. The most effective way to stop smoking is with an oral medication, such as bupropion or varenicline.

Less effective therapies that can be tried first are nicotine patches and gum.

Hypertension

All patients age >18 should have their blood pressure checked at every office visit.

Hyperlipidemia

Men age >35 and women age >45 should be screened for hyperlipidemia.

PART 3

Biostatistics and Epidemiology

Introduction

The amount of statistical analysis that you are expected to understand on USMLE Step 3 is increasing. This is because the Federation of State Medical Boards (FSMB) and the National Board of Medical Examiners (NBME) insist that licensed physicians understand both the statistical significance of the medical literature and the claims of drug manufacturers.

You must be prepared to calculate the following statistical measures on USMLE Step 3:

- Sensitivity
- Specificity
- Positive predictive value (PPV)
- Negative predictive value (NPV)
- Standard deviation (SD)
- Number needed to treat (NNT)
- Number needed to harm (NNH)

You must also be able to recognize concepts and applications to other statistical measures. However, USMLE will not ask you to do the calculations on these.

These topics include:

- Z-score
- T-score
- Analysis of variance (ANOVA)
- Chi-square
- Standard error of the mean (SEM)

Descriptive Statistics

The mode of a set of data points is the most frequently appearing measurement. For the following set of data points: 1, 2, 3, 4, 8, 8, 8, 20, 100, the mode is 8 because it is the most frequent measurement.

The mean is simply the average of all the data points. By using the earlier set of data points, the mean is 17. This data collection has 9 data points totaling 154.

To calculate the mean, simply divide the total sum (154) by the number of data points (9). In our example, the mean (average) is 17.

The median is the data point halfway between the highest and lowest in the collection of measurements. The median in this data set is 8 because it is the fifth of the 9 data points, which is exactly in the middle.

The range is the numerical distance between the highest value and the lowest. In the sample data set used here, the range is from 1 to 100. Notice that most of the data points in the sample set are under 10. This shows why the median can be a better assessment of groupings of data points than the mean. The mean is 17, but the median is 8. The median is a way of correcting for outliers in data sets.

Now consider the distribution of the same sample set: Is it normally distributed? No, it is not because 7 of 9 data points are under 10. This means the data set is skewed positively toward 100. A normal, or Gaussian, distribution of data forms a bell-shaped graph. In a normal distribution of data points, the mean (average), mode (most frequent measurement), and median (data point in the middle) are the same.

Here is what a normally distributed set of data points looks like when graphed:

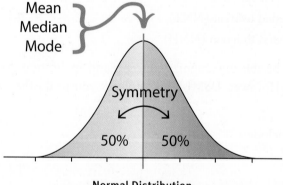

Normal Distribution

As already noted, our set of data (1, 2, 3, 4, 8, 8, 8, 20, 100) is positively "skewed"—that is, skewed to the right—because the single outlier at 100 extends the range of the data set out to the right. (Recall that larger numbers are represented farther to the right on the number line.) When the data in a set are skewed either negatively or positively, the mode, mean, and median are different points.

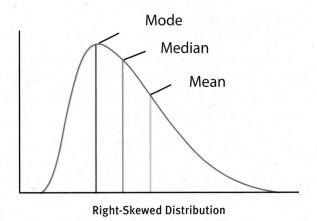

Right-Skewed Distribution

Types of Data

Nominal data is characterized by name only. There is no particular order to the naming, and the names are mutually exclusive. An example of nominal data is blood groups. The groups are A, B, AB, and O. It does not matter what order you put them in. Another example is hepatitis types: hepatitis A, B, C, D, and E. There is likewise no order in which to put hepatitis types, and they are not in a scale. Nor are they divided by another number to create a ratio. A final example is HIV status: HIV-positive status and HIV-negative status are nominal data.

A data set that does occur in a particular order is called ordinal data. Examples of ordinal data are students' class rank and the rank list for the match. Although ordinal data occur in a numerical list, there are no clear breakpoints. For instance, a pain scale is in a sequential order, but there are no clear breakpoints. By contrast, temperature has clear breakpoints at the freezing point and boiling point.

When there are clear breakpoints, or intervals, in a set of data points, you have interval data. Consider CD4: Monitor the CD4 count and stop MAI prophylaxis at 50 CD4 cells, and stop PCP prophylaxis when it rises above 200 CD4 cells. Thus the data for CD4 count has clear breakpoints, or intervals. Speed limit, temperature scales, and T-cell count are other examples of interval data.

Many biomedical markers are recorded as a ratio. Glucose is in milligrams per deciliter. Heart rate is in beats per minute. Hemoglobin is in grams per dL. Ratio data is like interval data in that it also has clear cutoff points. For instance, diabetes is diagnosed with glucose >126 mg/dL.

Incidence and Prevalence

In the context of epidemiology, incidence refers to the rate at which new diseases occur, measured in the number of new cases per unit time. For instance, there are 20,000 new diabetic patients per week in the United States and 750,000 cases of myocardial infarction per year.

Sometimes incidence can account for disease frequency as a ratio with the population, i.e., there is one new case of Creutzfeld-Jakob disease per 1 million people in the population every year or there is one new case of multiple sclerosis for every 1,000 people in the population every year.

Prevalence means the total number of cases in a population, i.e., there are 30 million people in the United States living with diabetes. Incidence and prevalence are directly related: The incidence of 20,000 new diabetes cases per week, or 1 million new cases per year, generates a prevalence of 30 million cases. Medical therapies that lower mortality do not change the incidence of disease. Rather, when there is less disease mortality, patients with a disease live longer and thus increase its prevalence.

Precision, Accuracy, and Reliability

As is defined in statistics, precision describes measurements that are immune from randomness. Precision means that the data points cluster around one point; it is the opposite of scattered or spread out.

Accuracy is equivalent to validity; it is the combination of sensitivity and specificity. If something is true, it is accurate. When people describe a test as the "gold standard," what they are saying is that it is the most accurate test.

Reliability indicates that a test can be reproduced: Reliable measurements will come out the same when repeated. Reliable results do not show a drug is effective on one measurement then ineffective on the next measurement. While a reliable measurement does not drift, it is not necessarily accurate. A reliable measurement comes out the same again and again—but bear in mind that you can have a sample come out reliably wrong. A test might be reliably inaccurate, or a treatment might be reliably ineffective.

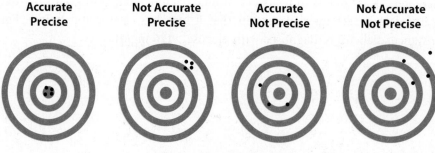

Accuracy Versus Precision

Standard Deviation (SD)

SD is a critical concept for understanding sets of data. It is a must-know concept for Step 3, but you do not have to perform SD calculations on the exam. The numbers used in this section are the real numbers for Step 3 scores.

The mean (average) score on Step 3 was recently 222. If your score is 238, the "deviation" from the mean for your score is 16. By itself, that does not tell you very much, but with additional data its significance becomes evident.

- The mean score on Step 2 CK was recently 240. A 238 was thus below average on Step 2 CK, whereas 238 was above average on Step 3.
- If you look at all the deviations from the mean of all test takers, you can go a step further and mathematically determine the standard of these deviations to tell you how good your score of 238 is on Step 3.

The SD for Step 3 is 16 points. We know that 68% of all scores are within one SD of the mean and 95% of all scores are within two SDs of the mean. Your score of 238 is 16 points above the mean. Here, one SD above the mean indicates that your score is better than 84% of test takers.

The same score on Step 2 CK is below average. The SD for Step 2 is 18 points, so you would have to score a 258 (mean 240 + 18) to be better than 84% of test takers.

Understanding these distinctions is critically important for applicants, who often feel embarrassed because they have a Step 3 score lower than their Step 2 score. The lower score is not a lesser score, however, because the mean is markedly different for each test.

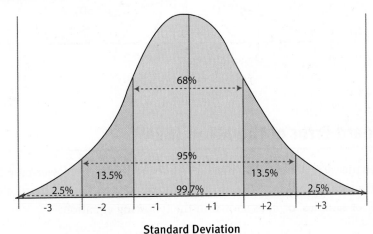

Standard Deviation

For Step 3, a score of 254 is two SDs above the mean (222 + 32). This puts you in the top 2.5% of all test takers. You are a genius! For Step 2, a score of 254 is one SD above average. When data is normally distributed, the following statements are true:

- 1 SD = 68% of scores
- 2 SD = 95% of scores
- 3 SD = 99.7% of scores

40,000 students take USMLE Step 3 each year. The mean score is 222 with an SD of 16. How many students scored above 254?

a. 10,000
b. 6,400
c. 1,000
d. 600
e. Cannot be calculated from the data given

Answer: **C.** There are 1,000 students who scored above 254 on Step 3. 254 is two SDs above the mean. This indicates that 2.5% were above 254. 2.5% of 40,000 is 1,000 students.

Following is a graphical representation of the effect of SD on how data is grouped around the mean. The tallest line on the graph shows the smallest SD. This is because the data clusters around the center point as dictated by the central limit theorem. The flattest line on the graph shows the largest SD. According to the central limit theory, when you collect more data it tends to cluster around the center of the graph.

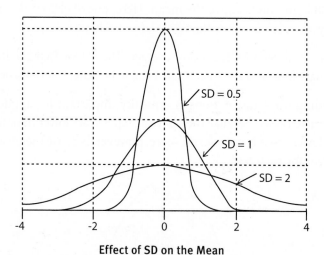

Effect of SD on the Mean

Standard Error of the Mean (SEM)

SEM is a measure of how tightly grouped a set of data is. The lower-case Greek letter σ (sigma) stands for SD. SEM is the SD divided by the square root of the number of samples, or *n*, as shown in the following equation:

$$\sigma_x = \frac{\sigma}{\sqrt{n}}$$

This means that as more samples are added to the data set, the grouping becomes narrower, or more precise.

You do not have to calculate SEM on Step 3. You just have to know that the smaller the SEM, the more precise the data.

Z-Score

The Z-score is a way of showing how far above or below your score is compared with the mean.

If you are one SD above the mean, your Z-score is 1.0. A score of 238 on Step 3, with a mean of 222 and SD 16, gives you a Z-score of +1.0, whereas a score of 254 on Step 3 gives a Z-score of +2.0.

For Step 2 CK, with a mean of 240 and SD 18, getting a 254 on the exam gives a Z-score of +0.78. This is because $\frac{14}{18} = 0.78$. If your Step 3 score is 230 with an SD of 12, this is 8 points or one-half SD above the mean. This means your Z-score is +0.5.

Confidence Intervals (CIs)

CIs give an indication of how precise a given collection of data is. Are the data points centralized around the mean, or are they scattered? The greater the scatter, the less the precision.

Consider the following statement: "On average, patients reported a 25% benefit from the drug." And observe that the following set of data points for this percentage of improvement could be: 0%, 0%, 0%, 100%. The average of these 4 figures is indeed 25%, but the CI ranges from 0.0 to 1.0.

When an outcome has a CI that crosses 1, the results are not significant. Suppose that a drug to prevent stroke from atrial fibrillation has a mean benefit of 30% relative risk (RR) reduction in stroke with a value of 0.7—this looks like a good drug. If the CI is listed as 0.5 to 1.5, however, this study had no validity. Why? Because these measures may mean that the average patient had a 30% reduction in stroke (RR 0.7) while some patients had a 50% increase in the risk of stroke as well (RR 1.5). When the CI crosses 1, it means the results are not precise enough to be useful.

The 95% CI that we use is basically 2 times SEM. SEM is equal to SD divided by the square root of n, or the number of measurements. Consequently, to double the precision of the test, you need to increase the sample size by 4 times. This is because you are dividing by a square root.

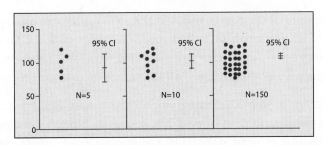

Confidence Intervals

Let's say you have a 95% CI of 4–8 with a mean of 6. This means 95% of measures are between 4 and 8. If you want to tighten this range and cut the CI in half to a range of 5–7, you would need to take 4 times the number of measurements. Both data groups have a mean of 6. The one with the narrower 95% CI is more precise.

Assessing Data for More Than One Group

Correlation Coefficient (*r*)

The correlation coefficient, or *r*, is what you use to give a numerical value to the level of connection or correlation between 2 variables or 2 groups. If there is a very strong correlation, the value is +1. If there is a strong inverse correlation, the value is −1. If there is no correlation, the value is 0.

For example, if you plot diabetes incidence on one axis, there will be a strong correlation over time with the development of stroke, blindness, and myocardial infarction, or +1. If you plot the rate of weight loss, exercise, and glucose control, there will be a strong inverse correlation with the rate of new end-organ damage, or −1.

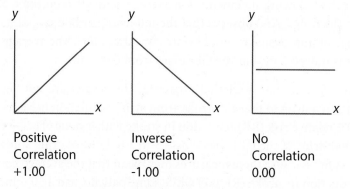

Correlation Coefficient Variation

T-Test (T-Score) and Analysis of Variance (ANOVA)

The t-test and ANOVA are used to assess different groups of data between different sets of data that are in more than one group. T-test is the answer when there are two groups of data to assess. ANOVA is used when there are three or more groups of data to assess.

The other feature of the t-tests and ANOVA is that they can analyze samples that are not in a normal, or bell-shaped, Gaussian distribution: They can assess more irregular data. They are also used when you have only a sample of measurements and do not know all the values in an entire population.

For example, in a Step 3 examination, all the results of all test takers are known and the distribution of data can be clearly plotted. By contrast, in a random screening of water samples in a municipal water supply, those taking samples do not know the water quality all the time, only what is in the samples taken at each particular time. T-test and ANOVA would be used if you were measuring the lead levels in water supplies from two or three or more outlets throughout a city and wanted to compare.

You do not need to be able to do the calculation for t-test and ANOVA for Step 3; you just need to know what they are for.

Chi-Square Test

The chi-square test also compares multiple groups and indicates whether or not they are statistically different. Whereas the t-test answers the question "Are the means between these groups different?", chi-square answers the question "Are these groups related (or not)?"

For example, to assess whether vaccination status is related to contracting a disease, you would use chi-square: People who get the polio vaccine are much less likely to contract polio, which means the polio vaccine is closely related to polio disease. In this case, the group of people who get the vaccine is different from the group of people who do not get the vaccine. A chi-square test is used when the data you are comparing comes in discrete categories.

Study Design, Analysis of Results, and Bias

Randomized Controlled Trial (RCT)

The most accurate type of study in biostatistics is the randomized controlled trial (RCT). Randomization means the persons, animals, or samples are sorted into different arms of the study by computer or a randomly generated list of assignments. This avoids selection bias on the basis of the patient being enrolled, on economic or insurance considerations, or by the investigating physician. For the purposes of sorting, all that matters is that at the end, the same number of patients ends up in each group of the trial.

The RCT is a prospective trial. This avoids many forms of bias. You cannot study the harmful effects of toxins and dangerous interventions prospectively and blindly. You cannot do an RCT on cigarettes where you have half the population smoke tobacco and the other half smoke fake tobacco and then see who develops cancer. You cannot induce diabetes in patients and then measure the rate of death in untreated diabetes. If clear harm or clear benefit is observed before the end of the RCT, an independent data monitoring group stops the study.

Cohort Study

A cohort study is undertaken in order to observe prospectively over time what happens to groups of patients with certain exposures or underlying illnesses. For example, to look at rates of heart and eye disease in those who smoke or have hypertension or diabetes, a study can observe these groups of patients, or "cohorts," over many years.

Cohort studies are observational and prospective. In other words, there is no intervention, and they take a look at a certain period of time. Cohort studies are used to assess the risk of disease. The relative risk calculation is used to assess the results.

Relative Risk (RR)

RR looks at the risk of a disease based on who was exposed to a potential danger in the past. RR for a cohort study starts with an asymptomatic group and calculates the comparative risk of developing disease either with the exposure or without the exposure. For example, RR might assess the risk of heart disease in a diabetic population and compare it with that of a nondiabetic population to see what the risk of developing heart disease is in people who do not have diabetes. RR starts with the risk, then looks for disease.

$$RR = \frac{a/(a+b)}{c/(c+d)} \quad \text{where}$$

	Cancer	
	✔	✗
Exposure ✔	a	b
Exposure ✗	c	d

Relative Risk Calculation

Case Control Studies

A case control study is a retrospective study looking for the odds of a previous exposure on the development of a rare disease manifestation. Case control studies start with people who have a disease and look backward at other groups that are otherwise matched to assess for risks of exposure. Case control studies are subject to recall bias about what people may have been exposed to in the past.

Odds Ratio

Odds ratio assesses case control studies. Odds ratio starts with those who have a disease and then looks for the chance of having an exposure, as shown in the following graph and formula:

	Cancer	
	✔	✗
Exposure ✔	a	b
Exposure ✗	c	d

Odds Ratio

$$\text{Odds ratio} = \frac{\text{Cases exposed/Cases not exposed}}{\text{Controls exposed/Controls not exposed}} = \frac{a/c}{b/d}$$

Selection Bias

Selection bias occurs, for instance, when an investigator chooses less ill patients for the drug side of the trial and sicker patients for the placebo side of the trial—constructing outcomes that make the drug look more successful than it really is. For instance, a trial of antidepressants in which previously suicidal patients or those with psychiatric hospitalization are chosen for the drug side can make the drug look less successful if compared to less depressed persons.

Berkson Bias

Here, hospitalized patients are used as trial subjects instead of the general population. This type of bias is solved by random selection of trial subjects.

Hawthorne Effect

In this type of study bias, those being studied know they are being watched for the effect of a drug or intervention. This problem is solved by using a placebo control and blinding both the investigator and the participants.

Lead-Time Bias

In this bias, early detection is confused with increased survival based on treatment. For instance, early detection of minor cancerous cells such as prostate cancer can make it look like screening was a benefit.

Null Hypothesis and the Meaning of P-Value

Investigation begins with forming a hypothesis. The hypothesis is then accepted or rejected.

The first challenge is with the phrases, "Accepting the null hypothesis" and "Rejecting the null hypothesis" because our tendency is to use the terms prove or disprove in relationship to the hypothesis. When analyzing data, we are supposed to speak of the "probability" of the hypothesis being true or not true.

This is what P-value means. If the P-value is 0.05, this means there is a 95% chance that the alternate hypothesis is true. That is not the same thing as saying "proven" or "disproven." Although we generally acknowledge a P-value of 0.05 as being sufficient, this still means there is a 1 in 20 chance the data is random.

A P-value of 0.05 means that if the study were repeated, there is a 95% chance it would reproduce findings consistent with the current findings. In other words, the same results could be replicated 95% of the time.

The other challenge is using the term null to describe a hypothesis. If we are studying a new medication to help people, the null hypothesis is that there is no benefit of the drug. We want to reject this null hypothesis and say that the new drug works. When studying a new treatment, we start by saying the null hypothesis is that there is no greater difference between the new drug and placebo than would occur by random chance. The alternate hypothesis is that the new drug works. If, after data analysis, the drug works with a P-value of <0.05, we say the null hypothesis is rejected. This is because there is less than a 5% chance that the data is due to random factors. If the P-value is <0.001, there is less than a 1 in 1,000 chance the data are random.

If the null hypothesis is true, the drug is no better at effecting a curve than random chance. The alternative to a null hypothesis is that the drug or test is really effective.

Rejecting the null hypothesis = New drug works

Rejecting the null hypothesis = Alternative hypothesis is true = New drug works

Type I Error and Type II Error

Type I error (or alpha error) is a false-positive result. Here are some examples of type I error:

- Rejecting the null hypothesis when it really is true
- Saying "The new drug works" when it really doesn't
- Accepting the alternate hypothesis when it isn't really true
- Saying there is a statistically significant difference in the data when there really isn't
- Saying a drug or test helps or makes a difference when it really doesn't

Type II error (or beta error) is a false-negative result. Here are some examples of type II error:

- Accepting the null hypothesis when you should reject it
- Saying "The drug doesn't work" when it really does
- Concluding that the drug is ineffective when it actually helps
- Rejecting the alternative hypothesis when it's actually true
- Saying there is no statistically significant difference in the data when there really is

Accepting the null hypothesis = New drug doesn't work

Accepting the null hypothesis = Alternative hypothesis is false = Drug is no different from a placebo

Sensitivity and Specificity

Sensitivity and specificity are qualities of diagnostic tests. The sensitivity and specificity of a test do not change based on the prevalence, or rate of a disease in a community.

Sensitivity = likelihood that a test will detect all the people with the disease

- All the people with a disease should have a positive test.
- A negative result of a sensitive test will exclude that disease in a population.

- If the test is perfectly sensitive, there will be no false negatives.
- A negative test rules a disease out.
- Sensitive: If you have the disease, will you have a positive test?
- $TP/(TP + FN)$ = Sensitivity

Specificity = likelihood that people without a disease are correctly identified as disease-negative

- Those with no disease will have a negative test.
- All the people with a positive test will have the disease.
- A positive specific test means you really have the disease.
- If the test is perfectly specific, there will be no false positives.
- A positive test rules a disease in.
- Specific: If you DON'T have a disease, will you have a negative test?
- $TN/(TN + FP)$ = Specificity

	Disease	
	Present	**Absent**
Test Positive	True positive *TP*	False positive *FP*
Test Negative	False negative *FN*	True negative *TN*

Sensitivity and Specificity

Negative and Positive Predictive Values

Negative predictive value (NPV) and positive predictive value (PPV) change with the prevalence of a disease in a community of a population. NPV and PPV start with the test.

- NPV: If you have a negative test, what is the likelihood you really DON'T have the disease?
- PPV: If you have a positive test, what is the likelihood you really DO have the disease?
- Sensitivity: If you DO have the disease, what is the likelihood you will have a positive test?
- Specificity: If you DON'T have the disease, what is the likelihood you will have a negative test?

	Disease		Measures
	Present	**Absent**	
Test **Positive**	True positive *TP*	False positive *FP*	Positive predictive value (PPV) $\dfrac{TP}{TP + FP}$
Negative	False negative *FN*	True negative *TN*	Negative predictive value (NPV) $\dfrac{TN}{FN + TN}$
Measures	Sensitivity $\dfrac{TP}{TP + FN}$	Specificity $\dfrac{TN}{FP + TN}$	Accuracy $\dfrac{TP + TN}{TP + FP + FN + TN}$

Negative and Positive Predictive Values

The greater the prevalence of a disease, the greater the PPV.

The lesser the prevalence of a disease, the greater the NPV.

Absolute and Relative Risk Reduction

Absolute risk reduction (ARR) is the percentage decrease in the risk of death or disease from a treatment compared with 100% of the people in a population.

For example, the mortality for an anterior wall myocardial infarction (MI) with no treatment is 40%; in other words, 40 out of 100 will die of anterior MI. With the use of angioplasty in the first 90 minutes of arriving at the hospital, however, only 20 out of 100 will die within a year after the MI. Since 40 of 100 (40%) die without angioplasty and 20 of 100 (20%) die with angioplasty, the absolute risk reduction (ARR) is 20%.

This means we only have to perform 5 angioplasties to save one life. The ARR is 20%, or 0.2. The NNT is $\dfrac{1}{\text{ARR}} \times \dfrac{1}{0.2} = 5$.

The practice of medicine also results in harm to patients. For every 100 angioplasty procedures performed, one person has major bleeding leading to death. The rate or attributable risk of fatal complications of angioplasty is 1% or 0.01. This means that for every 100 people we treat, we harm one person. The attributable risk (AR) is 1% or 0.01. The NNH is $\dfrac{1}{\text{AR}}$ or $\dfrac{1}{0.01} = 100$.

Relative risk reduction (RRR) always seems to be a much larger number. Since the risk of death from MI goes from 40% to 20%, the RRR is 50%. Relative to no treatment, the risk of death after the use of angioplasty is half, or 50%.

RRR can be used to exaggerate the effectiveness of medications.

- In patients without heart disease with high LDL, the use of statins may reduce mortality.
- In generally healthy persons whose only abnormality is elevated LDL, there is about a 3% mortality rate from cardiovascular disease over 5 years.
- With the use of statin medications for 5 years, this is reduced to 2% mortality, a difference of 1%; this is an ARR of 1%. In other words, you must treat 100 people for 5 years to save one life.

However, the RRR in this example looks much more impressive. Going from 3% mortality to 2% mortality is an RRR of 33%. And thus the benefit of statins in those without coronary disease or diabetes can be exaggerated by saying, "statins result in a 33% reduction in mortality." Yes, there is a 33% RRR in mortality, but only 1% ARR. Meanwhile, the risk of serious liver toxicity is at least 3%. So, a statin of 33 is the NNH, and 100 is the NNT one person.

Another way to say it is, for every person you help with a statin in the generally healthy hyperlipidemic population, you harm 3 people.

PART 4

Dermatology

Bullous and Blistering Diseases

Pemphigus Vulgaris

This is an autoimmune disease of unclear etiology in which the body becomes, essentially, allergic to its own skin. Antibodies are produced against antigens in the intercellular spaces of the epidermal cells. Its causes are idiopathic; ACE inhibitors; and penicillamine.

- Acts like a burn, because the bullae occur from destruction within the epidermis and so are relatively thin and fragile
- Oral lesions are more specific for vulgaris
- Nikolsky sign is present, the easy removal of skin with just a little pressure (examiner's finger pulls it off like a sheet)
- Lesions that are painful, not pruritic

The **most accurate diagnostic test** is a biopsy of the skin.

Treatment is glucocorticoids such as prednisone. If steroids are ineffective, use azathioprine; mycophenolate; or cyclophosphamide. For refractory pemphigus, use IVIG.

> Nikolsky sign is seen in pemphigus vulgaris, staphylococcal scalded skin syndrome, and toxic epidermal necrolysis.

Bullous Pemphigoid

Pemphigoid can be drug-induced by sulfa drugs and others.

- The fracture of the skin causing the blisters is relatively deep
- Bullae are thicker walled and much less likely to rupture than the bullae of pemphigus vulgaris, so no Nikolsky sign
- Oral lesions are rare
- Because the bullae are tense and intact, the skin is better protected (there is no dressing for skin as good as the skin; hence, there is much less fluid loss and infection is much less likely as compared with pemphigus vulgaris)

The **most accurate diagnostic test** is biopsy with immunofluorescent antibodies.

Treatment is systemic steroids such as prednisone. Alternatives to steroids include tetracycline and erythromycin with nicotinamide (not niacin).

The table compares pemphigus vulgaris and bullous pemphigoid.

> Mortality is much more likely with pemphigus vulgaris and much less likely with bullous pemphigoid.

	Pemphigus Vulgaris	**Bullous Pemphigoid**
Age range	30s and 40s	70s and 80s
Severity	Life-threatening	Resolves
Bullae	Thin and fragile	Thick and intact
Mouth involved	Yes	No
Other features	Nikolsky sign	

Pemphigus Foliaceus

This blistering disease is associated with other autoimmune diseases, or it can be drug-induced by ACE inhibitors or NSAIDs.

Foliaceus is much more superficial than pemphigus vulgaris and bullous pemphigoid, and intact bullae are not seen because they break so easily.

There are no oral lesions.

Diagnostic test is biopsy. Treatment is steroids in the same fashion as pemphigus vulgaris.

Porphyria Cutanea Tarda (PCT)

This is a disorder of porphyrin metabolism resulting in a photosensitivity reaction to an abnormally high accumulation of porphyrins. It is associated with the following:

- Alcoholism/liver disease/chronic hepatitis C (liver disease, e.g., chronic hepatitis or hemochromatosis PCT, is associated with increased liver iron stores)
- OCPs
- Diabetes (25% of patients)

Symptoms include:

- Nonhealing blisters on the sun-exposed parts of the body, such as the backs of the hands and the face
- Hyperpigmentation of the skin
- Hypertrichosis of the face

The **best diagnostic test** is urinary uroporphyrins (will be elevated 2–5× above the coproporphyrins).

Treatment is to stop all alcohol and estrogens; use barrier sun protection; phlebotomy to remove iron (alternative is deferoxamine); and chloroquine to increase the excretion of porphyrins.

Drug Eruptions/Hypersensitivity

Urticaria

Acute urticaria is a hypersensitivity reaction, most often mediated by IgE and mast cell activation, which results in evanescent wheals and hives. It is a type of localized, cutaneous anaphylaxis, but without hypotension and hemodynamic instability. The onset of the wheals and hives is usually within 30 minutes and lasts <24 hours. Itching is prominent.

Urticaria is most often caused by medication (aspirin, NSAIDs, morphine, codeine, penicillins, phenytoin, quinolones); insect bite; food (peanuts, shellfish, tomatoes, strawberries); emotions (occasionally); and contact with latex (in any form)

Chronic urticaria is associated with:

- Pressure on the skin (pressure on the skin resulting in localized urticaria is known as dermatographism)
- Cold
- Vibration

Treatment is as follows:

- H1 antihistamines (older medications i.e., diphenhydramine, hydroxyzine, or cyproheptadine) for severe, acute urticaria
- Systemic steroids for life-threatening reactions
- Newer, nonsedating antihistamines (loratadine, desloratadine, fexofenadine, or cetirizine) for chronic disease
- Desensitization when the trigger cannot be avoided (e.g., a bee sting in a farmer; beta blockers must be stopped prior to desensitization because they inhibit the epinephrine that may be used if there is an anaphylactic reaction)

Morbilliform Rash

Morbilliform rash is a milder version of a hypersensitivity reaction than urticaria. This is the "typical" type of drug reaction and is usually secondary to medications to which the patient is allergic, such as penicillin, sulfa, allopurinol, or phenytoin.

The rash resembles measles; it is a generalized maculopapular eruption that blanches with pressure. The reaction can appear a few days after the exposure and may begin even after the medication has been stopped.

Morbilliform rash is lymphocyte-mediated and is treated with antihistamines. Steroids are rarely necessary.

Erythema Multiforme (EM)

Erythema multiforme is caused by penicillins; phenytoin; NSAIDs; sulfa drugs; or an infection with herpes simplex or mycoplasma.

It presents with target-like lesions, seen especially on the palms and soles. These lesions can also be described as "iris-like." Bullae are not uniformly found. EM of this type usually does not involve mucous membranes.

Treatment is antihistamines and treatment of the underlying infection.

It can be difficult to distinguish SJS from TEN; they may be considered as the same disorder but on different spectrums of severity.

Stevens-Johnson Syndrome and Toxic Epidermal Necrolysis

Both Stevens-Johnson syndrome (SJS) and toxic epidermal necrolysis (TEN) may arise as a hypersensitivity response to the same set of medications (i.e., penicillins, sulfa drugs, NSAIDs, phenytoin, and phenobarbital).

For both SJS and TEN, manage patients in a burn unit. Death occurs from a combination of infection, dehydration, and malnutrition.

- **SJS**
  - Involves <10–15% of total body surface area
  - Overall mortality <5–10%
  - Mucous membrane involvement, most often of the oral cavity and conjunctivae
  - Possible extensive involvement of the respiratory tract, maybe so severe as to require mechanical ventilation
  - Treatments of possible value are IV immunoglobulins, cyclophosphamide, cyclosporine, and thalidomide; steroids have no proven benefit
- **TEN** (most serious version of cutaneous hypersensitivity reaction)
  - Involves 30–100% of total body surface area
  - Overall mortality up to 40–50%
  - Nikolsky sign is present
  - Skin easily sloughs off (similar to staphylococcal scalded skin syndrome; however, TEN is drug-induced, not caused by a toxin coming from an organism)
  - Sepsis is most common cause of death, but prophylactic systemic antibiotics are not indicated
  - **Best diagnostic test** is a skin biopsy
  - Systemic steroids are not an effective treatment and may even reduce chance of survival

Fixed Drug Reaction

This is a localized allergic drug reaction that recurs at precisely the same anatomic site on the skin with repeated drug exposure. Fixed drug reactions are generally round, sharply demarcated lesions that leave a hyperpigmented spot at the site after they resolve.

Fixed drug reactions can be treated with topical steroids.

Erythema Nodosum

This condition presents with painful, red, raised nodules on the anterior surface of the lower extremities. Nodules are tender to palpation; they last about 6 weeks and do not ulcerate.

Erythema nodosum is secondary to a recent infection or inflammatory condition, including the following:

- Pregnancy
- Recent streptococcal infection
- Coccidioidomycosis
- Histoplasmosis
- Sarcoidosis
- Inflammatory bowel disease
- Syphilis
- Hepatitis
- Enteric infections, such as *Yersinia*

Treatment is analgesics and NSAIDs, and treatment of the underlying disease.

Infections

Fungal Infections

Fungal infections include tinea pedis; tinea cruris; tinea corporis; tinea versicolor; tinea capitis; and onychomycosis.

Potassium hydroxide (KOH) test of the skin is the **best initial test**. The leading edge of the lesion on the skin or nails is scraped with a scalpel to remove some of the epithelial cells or some of the nail and hair. KOH has the ability to dissolve the epithelial cells and collagen of the nail but not the fungus.

Culture of the fungus is the **most accurate test.** Molds that grow on the skin (dermatophytes) take up to 6 weeks to grow, even on specialized fungal media. A specific species usually does not need to be isolated in most cases, unless the infection is of the hair or nails.

Treatment includes:

- Oral terbinafine, itraconazole, or efinaconazole for onychomycosis (nail infection) and hair infection (tinea capitis); use 6 weeks for fingernails and 12 weeks for toenails
  - Terbinafine is potentially hepatotoxic so monitor LFTs
  - Efinaconazole is less effective but topical: it can be used in a patient with liver damage
  - Griseofulvin must be used for 6–12 months and has much less antifungal efficacy than terbinafine

- Ketoconazole; clotrimazole; econazole; terbinafine; miconazole; sertaconazole; sulconazole; tolnaftate; or naftifine for all the other fungal infections of the skin that do not involve the hair or nails
  - When used topically, there is no clear difference in efficacy or adverse effects among these agents
  - When used systemically, ketoconazole can cause hepatotoxicity and gynecomastia; this is why ketoconazole is not used for onychomycosis
  - There is no topical form of fluconazole, and when used systemically it is less effective for dermatophytes of the nails

Bacterial Infections

Bacterial infections include impetigo; erysipelas; cellulitis; folliculitis; furuncles; carbuncles; necrotizing fasciitis; and paronychia.

Bacterial skin infections in general (including impetigo, erysipelas, cellulitis, folliculitis, furuncles, and carbuncles) are treated as follows:

- Dicloxacillin, cephalexin, or cefadroxil (the IV equivalent of dicloxacillin is oxacillin or nafcillin and the IV equivalent of cefadroxil is cefazolin)
- With penicillin allergy but the reaction is only a rash: use cephalosporins (there is far less than 1% cross-reaction between penicillins and cephalosporins, i.e., estimated to be 0.1%.)
- With penicillin allergy but the reaction is anaphylaxis: do not use cephalosporins but rather macrolides (erythromycin, azithromycin, clarithromycin) or the newer fluoroquinolones (levofloxacin, gatifloxacin, moxifloxacin)
  - Ciprofloxacin will not adequately cover the skin.
  - Vancomycin is only for IV use for skin infections; oral vancomycin is not absorbed and is used only for *Clostridium difficile* intestinal infection
  - Consider IV vancomycin if you suspect methicillin-resistant *Staphylococcus aureus* (MRSA) (i.e., those in a nursing home or in-patient for a long time); the oral alternative would be linezolid or TMP/SMX

Impetigo

This is a superficial bacterial infection of the skin limited largely to the epidermis and not spreading below the dermal-epidermal junction. The infection is described as "weeping," "oozing," "honey-colored," or "draining." It is seen in warm, humid conditions, particularly when there is poverty and crowding of children. It is both contagious and autoinoculable. Impetigo can cause glomerulonephritis, but it will not cause rheumatic fever.

Impetigo is more often caused by Staphylococcus but is sometimes caused by Streptococcus pyogenes, also known as group A *Streptococcus*.

Treatment is a topical antibiotic, such as mupirocin. If not effective, use an antistaphylococcal oral antibiotic.

Erysipelas

Erysipelas involves both the dermis and epidermis and is most commonly caused by group A Streptococcus (pyogenes). Erysipelas is more likely than other bacterial infections to result in the following:

- Fever, chills, and bacteremia
- Bright red, angry, swollen appearance to the face

Treatment is as follows:

- Use the systemic oral or IV antibiotics previously described
- If culture confirms the organism as *Streptococcus,* use penicillin G or ampicillin

Cellulitis

This is a bacterial infection of the dermis and subcutaneous tissues with *Staph* and *Strep.*

Cellulitis is treated with the antibiotics previously described, based on the severity of the disease.

- If there is fever, hypotension, or signs of sepsis (or if oral therapy has not been effective), give IV therapy.
- Oxacillin, nafcillin, or cefazolin is the best therapy; oral cephalexin is the microbiologic equivalent of cefazolin. Treatment failure needs a MRSA drug such as vancomycin. Dalbavancin and oritavancin last for 1–2 weeks after a single IV dose.
- Treatment is generally empiric because injecting and aspirating sterile saline for a specific microbiological diagnosis has only a 20% sensitivity.
- For minor skin infections with MRSA, use TMP/SMX, doxycycline, or clindamycin.

Folliculitis, Furuncles, and Carbuncles

These 3 disorders represent different degrees of severity of staphylococcal infection occurring around a hair follicle.

- Occasionally, folliculitis can occur from *Pseudomonas* in those who contract it in a whirlpool or hot tub.
- As folliculitis worsens from a simple infection superficially around the hair follicle, it becomes a small collection of infected material known as a furuncle.
- When several furuncles become confluent into a single lesion, it becomes known as a carbuncle, essentially a localized skin abscess that must be drained.
- Folliculitis is rarely tender, while furuncles and carbuncles are often extremely tender.

Treatment is as follows:

- Topical mupirocin for folliculitis
- Systemic antistaphylococcal antibiotics, e.g., dicloxacillin or cefadroxil, for furuncles and carbuncles

Necrotizing Fasciitis

This is an extremely severe, life-threatening infection of the skin. It starts as a cellulitis that dissects into the fascial planes of the skin. *Streptococcus* and *Clostridia* are the most common organisms involved, because they produce a toxin that worsens the damage to the fascia. Without adequate therapy, mortality is 80%.

Necrotizing fasciitis presents as follows:

- Very high fever
- Portal of entry into the skin
- Pain out of proportion to the superficial appearance
- Bullae
- Palpable crepitus

Diabetes increases the risk of developing fasciitis.

Diagnostic tests include elevated CPK and x-ray/CT/MRI showing air in the tissue or necrosis. However, since those methods lack both sensitivity and specificity, the best way to confirm diagnosis—and the mainstay of therapy—is surgical debridement.

Treatment is vancomycin or daptomycin + clindamycin + a beta lactam/beta lactamase + a beta lactam/beta lactamase combination medication:

- Ampicillin/sulbactam
- Ticarcillin/clavulanate
- Piperacillin/tazobactam
- Or a carbapenem

If there is a definite diagnosis of group A Streptococcus (pyogenes), then the treatment is clindamycin and penicillin. IVIG helps everyone.

Paronychia

This is an infection loculated under the skin surrounding a nail.

It is generally treated with a small incision to allow drainage and antistaphylococcal antibiotics as previously described.

Viral Infections

Herpes Simplex

Herpes simplex infections of the genitals are characterized by multiple, painful vesicles. They are usually obvious by examination, and you should proceed directly to therapy with acyclovir, famciclovir, or valacyclovir.

> If presented with an obvious clinical case with **crepitus**, pain, high fever, and a portal of entry and asked "What is the best initial step?", select **surgery**, not a diagnostic test such as x-ray.

> Clindamycin decreases toxin production in necrotizing fasciitis.

> For **necrotizing fasciitis**, treat with:
>
> Vancomycin **or** daptomycin
>
> **and**
>
> Carbapenem **or** beta lactam/lactamase
>
> **and**
>
> Clindamycin

If the diagnosis is not clear or the lesions have become confluent into an ulcer, the best initial test is a Tzanck smear.

- Similar in technique to a Pap smear; a scraping of the lesion is immediately placed on a slide and sprayed with fixative
- Nonspecific in that it will only determine that the infection is in the herpes virus family
- Detects multinucleated giant cells

The **most accurate test** is PCR, more accurate than viral culture.

Treatment is oral acyclovir, famciclovir, or valacyclovir.

- Topical acyclovir has extremely little efficacy.
- Topical penciclovir has some utility for oral herpetic lesions, but it must be used every 2 hours.
- Treat acyclovir-resistant herpes with foscarnet.

> The most common wrong answer is serology. Serology is not useful in the diagnosis of an acute herpes infection.

Herpes Zoster/Varicella

Chickenpox is primarily a disease of children. It is generally not treated with antivirals. If the child is immunocompromised or the primary infection occurs in an adult, then use acyclovir, valacyclovir, or famciclovir.

Complications of varicella are pneumonia; hepatitis; dissemination; and encephalitis.

Outbreaks of shingles, also known as dermatomal herpes zoster, occur more frequently in the elderly and those with defects of the lymphocytic portion of the immune system, such as leukemia, lymphoma, or HIV, or those on steroids. The vesicles are 2–3 mm in size at all stages of development and are on an erythematous base.

Although Tzanck prep and PCR are useful diagnostic tests, they are generally not necessary because little else will produce a band of vesicles in a dermatomal distribution besides herpes zoster. PCR is more accurate than viral culture. The **most accurate test** is PCR of a swab of the lesions.

Treatment is as follows:

- Steroids: not clearly beneficial, although the best evidence for their efficacy is in elderly patients with severe pain
- Rapid administration of acyclovir has best efficacy for reducing the risk of postherpetic neuralgia
- Gabapentin (most effective analgesic specifically for postherpetic neuralgia); tricyclic antidepressants; and topical capsaicin to manage the pain
- Nonimmune adults exposed to chickenpox should receive varicella zoster immune globulin within 96 hours of exposure for it to be effective

Sexually Transmitted Diseases (STDs)

Human Papillomavirus (HPV)

Warts caused by HPV, or condylomata acuminata, present as heaped up, translucent, white or flesh-colored lesions on mucous surfaces.

- No form of testing routinely necessary
- No definite benefit to biopsy, scraping, smears, and serology
- No benefit to routine subtyping of specific strain of papillomavirus

Treatment can be approached in the following ways:

- Mechanical removal: cryotherapy with liquid nitrogen, laser removal, or trichloroacetic acid to melt away the warts
- Imiquimod, a local immunostimulant that sloughs off the warts after several weeks; resolution is slower but there is neither damage to the surrounding normal tissue nor pain
- Podophyllin resin (but potentially teratogenic and should be scrupulously avoided in pregnancy)

Syphilis

Both primary and secondary syphilis present mainly with cutaneous disorders.

- Primary syphilis
  - Chancre is an ulceration with heaped-up indurated edges that is painless most of the time
  - **Best initial test** is a darkfield examination; this is because there is a false-negative rate of 25% for both the VDRL and RPR (in other words, these serologic tests need several weeks to become positive, and they are only 75% sensitive in primary syphilis)
- Secondary syphilis
  - Presents with a generalized copper-colored, maculopapular rash that is particularly intense on the palms and soles of the feet
  - Other manifestations are dermatologic as well: the mucous patch, alopecia areata, and condylomata lata
  - VDRL and RPR tests have nearly 100% sensitivity

Treatment for both primary and secondary syphilis is a single intramuscular dose of penicillin. For penicillin allergy, give oral doxycycline for 2 weeks.

Scabies and Pediculosis

Scabies

Scabies involves primarily the web spaces of the hands and feet but can also cause pruritic lesions around the penis and breast. The head is often spared. Itching can be extreme.

Because *Sarcoptes scabiei* is quite small, all that can be seen with the naked eye is the burrows and excoriations around small pruritic vesicles.

Scabies is confirmed by scraping out the organism after mineral oil is applied to a burrow.

Treatment is permethrin (lindane has equal efficacy but greater toxicity). An alternative (particularly for Norwegian scabies) is oral ivermectin.

Pediculosis (Lice and Crabs)

Pediculosis tends to include the head and is easily transmitted by sharing hats and hairbrushes. Both lice and crabs have an enormously high rate of transmission through sexual contact, with 90% transmission from a single contact.

Because pediculosis is caused by a much larger organism, scraping is not necessary. The organisms can be readily seen attached to hair-bearing areas, particularly under magnification. They are sometimes rust-colored from their ingestion of blood.

Treatment is permethrin. Lindane has equal efficacy but is more toxic. An alternative is over-the-counter pyrethrins.

Pediculosis	Scabies
• Larger • Hair-bearing areas, e.g., pubic area or axilla • Visible on the surface	• Small • Burrows in web spaces • Scrape and magnify
Treat with permethrin, pyrethrins, or lindane.	Treat with permethrin, lindane, or ivermectin.

Lyme Disease

More than 85% of patients who have Lyme disease develop a rash, usually 7–10 days after the tick bite.

The rash must have the following characteristics:

• Erythematous with central clearing
• At least 5 cm in diameter

Immunocompromised patients (e.g., those with HIV) are vulnerable to an extremely exuberant form of scabies with severe crusting known as "Norwegian scabies."

This rash is so characteristic of Lyme that it is more important than serological testing in terms of confirming a diagnosis.

If the rash is described, go straight to therapy with oral doxycycline, amoxicillin, or cefuroxime.

Without treatment, 70% of patients will develop joint disease. A smaller number will develop neurological or cardiac disease.

Toxin-Mediated Diseases

Toxic Shock Syndrome (TSS)

TSS is caused by *Staphylococcus* attached to a foreign body. Nasal packing, retained sutures, or any other form of surgical material retained in the body can promote the growth of the type of *Staph* that produces the toxin.

There is no single diagnostic test, so cases are a matter of definition as follows:
- Fever >38.9°C (>102.0°F)
- Systolic blood pressure <90 mm Hg
- Desquamative rash
- Vomiting
- Involvement of mucous membranes of the eye, mouth, and genitals

In addition, toxic shock is a systemic disease that:
- Raises creatinine, CPK, and LFTs
- Lowers platelet count
- Can cause CNS dysfunction, e.g., confusion

Treatment is vigorous fluid resuscitation; pressors (e.g., dopamine); and anti-staphylococcal medication (e.g., oxacillin, nafcillin, cefazolin). Since you do not know who has methicillin- (oxacillin-) resistant strains, add vancomycin. Clindamycin, which decreases toxin production, is often combined with a beta lactam antibiotic or vancomycin. If the exam question includes "Add IVIG" in the answer choices, then you should add IVIG.

Staphylococcal Scalded Skin Syndrome (SSSS)

SSSS is mediated by a toxin from *Staphylococcus*. It presents with loss of the superficial layers of the epidermis in sheets and Nikolsky sign.

SSSS differs from other conditions as follows:
- Presents with normal blood pressure and no involvement of the liver, kidney, bone marrow, or CNS (unlike TSS)
- Is caused by an infection (unlike TEN, which is caused by drug toxicity)
- Only splits off the superficial granular layer of skin and is not a full thickness split (as in TEN)

Treatment is management in a burn unit, use oxacillin, nafcillin, or another antistaphylococcal antibiotic such as cefazolin or vancomycin. IVIG is not essential in SSSS.

Anthrax

Bacillus anthracis is usually a cutaneous infection acquired from contact with infected livestock. It is an occupational hazard of wool sorters. Bioterrorism is also a potential source. A papule appears that later becomes inflamed and develops central necrosis that is black in color; hence the name anthrax, which is the Greek word for "coal." Of untreated cases, 20% are fatal.

Diagnosis is confirmed with Gram stain and culture of the lesion. Treatment is ciprofloxacin or doxycycline.

Malignant and Premalignant Diseases

Benign Lesions

The predominant way to distinguish between a benign and malignant lesion is by the shape and color of the lesion. Benign lesions, such as the junctional or intradermal nevus, have the following characteristics:

- Do not grow in size
- Smooth, regular borders
- Diameter usually <1 cm
- Homogenous in color, and the color remains constant

The **best diagnostic test** is biopsy. Benign lesions only need to be removed for cosmetic purposes.

Melanoma

These malignant lesions grow in size, have irregular borders, are uneven in shape, and have inconsistent coloring.

Biopsy diagnosis is best performed with a full thickness sample, because **tumor thickness is by far the most important prognostic factor**.

Treatment of melanoma is excision. Do sentinel node biopsy; if cancer is in it, give chemotherapy.

- All patients with melanoma should have their tumors assessed for specific mutations, which will allow targeted therapy; many of these agents can be effective against the frequent brain metastases of melanoma.
- Ipilimumab, vemurafenib, and dabrafenib target the V600 mutation in the BRAF gene.
- Cobimetinib and trametinib are inhibitors of mitogen extracellular kinase (MEK). MEK inhibitors are used in combination with BRAF inhibitors.
- Nivolumab and pembrolizumab restore programmed cell death, or apoptosis.

Ipilimumab: cytotoxic
T-lymphocyte drug

- Interferon provides no systemic benefit with melanoma. Targeted therapy with a BRAF inhibitor in combination with surgery and possible radiation is the right answer.
- Talimogene is a genetically modified herpes virus that attacks unresectable melanoma.

Seborrheic Keratosis

This is a benign condition with hyperpigmented lesions occurring in the elderly with a "stuck on" appearance. They appear most commonly on the face, shoulders, chest, and back. They have no malignant potential.

Removal of the lesions is done with liquid nitrogen or curettage only for cosmetic purposes. Seborrheic keratosis has no relationship to actinic keratosis or seborrheic dermatitis.

Actinic Keratosis

Actinic keratoses are precancerous lesions occurring on sun-exposed areas of the body in older persons. They occur more often in those with light skin color. Although they are usually asymptomatic, they can be tender to the touch.

Therapy includes sunscreen to prevent progression and recurrence. Lesions should be removed with cryotherapy, topical 5 fluorouracil (5FU), imiquimod, topical retinoic acid derivatives, or even curettage.

Squamous Cell Carcinoma

Of all skin cancers, 10–25% are squamous cell. Squamous cell carcinoma develops on sun-exposed skin surfaces in elderly patients. It is particularly common on the lip, where the carcinogenic potential of tobacco is multiplicative. Ulceration of the lesion is common. Metastases are rare (only 3–7% of patients).

Diagnosis is with a biopsy, and treatment is surgical removal.

Basal Cell Carcinoma

Of all skin cancers, 65–80% are basal cell (rate of metastases <0.1%). Basal cell carcinoma has a shiny or "pearly" appearance.

Diagnosis is confirmed by shave or punch biopsy.

Treatment is surgical removal. The greatest cure rate is with Mohs microsurgery; instant frozen sections are done to determine when enough tissue has been removed to give a clean margin.

Kaposi Sarcoma

These are purplish lesions found on the skin predominantly of patients with HIV and CD4 count <100. Human herpes virus 8 is the causative organism.

Treatment is ART to raise the CD4 count. When this is not effective, the specific chemotherapy for Kaposi sarcoma is liposomal adriamycin and vinblastine.

Scaling Disorders (Eczema)/Papulosquamous Dermatitis

Psoriasis

Silvery scales develop on the extensor surfaces. Psoriasis can be local or enormously extensive. Nail pitting is a common accompaniment. A Koebner phenomenon is the development of lesions to the site of an epidermal injury.

All patients should use an emollient, such as petroleum jelly or mineral oil. Salicylic acid is used to remove heaped-up collections of scaly material so the other therapies can make contact.

- For localized disease, use topical steroids.
- For severe disease, add coal tar or anthralin derivatives.
- To avoid the long-term use of steroids (can cause skin atrophy) and coal tars (messy), one can substitute a topical vitamin D and vitamin A derivative (oftentimes calcipotriene and tazarotene).
- If >30% of the body surface area is involved (and topical therapy cannot control disease), use ultraviolet light, the most rapid way to control extensive disease.
- Apremilast is a phosphodiesterase inhibitor that helps psoriasis.
- For the most severe, widespread, and progressive forms of the disease, consider methotrexate; however, this has the highest toxicity and may cause liver fibrosis.

The newest therapies are immunomodulatory biological agents, such as alefacept, efalizumab, etanercept, and infliximab.

IL-17 inhibitors (secukinumab, ixekizumab) have good results when TNF inhibitors don't work.

Xerosis/Asteatotic Dermatitis

Xerosis and dry skin are managed with humidifiers and emollients such as petroleum jelly or mineral oil. When skin is especially inflamed, topical steroids can be used briefly.

Atopic Dermatitis

This extraordinarily pruritic disorder presents with high IgE levels, and red, itchy plaques of the flexor surfaces.

Treatment involves preventive therapy, because patients are very sensitive to drying: keep the skin moist with emollients, avoid hot water and drying soap, and wear only cotton.

Active disease is treated with the following:

- Topical steroids
- Antihistamines
- Coal tars
- Phototherapy
- Antistaphylococcal antibiotics for impetiginization of the skin
- Topical immunosuppressants, such as tacrolimus and pimecrolimus, to reduce dependence on steroid use
- Crisaborole, a topical phosphodiesterase inhibitor, for psoriasis
- Doxepin (topical tricyclic) for pruritus

Every effort should be made to avoid scratching.

Seborrheic Dermatitis

An oversecretion of sebaceous material, as well as a hypersensitivity reaction to a superficial fungal organism, Pityrosporum ovale, underlies seborrheic dermatitis. These patients present with "dandruff," which may also occur on the face. Scaly, greasy, flaky skin is found on a red base on the scalp, around the eyebrows, and in the nasolabial fold.

Treatment is a low-potency topical steroid (e.g., hydrocortisone); topical antifungal (e.g., ketoconazole or selenium sulfide); and zinc pyrithione used as a shampoo.

Stasis Dermatitis

This is a hyperpigmentation that is built up from hemosiderin in the tissue. It occurs over a long period from venous incompetence of the lower extremities leading to the microscopic extravasation of blood in the dermis. Some respond to steroids.

Prevention of progression is with elevation of the legs and lower extremity support hose.

Contact Dermatitis

This is a hypersensitivity reaction to soaps, detergents, latex, sunscreens, or neomycin over the area of contact. Jewelry is a frequent cause, as is contact with the metal nickel from belt buckle and wristwatches. It can present as linear streaked vesicles, particularly when it is caused by poison ivy.

Diagnostic testing is patch testing.

Treatment is identification of the causative agent, then antihistamines and topical steroids.

Pityriasis Rosea

This is a pruritic eruption that begins with a "herald patch" 70–80% of the time. It is erythematous and salmon colored and looks like secondary syphilis, except that it spares the palms and soles, has a herald patch, and the VDRL/RPR is negative. The lesions on the back appear in a pattern like a Christmas tree (if the observer is especially imaginative).

It is mild and self-limited and usually resolves in 8 weeks without scarring. Treatment for lesions that are very itchy is topical steroids.

Acne

Pustules and cysts occur and rupture, releasing free fatty acids that cause further irritation. The contributing organism is *Propionibacterium acnes*. The discharge, although purulent, is odorless.

Treatment depends on the extent of the disease.

- **Mild disease:** topical antibiotic (clindamycin, erythromycin, sulfacetamide) plus the bacteriostatic agent benzoyl peroxide and dapsone gel. If those agents cannot control the load of bacterial locally, use topical retinoids.
- **Moderate disease:** benzoyl peroxide, plus a retinoid (tazarotene, tretinoin, adapalene). Adapalene is the only retinoid that does not require a prescription.
- **Severe cystic acne:** oral antibiotic (minocycline, tetracycline, clindamycin, isotretinoin) but use great caution because oral retinoic acid derivatives are strong teratogens. Do a urine pregnancy test and **make sure women of childbearing age are taking oral contraceptives.**

Rosacea

The inflammatory pustules of rosacea can be confused with acne; to differentiate, look for redness of the nose and cheeks in rosacea.

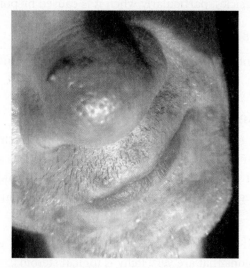

Rosacea (source: WikiCommons)

Treat with:

- UV light and laser
- Topical brimonidine (alpha-2 agonist) to constrict vessels
- Topical metronidazole, azelaic acid (an anti-inflammatory also used for acne), and oral doxycycline
- Ivermectin cream

PART 5

Surgery

Contributing author Niket Sonpal, MD

Trauma

Airway

Establishing and securing the airway is always the first step in management in any patient with acute trauma or change in mental status. Altered mental status is the most common indication for intubation in the trauma patient (unconscious patients can't maintain their airways). The exam will want you to know the best step in securing an airway.

- Orotracheal intubation (**best way to secure an airway**)
- If there is trauma with cervical spine injury, orotracheal intubation can still be used with manual cervical immobilization (**best answer** is a flexible bronchoscope)
- If there is extensive facial trauma and bleeding into the airway (listen for gurgling sounds), the **best answer** is cricothyroidotomy.

Breathing

Always check oxygen saturation. If saturation <90%, obtain an arterial blood gas (ABG) and determine likely causes of hypoxia based on the history.

> Normal PCO_2 = 40
> Normal bicarb = 24

A 55-year-old woman presents with profuse watery diarrhea of 4 days' duration and syncope 2 hours ago. She was recently treated with antibiotics for an uncomplicated UTI. She has 20 bowel movements per day without blood and feels light-headed. The patient does not remember losing consciousness and denies any postsyncope symptoms. Placement of Foley catheter in the ED yields no urine output. What is the most likely diagnosis?

a. Septic shock
b. Anaphylactic shock
c. Hemorrhagic shock
d. Hypovolemic shock
e. Cardiogenic shock

Answer: **D.** Common findings in a patient with hypovolemic shock are unstable vital signs; organ dysfunction such as low urine output; cold, clammy extremities; and light-headedness. This patient is in hypovolemic shock caused by intravascular volume loss. The lack of volume decreases the cardiac output (CO) because of lack of preload. The systemic vascular resistance (SVR) increases in an effort to compensate for the diminished cardiac output and maintain perfusion to the vital organs.

Circulation

Chest Trauma

Circulatory disturbances in the setting of trauma may have one of 3 major causes. On the exam, you will need to determine the likely cause quickly so that prompt therapy can be instituted.

- Hemorrhagic shock (**most common type of hypovolemic shock**)
  - Look for a source of bleeding; a large volume of blood may be lost in abdomen or thigh following diaphyseal fracture of the femur
  - In hypovolemic shock, right atrial pressure, pulmonary capillary wedge pressure, cardiac index, and mixed venous saturation are decreased; systemic vascular resistance is the only parameter that is elevated
- Pericardial tamponade involves the following:
  - Perform pericardiocentesis immediately; if unsuccessful, proceed with pericardial window
  - Electrical alternans on EKG
  - Pulsus paradoxus on vital signs
- Tension pneumothorax
  - Look for respiratory distress, tracheal deviation, absent breath sounds, and hyperresonance to percussion
  - Place a large-bore needle or IV catheter immediately into the pleural space at the second intercostal space; then place a chest tube
  - Never wait for a chest x-ray for diagnosis.

> Pericardial tamponade and tension pneumothorax can both result from thoracic trauma. Distended neck veins or a high central venous pressure (CVP) are seen.

> Do not be distracted by head trauma or dilated pupils in a hypotensive trauma patient. Intracranial bleed is never the cause of hypotensive shock.
>
> The first step in management is to identify and control the site of bleeding.

Basic Science Correlate

Must-know formulas for the USMLE Step 3:

Cardiac output = Stroke volume × Heart rate

and

Stroke volume = End-diastolic volume – End-systolic volume

thus:

Cardiac output = (End-diastolic volume – End-systolic volume) × Heart rate

and

Total peripheral resistance = Mean arterial pressure – Mean venous pressure

therefore:

Blood pressure = Cardiac output × Total peripheral resistance

Abdominal Trauma

A 24-year-old man presents to the ED with 3 stab wounds to the abdomen. He was intubated in the field for airway protection. Blood pressure is 70/30 mm Hg and pulse 140/min. On examination, 3 penetrating wounds covered by abdominal pressure pads are noted. What is the best next step in management?

a. Direct pressure to the abdomen
b. Abdominal x-ray
c. IV fluids
d. IV antibiotics
e. Obtain consent for surgery

Answer: C. This patient is in hemorrhagic shock and requires immediate resuscitation. Of the choices listed, the best next step is IV fluids after obtaining venous access. The best form of venous access is 2 large-bore IVs in the periphery and/or central venous access. Applying direct pressure to the abdomen does not treat the underlying cause. Getting an abdominal x-ray will take too long with this rate of blood loss. IV antibiotics may be needed later, but stabilizing blood pressure is the more urgent need now. Surgical consent is implied in a life-threatening emergency in which a patient cannot communicate his wishes.

Basic Science Correlate

Hemodynamic measurements in hemorrhagic shock:

- Pulmonary capillary wedge pressure is decreased.
- Cardiac output is decreased.
- Mixed venous oxygen saturation is decreased.
- Systemic vascular resistance is increased.

Management of circulatory disturbances in cases of abdominal trauma involves the following:

- Apply direct local pressure when site is visible (e.g., extremity)
- Fluid resuscitation (**best next step if patient is hemodynamically unstable**)
- Do several things at once in preparation for immediate exploratory laparotomy:
  - Set up 2 large-gauge IV lines
  - Give fluids and blood products
  - Type and screen
  - Insert Foley catheter
  - Administer IV antibiotics
- If surgery isn't needed (e.g., blunt trauma), fluid resuscitation is the first step in management and is also diagnostic (if patient responds promptly, he is probably no longer bleeding).

> Intraosseous cannulation in the proximal tibia is used in children (generally age <6). Give an initial bolus of Ringer lactate at 20 mL/kg of body weight.

A 9-year-old child is brought to the ED by his school teacher. The child is in severe respiratory distress, has difficulty swallowing, has swollen eyes and lips, and is unable to speak. The child's teacher says he was throwing rocks at a beehive outside during recess. His blood pressure is 88/40 mm Hg and heart rate is 120 beats/min. Physical exam reveals bilateral wheezing and tachycardia. What is the most likely diagnosis?

a. Anaphylactic shock
b. Sepsis
c. Pulmonary embolus
d. Myocardial infarction
e. Medication side effect

Answer: **A.** The acute onset of an illness involving the skin and mucosa combined with respiratory compromise, reduced blood pressure, and subsequent end-organ dysfunction is anaphylactic shock. The trigger for this child is most likely a bee sting. It cannot be sepsis as there is no fever and onset was too sudden. Pulmonary embolism would have a normal lung exam, and the odds are against a child with this clinical picture having a myocardial infarction. He requires urgent intramuscular epinephrine and observation.

Vasomotor Shock

Vasomotor shock is the cause of hypotension and tachycardia in patients who are warm and flushed (rather than pale and cold). Look for a history of medication use (e.g., penicillin that may have triggered a penicillin allergy), spinal anesthesia, or exposure to allergen (e.g., bee sting).

> ### Basic Science Correlate
>
> On exposure to a foreign substance:
> - IgE binds to the antigen, forming an antigen-antibody complex.
> - This complex activates the high-affinity receptor for the Fc region of immunoglobulin E (FcεRI), leading to mast cell and basophil degranulation and the release of inflammatory mediators such as histamine.
> - These mediators cause vasodilation, bronchoconstriction, tachycardia, and swelling.

The first step in management is to administer vasoconstrictors and fluids.

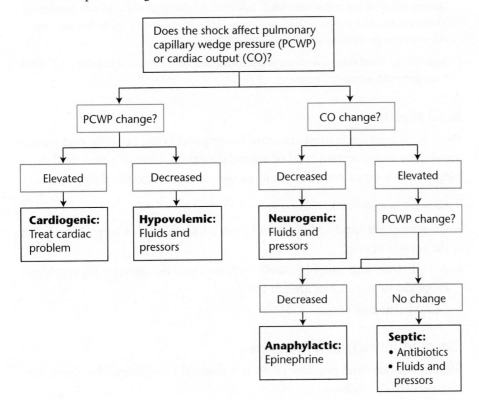

Trauma to Localized Sites

All patients with damage to internal organs need to go to the OR. If the case describes an object embedded in the patient, never remove it at the scene of the accident or in the ER. All impaled objects are to be removed in the OR under a controlled setting.

Head Trauma

A man was hit over the head with a baseball bat during a mugging. He has a scalp laceration and a linear skull fracture on CT scan. He denies loss of consciousness. There are no neurological signs on exam. Is surgery indicated?

Answer: No surgical intervention is needed for an asymptomatic head injury with a closed skull fracture (no overlying wound) alone. The next step in management is to clean any lacerations.

A woman was hit over the head with a baseball bat during a mugging. She has a scalp laceration, and a comminuted, depressed fracture is seen on CT scan. She denies loss of consciousness. There are no neurological signs on exam. Is surgery indicated?

Answer: Surgery (repair or craniotomy) is considered for comminuted or depressed skull fracture, even if the patient is asymptomatic. Send the patient to the OR.

Give **tetanus toxoid** and **prophylactic antibiotics** to all patients with open skull fractures.

A man is hit over the head with a baseball bat during a mugging. He reports "being out of it for a few seconds," but then he came to without any symptoms. There are no neurological signs on exam. What is the next step in management? He wants to go home—what will you tell him?

Answer: For head trauma and loss of consciousness, the first step is to order a CT of the head and neck without contrast.

Basal Skull Fracture

Basal skull fracture is most common in temporal bone. Look for ecchymosis around the eyes (raccoon eyes) or behind the ear (Battle sign); clear fluid dripping from the ear or nose (CSF leak); or hemotympanum (bleeding in the ear).

Treatment is as follows:

- CT scan of the head and neck (will show a basal skull fracture). X-ray is not the correct answer.
- A CSF leak will stop by itself and requires no specific management. Prophylactic antibiotics are not indicated.
- Facial palsy may occur.

Elevated Intracranial Pressure

Elevated intracranial pressure (ICP) is a medical emergency. The classic history proceeds as follows:

1. Briefly depressed consciousness after head trauma
2. Improvement
3. Progressive drowsiness

Do not think about doing a lumbar puncture without first getting a head CT. If lumbar puncture is done on a person with increased ICP, you will herniate the brain, kill the patient, and fail the exam.

Diagnostic testing includes:

- Gradual dilatation of one pupil and a decreasing responsiveness to light indicates clot expansion on the ipsilateral hemisphere (important sign)
- Head CT: look for midline shift or dilated ventricles

Basic Science Correlate

Hyperventilation causes vasoconstriction and decreased blood volume in the brain, lowering ICP.

Treatment is head elevation; hyperventilation; hypertonic saline; barbiturates; and sedation/hypothermia to lower oxygen demand. Avoid fluid overload. Use mannitol to reduce cerebral perfusion.

> **Basic Science Correlate**
>
> Mannitol is filtered by the glomeruli but not reabsorbed from the renal tubule. The result is decreased water and Na+ reabsorption, which subsequently leads to decreased extracellular fluid volume.

Lowering ICP is not the ultimate goal; preserving brain perfusion is. Systemic hypotension or excessive cerebral vasoconstriction may be counterproductive.

A 55-year-old woman presents with a droopy left eyelid. She says she first noticed it about 2 months ago. She denies headache, fever, and neck pain. A head CT without contrast shows no bleed. On physical examination the patient has a ptosis of the left eye and the pupils are unequal in size. What is the most likely diagnosis?

a. Third cranial nerve palsy
b. Normal variant
c. Diabetic neuropathy
d. Myasthenia gravis
e. Stroke

Answer: **A.** The symptoms most likely result from third cranial nerve palsy caused by a posterior communicating artery aneurysm. The most common findings are anisocoria, palsy of the rectus muscles of the eyes, and weakness of levator palpebrae superioris. MRI of the brain with angiography is the best initial test in a patient who presents with isolated third cranial nerve findings. Embolization through endovascular repair has been found to be superior to surgical clipping and is the most appropriate therapy.

General Surgery

Acute Abdomen

The main causes of an acute abdomen are perforation, obstruction, inflammatory reaction/infection, and ischemia.

Nonsurgical causes of an acute abdomen are the following:

- Myocardial infarction, acute pericarditis
- Lower lobe pneumonia, pulmonary infarction
- Hepatitis, GERD
- DKA, adrenal insufficiency
- Sickle cell crisis
- Acute porphyria

When is **medical treatment** the answer?

- When there is pancreatitis, cholangitis, or ruptured ovarian cyst
- Things that can mimic an acute abdomen include lower lobe pneumonia (look for infiltrate on chest x-ray), myocardial ischemia (look for EKG changes), and pulmonary embolism (suspect this in any immobilized patient)

Perforation

GI Perforation

GI perforation involves acute abdominal pain that is sudden, severe, constant, and generalized. Pain is excruciating with any movement (it may be blunted in elderly patients). The most common causes include the following:

- **Diverticulitis:** elderly patient with lower abdominal pain and fever (most common cause of colonic perforation in elderly)
- **Perforated peptic ulcer (PUD):** epigastric pain that classically wakens patient at night and may include referred pain to scapula

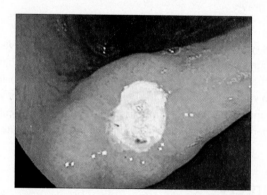

Peptic Ulcer (source: Niket Sonpal, MD)

Diagnose with an erect chest x-ray (free air under diaphragm, or falciform ligament) or left lateral decubitus x-ray if patient is too sick to stand up.

Treatment is as follows:

- Order nothing by mouth (NPO) and IV fluid hydration
- IV antibiotics
- Emergency surgery

Basic Science Correlate

Metronidazole covalently binds to DNA. This disrupts its helical structure, inhibits bacterial nucleic acid synthesis, and results in bacterial death.

Esophageal Perforation

The most common cause of esophageal perforation is iatrogenic. The classic presentation is after endoscopy.

Symptoms include:

- Pain in chest or upper abdomen
- Dysphagia or odynophagia
- Subcutaneous emphysema shortly after endoscopy

Diagnose with water-soluble contrast esophagram.

Treatment is endoscopic placement of stents and antibiotics for small perforations, and surgery for large perforations.

In a CCS case, order antibiotics because of high risk of mediastinitis.

Obstruction

Suspect obstruction in patients with the following symptoms:

- Severe colicky pain
- Absence of flatus or feces
- High-pitched bowel sounds
- Nausea and vomiting in patients with these risk factors:
  - Prior surgery (think adhesions, most common cause in United States)
  - Elderly patient with weight loss and anemia or melanotic stools (think tumor)
  - History of recurrent lower abdominal pain (think diverticulitis)
  - History of hernia (incarcerated hernia)
  - Sudden abdominal pain in elderly patient (don't forget about volvulus)
  - Vascular events such as ischemia, perforation/diverticulitis, AAA, or dissection
- Constant movement, as the patient tries to find a position of comfort

Diagnostic tests include:

- CBC and lactate level (elevated)
- Supine and erect abdominal x-ray (**best initial test**) (look for dilated loops of bowel, air-fluid levels, absence of gas in rectum, bird's beak sign for volvulus)
- CT scan of the abdomen and pelvis with contrast (**most accurate test**) may reveal a transition point, i.e., the location at which the obstruction has occurred.

> In a patient with a hernia, immediate surgery is the answer if the case describes fever, leukocytosis, constant pain, and signs of peritoneal irritation (think strangulated obstruction).

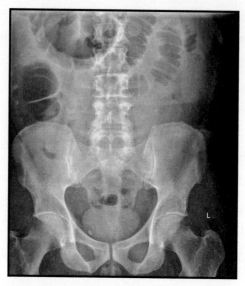

X-ray Showing Multiple Dilated Loops of Bowel
(source: Niket Sonpal, MD)

Treatment is NPO, nasogastric suction, and IV fluid hydration. Consider gastrografin contrast study until perforation has been ruled out.

- Sigmoid volvulus: perform proctosigmoidoscopy; leave rectal tube in place; perform sigmoid resection for recurrent cases
- All other obstructions: emergency surgery

> **Basic Science Correlate**
>
> Gastrografin is water soluble, unlike barium, which is caustic if it extravasates.

Inflammation

Inflammatory causes of acute abdomen include acute diverticulitis, acute pancreatitis, and acute appendicitis. The question will describe the following:

- Gradual onset of constant abdominal pain that slowly builds up over several hours
- Initially ill-defined pain that eventually becomes localized to the site of inflammation

Acute Diverticulitis

Acute diverticulitis is one of the few infectious processes presenting with acute abdominal pain in the left lower quadrant.

Look for a patient in middle age or older with fever, leukocytosis, and peritoneal irritation in the left lower quadrant with a palpable tender mass. In women, think about fallopian tube and ovaries as potential sources.

> ### Basic Science Correlate
>
> The common location for diverticulosis is the sigmoid colon. This is because it has the smallest diameter and therefore the highest intraluminal pressure. Concurrently, the sigmoid has the highest degree of diverticulitis.

Diagnostic testing is as follows:

- CT with contrast (**most accurate test**) to look for abscess or free air; fat stranding is common around the inflamed bowel
- Urine pregnancy test when diagnosing acute diverticulitis in women of childbearing age
- Colonoscopy is absolutely contraindicated in acute diverticulitis, as it increases risk of perforation

Treatment is as follows:

- No peritoneal signs: manage as outpatient with ciprofloxacin and metronidazole
- Localized peritoneal signs and abscess: admit patient and order NPO, IV fluids, IV antibiotics, and CT-guided percutaneous drainage of the abscess
- Generalized peritonitis or perforation: emergency surgery
- Recurrent attacks of diverticulitis: elective surgery

Diverticular Abscess

Patients who have acute diverticulitis can develop an abscess, which occurs when pus collects in the pouch. Suspect a diverticular abscess in patients with uncomplicated diverticulitis who have no improvement in abdominal pain or a persistent fever despite 3 days of antibiotic treatment.

Diagnosis is made by CT scan of the abdomen.

Treatment is always percutaneous or surgical drainage. Start antibiotics to prevent spread of the infection.

Acute Pancreatitis

Suspect this in the alcoholic who develops acute (over several hours) upper abdominal pain, radiating to the back, with nausea and vomiting. Acute pancreatitis may be edematous; hemorrhagic; or suppurative (pancreatic abscess).

In addition to alcoholism, risk factors include gallstones; medication (didanosine, pentamidine, metronidazole, tetracycline, thiazides, furosemide); hypertriglyceridemia; trauma; and post-ERCP.

Late complications include pancreatic pseudocyst and chronic pancreatitis.

Diagnose with a serum or urinary amylase or lipase (serum from 12–48 hours, urinary from days 3–6). Amylase gives the highest sensitivity, and lipase gives the highest specificity. If diagnosis is uncertain, do a CT.

> Warning signs for **hemorrhagic pancreatitis** include:
>
> - Lower hematocrit that continues to fall the day after presentation
> - Very high WBC (>18,000), glucose, BUN
> - Very low calcium

> **Basic Science Correlate**
>
> Pancreatitis can lead to low calcium levels due to the insoluble calcium salts in the pancreas. The free fatty acids avidly chelate the salts, resulting in calcium deposition in the retroperitoneum.

Treatment is NPO, NG suction, and IV fluids. Complications can include:

- Abscess: appears 10 days after onset with persistent fevers and high WBC count; treat with surgical drainage
- Pseudocyst: appears 5 weeks after initial symptoms, when a collection of pancreatic juice causes anorexia, pain, and a palpable mass
- Chronic damage: causes diabetes and steatorrhea; treat with insulin and pancreatic enzyme supplements

Acute Appendicitis

Acute appendicitis classically begins with anorexia, followed by vague peri-umbilical pain.

- Several hours later, pain becomes sharp, severe, constant, and localized to the right lower quadrant of abdomen
- Tenderness, guarding, and rebound are found to the right and below the umbilicus (but not elsewhere in belly)

> **Rovsing sign:** palpation of LLQ increases the pain felt in RLQ

To diagnose, look for fever and leukocytosis 10,000–15,000, with neutrophilia and immature forms. If diagnosis is unclear by clinical history and exam, the best imaging study is CT scan; less optimal is abdominal ultrasound.

Treatment is determined by CT findings: IV antibiotic for perforated appendix and for phlegmon, drainage for abscess; and surgery for frank perforation.

Chronic Ulcerative Colitis

Ulcerative colitis extends from the anal verge in an uninterrupted pattern to the entire colon.

Chronic ulcerative colitis (CUC) is managed medically; however, toxic megacolon (abdominal pain, fever, leukocytosis, epigastric tenderness, massively distended transverse colon on x-ray with gas within the wall of the colon) requires emergent surgery.

Ischemia

The intestine is supplied by 3 major gastrointestinal arteries that arise from the abdominal aorta: celiac axis, superior mesenteric artery (SMA), and inferior mesenteric artery (IMA).

With ischemia, always consider the following:

- History of arrhythmia (atrial fibrillation)
- Coronary artery disease
- Recent MI

Acute Mesenteric Ischemia

Classically, pain is out of proportion to the exam. If ischemia is suspected, do not wait for lab findings (acidosis, elevated lactate); go straight to surgery or order angiography.

- If diagnosis is during surgery: perform embolectomy and revascularization or resection.
- If diagnosis is during angiography: give vasodilators or thrombolysis.

CCS Tip: When you think a patient has an acute (or near-acute) abdomen, get a surgical consult. The consult itself will not offer useful information; rather, you are being tested to see if you know the timing to consult surgery.

Basic Science Correlate

The most common vessel affected is the superior mesenteric artery, due to the acuity of its angle and because it is a direct branch off the aorta.

A 65-year-old woman comes to the office reporting 2 episodes of cramping abdominal pain followed by bloody diarrhea. The patient had just participated in a half-marathon and came in fifth place. She has some mild tenderness over the left upper and left lower quadrants. Otherwise, vital signs and physical exam are normal. What is the most likely diagnosis?

a. Acute mesenteric ischemia
b. Abdominal aortic aneurysm (AAA)
c. Ischemic colitis
d. Peptic ulcer disease
e. Chronic mesenteric ischemia

Answer: **C.** Ischemic colitis is a condition in which there is an ischemic injury of the large intestine resulting from inadequate blood supply. The most common symptoms are cramping abdominal pain caused by ischemia followed by bloody diarrhea. The bloody diarrhea is a mix of mucus and blood because the mucosal layer is the farthest from the bowel's blood supply.

Ischemic Colitis

CT scan of the abdomen is the **best initial** and **most accurate diagnostic test** for ischemic colitis. It will show thickening of the bowel in a segmental pattern.

Treatment is IV fluid hydration to restore adequate bowel perfusion and bowel rest; antibiotics are given to those who also have fever.

Chronic Mesenteric Ischemia

Chronic intestinal ischemia usually results from longstanding atherosclerotic disease of ≥ 2 mesenteric vessels.

- Upon eating, patient's intestinal demand for oxygen is unmet because of atherosclerotic obstruction of blood flow
- Causes excruciating pain, which over time leads to pain-induced anorexia
- Analogous to angina of the heart, but affects only the gut

Angiography is both **diagnostic and therapeutic**. Surgical correction requires, first, angiography to delineate the location of the lesions, and then stenting or bypass to reestablish blood flow.

Celiac Artery Compression Syndrome

Celiac artery compression syndrome (CACS) presents similarly to chronic mesenteric ischemia, but it usually results from external compression of the celiac trunk by the median arcuate ligament or celiac ganglion, not atherosclerotic disease. Symptoms include:

- Severe postprandial, ischemic abdominal pain, caused by the median arcuate compressing the celiac trunk
- Unrelenting nausea
- Anorexia and weight loss (development of symptoms after recent dramatic weight loss is a **classic clue**)

CACS is a diagnosis of exclusion and is confirmed by duplex ultrasonography to measure blood flow through the celiac artery.

Treatment is surgical decompression of the celiac artery.

Abscess

Intra-Abdominal Abscess

Consider the possibility of an abscess in any patient with a history of a previous operation, trauma, or intra-abdominal infection/inflammation. Abscess can occur anywhere in the abdomen or retroperitoneum.

Diagnose with a CBC and contrast CT of the abdomen/pelvis.

Treatment is drainage of an intra-abdominal abscess (surgically or percutaneously) and antibiotics to prevent the spread of infection. Note this does not cure the abscess.

Pyogenic Liver Abscess

Liver abscess (**most common type of visceral abscess**) is usually caused by a recent abdominal inflammatory process such as diverticulitis or cholangitis, which seeds an infection to the liver. Symptoms include:

- Fever
- Abdominal pain
- Elevated white blood cells
- Increased AST/ALT (in nonspecific pattern)
- Most commonly involves right lobe of the liver because it is larger and has greater blood supply than the left and caudate lobes

Diagnostic testing is ultrasound (**best initial** and **most accurate test**) and concurrent percutaneous aspiration (also therapeutic).

Treatment is antibiotics to cover gram negative and anaerobes. Most pyogenic liver abscesses are polymicrobial, but use the following guidelines:

- Enteric gram-negative bacilli (**most common finding**)
- *Klebsiella pneumoniae*: associated with colorectal cancer: do a colonoscopy
- *Staphylococcus aureus*: seen after transarterial embolization for HCC
- *Candida*: seen during recovery of neutrophil counts following a neutropenic episode
- *Burkholderia pseudomallei*: seen after recent travel to Southeast Asia
- *E. histolytica*: seen after recent travel to Central and South America with diarrhea

Hepatobiliary Disease

The question will describe an obese, premenopausal woman in her 40s with the following signs:

- Recurrent episodes of abdominal pain
- High alkaline phosphatase
- Dilated ducts on sonogram
- Nondilated gallbladder full of stones
- Direct hyperbilirubinemia

Basic Science Correlate

The common hepatic duct and cystic duct merge to form the common bile duct, which merges with the pancreatic duct and allows enzyme and bile exit through the sphincter of Oddi.

Obstructive Jaundice Caused by Tumor

In patients with progressive symptoms in preceding weeks and weight loss, suspect a tumor:

- Adenocarcinoma at the head of the pancreas
- Adenocarcinoma of the ampulla of Vater
- Cholangiocarcinoma arising in the common duct itself

Diagnostic testing is sonogram and CT scan, which will show a double duct sign (i.e., simultaneous dilatation of both the common bile duct and pancreatic duct).

- **If a lesion is seen on CT:** get tissue diagnosis via EUS
- **If no lesion is seen on CT:** order an MRCP (shows ampullary or common bile duct tumors not seen on CT) and get tissue diagnosis via EUS/ERCP

Treatment is surgical resection.

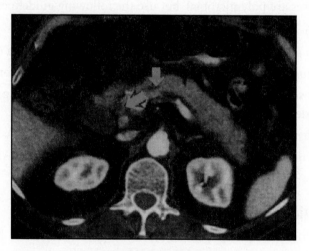

Double Duct Sign
(source: Niket Sonpal, MD)

Gallstones

Biliary Colic

Temporary occlusion of the cystic duct causes colicky pain in the right upper quadrant, radiating to the right shoulder and back, often triggered by fatty food. Episodes are brief (20 minutes), and there are no signs of peritoneal irritation or systemic signs.

Diagnosis is made with a sonogram. Treatment is elective cholecystectomy.

Acute Cholecystitis

Persistent occlusion of the cystic duct from a stone causes constant pain, as well as fever, leukocytosis, and peritoneal irritation in the right upper quadrant.

Murphy sign: pain on palpation of RUQ during inhalation

Diagnosis is made with a sonogram, which will show gallstones, a thick-walled gallbladder, and pericholecystic fluid. The **most accurate test** is a hepatobiliary iminodiacetic acid (HIDA) scan.

Treatment is NPO, IV fluids, and antibiotics, followed by cholecystectomy. If there is generalized peritonitis or emphysematous cholecystitis (suggestive of perforation or gangrene), emergency cholecystectomy is needed.

Acute Ascending Cholangitis

Obstruction of the common duct causes ascending infection. There is high fever and very high white blood cell count. Key findings are high levels of alkaline phosphatase and high levels of total bilirubin and direct bilirubin with mild elevation of transaminases.

> Reynolds pentad: jaundice, fever, abdominal pain, altered mental status, and shock

Treatment is IV antibiotics; emergency decompression of the common bile duct (lifesaving) (ideally by ERCP, alternatively through the liver by percutaneous transhepatic cholangiogram, and rarely by surgery); and eventual cholecystectomy.

Acalculous Cholecystitis

Acalculous cholecystitis is an inflammatory disease of the gallbladder without evidence of gallstones or cystic duct obstruction caused by bile stasis, ischemia, and bile salt concentration. Critically ill patients are more predisposed; patients do not eat and there is an absence of cholecystokinin-induced gallbladder contraction. It is most commonly seen in patients with sepsis or receiving TPN.

Once acalculous cholecystitis is established, secondary infection with enteric pathogens is common, e.g., *E. coli*, *Enterococcus faecalis*, *Klebsiella*, *Pseudomonas*, *Proteus*, and *B. fragilis*.

Diagnosis is made with clinical presentation and history. Imaging is used to exclude other conditions and is not specific enough for acalculous cholecystitis.

Treatment is cholecystostomy; surgery is reserved for those with gallbladder necrosis gallbladder perforation, and emphysematous cholecystitis.

Bile Leak

Biliary leakage should be suspected when patients present after cholecystectomy with fever, abdominal pain, and/or bilious ascites. The **most accurate test** is HIDA scan. Large loculated collections should be percutaneously drained with radiologic guidance. ERCP finds the leak, and a stent closes it.

Gallbladder Polyps

Gallbladder polyps are outgrowths of the gallbladder mucosal wall. They are usually found incidentally on ultrasound or after cholecystectomy. Management depends on the size of the polyps and symptoms. All symptomatic patients regardless of size should have a cholecystectomy.

Asymptomatic polyps:

- **Polyp >20 mm:** treated as malignant and should be surgically resected
- **Polyp 10–20 mm:** might be malignant and should be removed through laparoscopic cholecystectomy

- **Polyp 6–9 mm:** yearly ultrasound to demonstrate stability of polyp size; if it increases, should be removed surgically
- **Polyps ≤5 mm:** usually benign and most frequently represent cholesterolosis; ultrasound at 1 year to demonstrate stability of polyp size

Sphincter of Oddi Dysfunction (SOD)

The sphincter of Oddi is a muscular structure where the distal common bile duct and the pancreatic duct combine and penetrate the duodenal wall. Functional abnormalities of the sphincter of Oddi that cause biliary or pancreatic obstruction are known as SOD.

SOD is suspected in patients who have biliary-type pain without other apparent causes. All of the following conditions must be present for a diagnosis of SOD to be made:

- Pain located in the epigastrium and/or RUQ
- Episodes lasting ≥30 minutes and recurrent at irregular intervals (not daily)
- Pain that builds up to a steady level and severe enough to interrupt daily activities or prompt a visit to ED
- Pain not significantly related to bowel movements
- Pain not significantly relieved by postural change or acid suppression

Diagnose with sphincter of Oddi manometry (SOM) (most accurate test).

Treatment for symptomatic SOD is geared toward the elimination of pain and/or recurrent pancreatitis by improving the impaired flow of biliary and pancreatic secretions. Definitive management is based on the type of SOD.

Type	Characteristics	Management
Type I	Biliary-type pain, abnormal liver tests, dilated common bile duct	Endoscopic sphincterotomy WITHOUT preprocedure SOM (offers greatest relief for the patient)
Type II	Biliary-type pain plus: • Abnormal liver tests OR • Dilated common bile duct	SOM followed by endoscopic sphincterotomy (most common cause: sphincter of Oddi stenosis)
Type III	Biliary-type pain, normal liver tests, dilated common bile duct	Medical management WITHOUT endoscopic sphincterotomy

Anorectal Disease

Fecal Incontinence

Fecal incontinence is involuntary passage of bowel contents for at least 1 month in a patient age >3.

Diagnosis is made with clinical history and flexible sigmoidoscopy or anoscopy (**best initial test**). Patients with a history of anatomic injury should undergo endorectal manometry (**most accurate test**).

Initial treatment is bulking agents (e.g., fiber) plus biofeedback techniques (e.g., control exercises and muscle strengthening exercises). The best next step is endoscopic injection of dextranomer/hyaluronic acid in an effort to create a pseudo-sphincter (can reduce incontinence episodes by 50%). If this fails, colorectal surgery is needed.

Pilonidal Cyst

Pilonidal cyst is an acute or chronic abscess of the sacrococcygeal region, arising from an infection of the skin and subcutaneous tissue. Risk factors include poor hygiene, obesity, and the presence of a deep natal cleft.

- When sitting/bending, the natal cleft stretches, damaging or breaking hair follicles and opening a pore, or "pit," which collects debris (roots of hairs shed from the head, back, or buttocks).

- As movement draws the skin taut over the natal cleft, it creates negative pressure in the subcutaneous space that draws hair deeper into the pore, and the friction generates a sinus.

Symptoms include sudden onset of mild to severe pain in the intergluteal region while sitting or performing activities that stretch the skin overlying the natal cleft (e.g., bending, sit-ups). The patient may report intermittent swelling as well as mucoid, purulent, and/or bloody drainage in the area.

Treatment is incision and drainage. Recurrence is treated with sinus tract excision.

Anal Fissure

Anal fissure is a common benign anorectal disease that starts with a tear to the anoderm within the distal half of the anal canal. The tear then triggers cycles of recurring anal pain and bleeding, which leads to the development of a chronic anal fissure. It is most commonly a longitudinal tear and does not go beyond the dentate line.

Most anal fissures are primary (most commonly at the posterior midline) and are caused by local trauma such as constipation, diarrhea, vaginal delivery, and anal sex.

> **Anal Fissure Pain**
>
> Acute = <8 weeks
>
> Chronic = >8 weeks

Those with an acute anal fissure present with anal pain that is often present at rest but is exacerbated by defecation.

Diagnosis can be confirmed on physical exam by directly visualizing a fissure or reproducing the patient's presenting complaints by gentle digital palpation of the posterior (or anterior) midline anal verge.

Initial treatment is sitz baths, increased fiber intake/stool softeners, and topical vasodilators such as nitroglycerin. If there is no improvement after 8 weeks, the next step is lateral internal sphincterotomy. For older patients or multiparous women who are at high risk for developing fecal incontinence, botulinum toxin injection is used.

Preoperative and Postoperative Care

Preoperative Assessment

The most important aspect of preoperative assessment is being able to identify comorbidities that preclude surgery. Another aspect is to understand the modifications that may need to be instituted to prepare patients for surgery.

> A 42-year-old man with hepatitis C cirrhosis presents with a large umbilical hernia with intermittent pain. On examination he has large amounts of ascites. Surgical intervention is being considered. His bilirubin is 3.0, prothrombin time 32 seconds, INR 2.2, and serum albumin is 1.9. Which of the following is the best next step in management?
>
> a. Emergency surgery
> b. Vitamin K and then surgery
> c. Total parenteral nutrition and then surgery
> d. Albumin infusion and then surgery
> e. No surgery
>
> Answer: **E.** Do not do surgery in patients with multiple derangements in hepatic risk factors. Any one of the hepatic risks alone—bilirubin >2, albumin <3, prothrombin >16 sec, and encephalopathy (as suggested by altered mental status)—predicts a mortality >40%. If 3 of them are present, the risk is 85%; if all 4 risks are present, there is near 100% risk of mortality.

A 59-year-old man is scheduled for prostatectomy. He has a history of HTN, COPD, and diabetes mellitus. He takes atenolol for blood pressure, tiotropium and albuterol for COPD, and glipizide for diabetes. BP is 145/89 mm Hg and HgbA1c is 7.1. Recent pulmonary tests document FEV_1 1.3. Blood CO_2 is 47. This patient is most at risk of developing which of the following?

a. Intraoperative myocardial infarction

b. Pneumothorax

c. Postoperative pneumonia

d. Hypercapnic failure

e. Respiratory failure

Answer: **C.** Severe COPD (FEV_1 <1.5 l) increases surgical risk, mainly because patients have an ineffective cough and cannot clear secretions. they are subsequently at risk for postoperative pneumonia.

The table summarizes important principles in preoperative assessment.

Organ System	Risk Factor	Modifications/Interventions
Cardiac risk	Ejection fraction <35%	Prohibits noncardiac surgery
	Jugular venous distention (sign of CHF)	Optimize medications with ACE inhibitors, beta blockers, digitalis, and diuretics prior to surgery
	Recent myocardial infarction	Defer surgery for 6 months after MI
	Severe progressive angina	Perform cardiac catheterization to evaluate for possible coronary revascularization
Pulmonary risk	Smoking (compromised ventilation: high pCO_2, FEV_1 <1.5)	• Order PFTs to evaluate FEV1 • If FEV1 is abnormal, obtain blood gas • Cessation of smoking for 8 weeks prior to surgery
Hepatic risk	Bilirubin >2.0 Prothrombin time >16 Serum albumin <3.0 Encephalopathy	• 40% mortality with any single risk factor • 80–85% mortality is predictable if ≥3 risk factors are present
Nutritional risk	Loss of 20% of body weight over several months Serum albumin <3.0 Anergy to skin antigens Serum transferrin <200 mg/dl Diabetic coma	• Provide 5–10 days of nutritional supplements (preferably via gut) before surgery • Absolute contraindication to surgery; first stabilize diabetes; rehydrate and normalize acidosis prior to surgery

The table shows the calculation of the cardiac risk index in noncardiac surgery.

Cardiac Risk Index in Noncardiac Surgery		
Criterion	**Finding**	**Points***
Age	>70	5
Cardiac status	MI within 6 months	10
	Ventricular gallop or jugular venous distention (signs of heart failure)	11
	Significant aortic stenosis	3
	Arrhythmia other than sinus or premature atrial contractions	7
	≥5 premature ventricular contractions/minute	7
General medical condition	pO_2 <60 mm Hg, pCO_2 >50 mm Hg, K <3 mmol/L, HCO_3 <20 mmol/L, BUN >50 mg/dL, serum creatinine >3 mg/dL, elevated AST, a chronic liver disorder, or bedbound	3
Type of surgery needed	Emergency surgery	4
	Intraperitoneal, intrathoracic, or aortic surgery	3
*Risk is based on total number of points: Level I: 0–5 Level II: 6–12 Level III: 13–25 Level IV: >25		
Adapted from Goldman L, Caldera DL, Nussbaum SR, et al. Multifactorial index of cardiac risk in noncardiac surgical procedures. *New England Journal of Medicine.* 1997; 297 (lb): 845–850.		

Postoperative Complications

In each of the following cases, which diagnostic tests will likely show the cause of the patient's postoperative fever?

1. A patient who had major abdominal surgery is afebrile during the first 2 post-operative days but on Day 3 has a fever to 103°F.
2. A patient who had major abdominal surgery is afebrile during the first 4 post-operative days but on Day 5 has a fever to 103°F.
3. A patient who had major abdominal surgery is afebrile during the first 6 post-operative days but on Day 7 has a fever to 103°F.

   a. Chest x-ray
   b. CT of the abdomen
   c. CT of the chest
   d. Doppler of the lower extremities
   e. Urinalysis

Answers:

1. **E.** Urinalysis
2. **D.** Doppler of the lower extremities
3. **B.** CT of the abdomen

Every potential source of post-op fever must be investigated, but the timing of the first febrile episode gives a clue as to the most likely source. While not a hard-and-fast rule, the "four Ws" mnemonic gives a clue to the likely cause of the fever:

- "**Wind**" for atelectasis, common post-op day 1: order a **chest x-ray**
- "**Water**" for UTI, common post-op day 3: order **urinalysis, urine culture**, and **early removal of Foley**
- "**Walking**" for thrombophlebitis, common post-op day 5: order a **Doppler**
- "**Wound**" for wound infections, common post-op day 7: conduct a **complete physical exam** and consider **CT scan** to evaluate for deep infections

A 46-year-old woman with medical history significant for large fibroids and anemia becomes disoriented 18 hours after an uncomplicated hysterectomy. What is the next step in management?

a. Arterial blood gas
b. CT scan of the pelvis
c. IV fluids
d. Lorazepam
e. Blood transfusions

Answer: **A.** There is a long list of causes for post-op disorientation, but the most lethal one if not recognized and treated early is hypoxia. Unless the vignette clearly identifies other possible metabolic causes of disorientation—uremia, hyponatremia, hypernatremia, ammonium, hyperglycemia, delirium tremens, or iatrogenic medications—the safest thing is to obtain a blood gas first.

Postoperative Ileus

Postoperative ileus refers to obstipation and intolerance of oral intake following surgery, most often due to electrolyte abnormalities; prolonged abdominal/pelvic surgery; sepsis; or perioperative opioid use. Symptoms include oral intolerance, nausea and vomiting, obstipation, and lack of flatus. Physical exam shows decreased or absent bowel sounds.

The best initial test for postoperative ileus is abdominal x-ray showing air fluid levels. The most accurate test is CT scan demonstrating a lack of a transition zone as seen in SBO. Treat with supportive care, electrolyte replacement, and elimination of the offending medication.

The table summarizes the features and management of postoperative complications.

Postoperative Complication	Features	Management
Fever		
Malignant hyperthermia exceeding 40.0°C (104.0°F)	Shortly after the onset of the anesthetic (halothane or succinylcholine) Treat with IV dantrolene, 100% oxygen, correction of the acidosis, and cooling blankets.	Watch for development of myoglobinuria.
Bacteremia exceeding 40.0°C (104.0°F)	Within 30–45 minutes of invasive procedures	Blood cultures Start empiric antibiotics.
Postoperative fever in the usual range 38.3–39.4°C (101.0–103.0°F)	Atelectasis (Day 1)	Incentive spirometry
	Pneumonia (Day 3)	CXR: Infiltrate Sputum culture Antibiotics (hospital-acquired pneumonia)
	UTI (Day 3)	Urinalysis Antibiotics
	Deep venous thrombophlebitis (Day 5)	Doppler ultrasound of deep veins of legs and pelvis Anticoagulation
	Wound infection (Day 7)	Antibiotics if only cellulitis. Incision and drainage if abscess is present.
	Deep abscesses (subphrenic, pelvic, or subhepatic) (Days 10–15)	CT scan of the appropriate body cavity is diagnostic. Percutaneous radiologically guided drainage is therapeutic.
Perioperative myocardial infarction	Precipitated by hypotension when intraoperative.	Mortality rate is higher than for non-surgery-related MI.
Pulmonary embolus (Day 7)	Tachycardia, shortness of breath, hypoxia, increased A-a gradient	CTA (CT angiogram) Anticoagulate IVC filter if recurrent PE
Aspiration	Shortness of breath, hypoxia, infiltrate on x-ray	Lavage and remove gastric contents. Bronchodilators and respiratory support Steroids do not help.
Intraoperative tension pneumothorax	Positive-pressure breathing; patient becomes progressively more difficult to "bag" BP steadily declines, and CVP steadily rises.	Insert needle to decompress and place chest tube later.
Postoperative confusion	Suspect hypoxia first. Consider sepsis.	Check blood gases. Get blood cultures and CBC.
Acute respiratory distress syndrome (ARDS)	Bilateral pulmonary infiltrates and hypoxia, with no evidence of CHF	Positive end-expiratory pressure (PEEP)

Pediatric Surgery

Conditions Requiring Surgery at Birth

Congenital anomalies constitute the conditions that need surgery at birth. On the Step 3 exam, the most important first step before surgery is to **r**ule out other associated congenital conditions. In any of the following presentations, look for other associated elements of the **VACTER** (vertebral, anal, cardiac, tracheal, esophageal, renal, and radial) constellation:

- Look at anus for imperforation.
- Check the x-ray for vertebral and radial anomalies.
- Do echocardiogram looking for cardiac anomalies.
- Do sonogram looking for renal anomalies.

Esophageal Atresia

Excessive salivation is noted shortly after birth, or choking spells are noticed when first feeding is attempted.

> **Basic Science Correlate**
>
> Ventrally displaced location of the notochord in an embryo can lead to a failure of apoptosis in the developing foregut and cause esophageal atresia.

Confirm the diagnosis with an **NG tube,** which becomes coiled in the upper chest on x-ray.

Primary **surgical repair** is indicated.

Anal Atresia

This is indicated by an absence of flatus or stool. The anal canal is absent on exam.

Treatment starts with looking for a fistula nearby (to vagina or perineum).

- If **present,** delay repair until further growth (but before toilet training time).
- If **not present,** a **colostomy** needs to be done for high rectal pouches.

Congenital Diaphragmatic Hernia

Dyspnea is noted at birth, and loops of bowel in left chest are seen on x-ray. The primary abnormality is the hypoplastic lung with fetal-type circulation.

> **Basic Science Correlate**
>
> Left-sided hernias allow herniation of intra-abdominal organs into the thoracic cavity, while right-sided hernias allow the liver to herniate.

> **VACTERL syndrome =** association of:
>
> **V**ertebral anomalies
>
> **A**nal atresia
>
> **C**ardiovascular anomalies
>
> **T**racheo**E**sophageal fistula
>
> **R**enal (kidney) and/or radial anomalies
>
> **L**imb defects

Treat with endotracheal intubation, low-pressure ventilation, sedation, and NG suction. Delay repair 3–4 days to allow lung maturation.

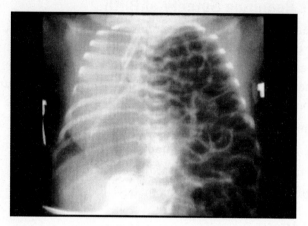

Congenital Diaphragmatic Hernia

Gastroschisis and Omphalocele

In **gastroschisis**, the umbilical cord is normal (it reaches the baby); the defect is to the right of the cord, where there is no protective membrane and the bowel looks angry and matted.

In **omphalocele**, the umbilical cord goes to the defect, which has a thin membrane under which one can see normal-looking bowel and a little slice of liver. Edward syndrome (Trisomy 18) and Patau syndrome (Trisomy 13) are both associated with omphalocele.

Treat as follows:

- **Small defects:** close small defects primarily
- **Large defects:** silastic "silo" to protect the bowel and **manual replacement of the bowel daily** until complete closure (in ~1 week); until then, give parenteral nutrition (the bowel will not work in gastroschisis) and IV antibiotics

A newborn is vomiting greenish liquid material. A "double-bubble" is seen on x-ray. What is the diagnosis?

a. Annular pancreas
b. Congenital diaphragmatic hernia
c. Gastroschisis
d. Imperforated anus
e. Intestinal atresia

Answer: **A.** Don't be fooled into thinking that only duodenal atresia presents with double-bubble sign. Annular pancreas and malrotation also present with double-bubble sign. All of these anomalies require surgical correction, but malrotation is the most dangerous because the bowel can twist on itself, cut off its blood supply, and become necrotic.

> ### Basic Science Correlate
>
> **Embryology and Omphalocele**
>
> Incomplete fusion during the fourth week of development results in a defect that allows abdominal viscera to protrude through the anterior body wall, which is made when the lateral body folds move ventrally and fuse in the midline.

Intestinal Atresia

Like annular pancreas, this condition also presents with green vomiting. But instead of a double-bubble, there are multiple air-fluid levels throughout the abdomen. There is no need to suspect other congenital anomalies, because this condition results from a vascular accident in utero.

Surgical Conditions in First 2 Months of Life

Necrotizing Enterocolitis

This shows up as feeding intolerance in premature infants when they are first fed. There is abdominal distention and a rapidly dropping platelet count (in babies, this is a sign of sepsis). Pneumatosis intestinalis refers to the presence of gas within the wall of the small or large intestine.

The most common pathogens are *E. coli* and *Klebsiella pneumonia.*

Treatment is to stop all feedings and give broad-spectrum antibiotics, IV fluids, and nutrition. If there are signs of necrosis or perforation (abdominal wall erythema, portal vein gas, or gas in the bowel wall), surgery will be required.

Meconium Ileus

Symptoms are feeding intolerance and bilious vomiting in a baby with cystic fibrosis (look for cystic fibrosis in family history).

> ### Basic Science Correlate
>
> Cystic fibrosis, an autosomal recessive disease, results from a point mutation at position 508 of the CFTR gene that causes the mistranslation of phenylalanine.

Diagnose with x-ray, which shows multiple dilated loops of small bowel and a ground-glass appearance in the lower abdomen.

Gastrografin enema is both:

- Diagnostic (microcolon and inspissated pellets of meconium in the terminal ileum); and
- Therapeutic (gastrografin draws fluid in and dissolves the pellets); if this fails, consider surgery.

Hypertrophic Pyloric Stenosis

This shows up as nonbilious projectile vomiting after each feeding at approximately 3 weeks of age. Look for gastric peristaltic waves and a palpable "olive-size" mass in the right upper quadrant.

Diagnose with a sonogram, which shows a target sign in hypertrophic pyloric stenosis.

Treatment is to first correct dehydration and associated hypochloremic, hypokalemic metabolic alkalosis. Then, proceed with pyloromyotomy.

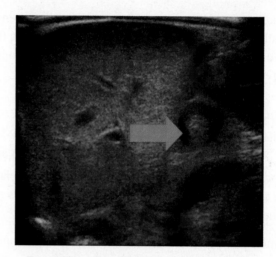

Target Sign in Hypertrophic Pyloric Stenosis
(source: Niket Sonpal, MD)

Biliary Atresia

This appears in 6- to 8-week-old babies who have persistent, progressively increasing jaundice (conjugated bilirubin).

Diagnose with serologies and sweat test to rule out other problems, and then proceed to ultrasound (**best initial test**). The most accurate test is MRCP.

Treatment is a Kasai procedure—hepatoportoenterostomy.

Hirschsprung Disease (Aganglionic Megacolon)

The most important clue to diagnosis is **chronic constipation.** A rectal exam may lead to explosive expulsion of stool and flatus with relief of abdominal distention.

Definitive diagnosis is made with a full thickness rectal biopsy, which may be supported by findings on abdominal x-ray, contrast enema, or anorectal manometry.

Basic Science Correlate

Hirschsprung disease occurs when the neural crest fails to migrate, resulting in the absence of ganglion cells.

Surgical Conditions Later in Infancy

Intussusception

Intussusception is the most common cause of obstruction in infants age 6–36 months. It presents in chubby, healthy-looking infants with brief episodes of colicky abdominal pain that makes them "double up and squat." The following are also present:

- Vague mass on the right side of the abdomen
- "Empty" right lower quadrant
- "Currant jelly" stools

Diagnose with ultrasound (**best test**), showing a "bull's eye" sign. A barium or air enema is therapeutic.

Treatment is enema to achieve reduction. If that fails, perform surgery.

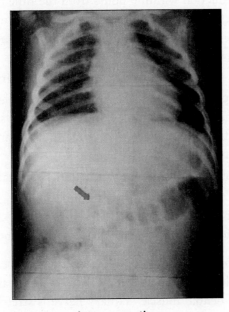

Intussusception

Meckel Diverticulum

Meckel diverticulum is a true diverticulum consisting of all 3 layers of the bowel wall: mucosa, submucosa, and muscularis propria. It presents as lower GI bleeding in a child of pediatric age.

Diagnosis is with a radioisotope scan (Meckel scan), which looks for gastric mucosa in the lower abdomen.

Treatment is surgical resection.

Orthopedics

Orthopedic Injury

When a fracture is suspected, order 2 views at 90° to one another. Make sure to include the joints above/below the broken bone and other sites in the "line of force" (e.g., lumbar spine for someone who falls and lands on the feet; hips for someone who has been in a car accident with force of knees against the dashboard).

- **Closed reduction** is the answer for fractures that are not badly displaced or angulated.
- **Open reduction and internal fixation** is the answer when the fracture is severely displaced or angulated or cannot be aligned.
- Open fractures (broken bone sticking out through a wound) require cleaning in the OR and reduction within 6 hours from the time of the injury. Open femoral shaft fracture is an orthopedic emergency and can result in massive blood loss and a high rate of infection. Immediate surgery and cleaning within 6 hours are needed.
- Perform cervical spine films in any patient with facial injury.
- Fat embolism is caused by the release of large fat droplets into the venous system, where they obstruct capillary beds. It is seen secondary to long-bone trauma, often with femoral shaft fracture. It can also result from parenteral lipid infusion or burns.
  - Patients present with neurologic dysfunction, petechial rash, and respiratory distress.
  - Management is stabilization of the fracture within 24 hours (show to reduce the incidence of respiratory distress from embolic phenomena).

Anterior dislocation is the most common shoulder dislocation. Look for an arm held close to the body but an externally rotated forearm and associated numbness over the deltoid muscle (axillary nerve is stretched). In **posterior dislocation**, the arm is held close to the body and the forearm is internally rotated.

A 27-year-old woman with a known seizure disorder has a grand mal seizure. She complains of left shoulder pain. PA and lateral x-rays are obtained and fail to reveal fracture or dislocation. She is given ibuprofen for pain. She returns 3 days later with persistent pain with her arm held close to her side. She reports that she is unable to move the left arm. What is the next step in management?

a. Axillary radiograph of the left shoulder
b. Change analgesic to Percocet
c. CT of the left shoulder
d. MRI of the left shoulder
e. Ultrasound of tendon insertion sites

Answer: **A.** Although **anterior shoulder dislocation** is easily seen on erect posteroanterior (PA) and lateral films—look for adducted arm and externally rotated forearm with numbness over deltoid (axillary nerve is stretched)—posterior shoulder dislocation is often missed. Suspect posterior shoulder dislocation in a patient with a recent seizure or electrical burn and shoulder injury or pain. Order axillary or scapular views of the affected shoulder.

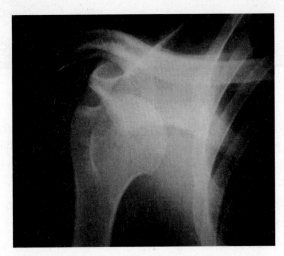

Anterior Dislocation of the Shoulder

Management is done as follows:

- Colles fracture: closed reduction and casting (common in elderly women who fall on an outstretched hand; look for a painful wrist with a "dinner-fork" deformity)

- Direct blow to the ulna (Monteggia fracture) or radius (Galeazzi fracture) results in a combination of diaphyseal fracture and displaced dislocation of the nearby joint. Open reduction and internal fixation is needed for the diaphyseal fracture, and closed reduction for the dislocated joint.

- Fall on an outstretched hand with persistent pain in the anatomical snuffbox is a scaphoid fracture until proven otherwise (takes >3 weeks to be seen on x-ray). Place thumb spica cast to help prevent nonunion.

- Consider a hip fracture in any elderly patient who sustains a fall. Look for externally rotated and shortened leg.

  - Femoral neck fracture is at high risk of avascular necrosis (tenuous blood supply) and is best treated with femoral head replacement.

  - Intertrochanteric fracture is treated with open reduction and pinning.

  - Femoral shaft fracture is treated with intramedullary rod fixation. Be aware of a high risk for fat emboli.

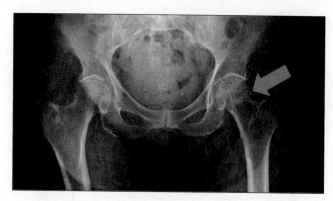

Hip Fracture
(source: Niket Sonpal, MD)

- Trigger finger (woman who awakens at night with an acutely flexed finger that "snaps" when forcibly extended) and De Quervain tenosynovitis (young mother carrying baby with flexed wrist and extended thumb to stabilize the baby's head): Steroid injection is the best initial therapy.

- Dupuytren contracture (contracture of the palm with palmar fascial nodules): Surgery is the treatment if collagenase fails.

- Posterior dislocation of the hip (history of head-on car collision where the knees hit the dashboard) is an orthopedic emergency. Differentiate it from hip fracture by an internally rotated leg (the leg is also shortened). Emergency reduction is needed to avoid avascular necrosis.

- Knee injuries
  - Medial/lateral collateral ligament injury (caused by a direct blow to the opposite side of the joint): Casting if isolated ligament injury; surgical repair if multiple ligaments injured.
  - Anterior/posterior cruciate ligament injuries (swelling pain and anterior/posterior drawer sign): Young athletes need arthroscopic repair. Older patients may be treated with immobilization and rehabilitation.
  - Meniscal injury (prolonged pain and swelling with "catching" and "locking" during ambulation). Treat with arthroscopic repair.

- Tibial stress injury (e.g., history of military or cadet marches): x-ray may be negative initially. Treat with cast, order the patient not to bear weight, and repeat films in 2 weeks.

- Rupture of the Achilles tendon (middle-aged man "overdoes it" at tennis or basketball, or patient with history of fluoroquinolone use, complaining of sudden "popping" and limping): Treat with casting in equinus position or surgical repair.

Total Knee Replacement

A 58-year-old woman presents to her primary care doctor for evaluation of left knee pain. The pain has been present in both knees for approximately 10 years and has steadily worsened to the point where she can no longer walk. She requires pain medications daily and has difficulty walking as far as the bathroom. On physical exam she has an antalgic gait. What is the most likely diagnosis?

a. Osteoarthritis
b. Rheumatoid arthritis
c. Knee trauma
d. Baker cyst
e. DVT

Answer: **A.** Osteoarthritis of the knee is a chronic, noninflammatory arthritis of the synovial joints caused by wear and tear. Patients classically present with **joint pain, crepitus, and difficulty bearing weight** on the affected joints. Rheumatoid arthritis would be symmetrical and affect multiple joints. While knee trauma actually may precipitate osteoarthritis as the nidus event, it takes many years to develop. DVT would have a painful swollen calf, which is not the case here.

Diagnosis of osteoarthritis of the knee is made with history and physical and confirmed with x-ray. Steps in conservative management include physical therapy, analgesics, and intraarticular injections; however, most patients ultimately require knee replacement.

When a patient develops severe osteoarthritis symptoms (difficulty walking, inability to perform ADLs, or bone-on-bone disease seen on x-ray), an elective knee replacement is indicated.

Compartment Syndrome

This is most frequent in the lower leg. Look for a history of prolonged ischemia followed by reperfusion, crushing injuries, or other types of trauma. There is pain, and the affected area feels tight and tender to palpation. The classic sign is excruciating pain with passive extension.

When assessing for neurovascular integrity, remember the 5 P's: **p**allor, **p**ain, **p**ulse, **p**aralysis, and **p**aresthesia.

When a patient complains of pain at the site of a cast, always remove the cast and examine for compartment syndrome.

The first step in management is emergency fasciotomy.

Neurovascular Injury

The table summarizes injuries that involve neurovascular complications.

Primary Injury	Neurovascular Complication	Signs/Symptoms	Next Step in Management
Oblique distal humerus	Radial nerve	Unable to dorsiflex (extend) the wrist Function regained after reduction	Surgery is indicated if paralysis persists after reduction
Posterior dislocation of the knee	Popliteal artery injuries	Decreased distal pulses	Doppler studies or arteriogram Prophylactic fasciotomy if reduction is delayed

Thoracic Outlet Syndrome

Thoracic outlet syndrome (TOS) is a condition in which there is compression of the nerves, arteries, or veins in the passageway from the lower neck to the armpit. The most common cause is a congenital cervical rib, which is an extra rib that arises from the seventh cervical vertebra.

There are 3 main types: neurogenic, venous, and arterial:

- **Neurogenic type** (most common) presents with pain, weakness, and thenar atrophy.
- **Venous type** results in swelling, pain, and cyanosis of the arm.
- **Arterial type** results in pain, coldness, and pallor of the arm.

Some patients may have Adson's sign, which is the loss of the radial pulse in the arm by rotating head to the ipsilateral side with extended neck following deep inspiration.

The best initial test is a **Doppler ultrasound** of the subclavian vessels. The most accurate test is a **magnetic resonance angiography.**

Treatment is indicated only for symptomatic patients, and incidentally found asymptomatic cervical ribs should be observed. Neurogenic TOS should initially be managed with physical therapy. Thoracic outlet decompression is indicated for symptomatic patients with vascular symptoms of TOS or neurologic weakness/disabling pain and paresthesia.

Back Pain

Disc Herniation

A sluggish ankle jerk reflex is suggestive of pathology at **S1/S2**. A sluggish patellar reflex is suggestive of pathology at **L4/L5**.

A 45-year-old man with a history of back pain for several months presents with sudden-onset severe back pain that came on when he was moving a television. He describes an "electrical shock" that shoots down his leg, which is worse when he coughs or strains and is partially relieved by flexing his legs. The pain has prevented him from ambulating. Straight leg raising gives excruciating pain. What is the next step in management?

a. CT of the spine
b. Dexamethasone
c. Immediate surgery
d. Ibuprofen and brief bed rest
e. MRI of the spine

Answer: **D.** This is the classic presentation of **lumbar disc herniation.** It occurs almost exclusively at L4–L5 or L5–S1. Peak age is 43–46. Anti-inflammatories and brief bed rest are all that is needed at this stage. Immediate surgical compression is needed if the history suggests **cauda equina syndrome** (look for bowel/bladder incontinence, flaccid anal sphincter, and saddle anesthesia). MRI can confirm both disc herniation and cauda equina, but do not answer MRI in classic cases of disc herniation. Trial of anti-inflammatories is also the first step in management.

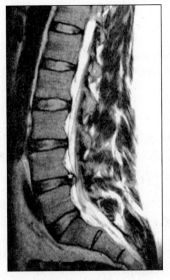

Lumbar Disc Herniation

Skin Conditions

Hidradenitis Suppurativa (HS)

HS is a chronic inflammatory condition involving occluded apocrine glands and hair follicles. It is characterized by painful cutaneous draining lesions, abscesses, and sinuses. The exact pathogenesis is not fully known, but multiple risk factors play a role, including obesity, smoking, and family history. HS can affect the axillae (most common site), inguinal area, inner thighs, perianal, and perineal areas.

A diagnosis of HS is straightforward in patients who demonstrate the constellation of recurrent inflammatory nodules, sinus tracts, and hypertrophic scarring in intertriginous areas.

Initial management is tobacco cessation, weight loss, topical antibiotics, and measures to keep the skin clean and friction-free. If those do not help, give a short course of antibiotics (e.g., tetracycline). For antibiotic-refractory or worsening disease, consider TNF alpha inhibitors and surgery.

Urology

A 24-year-old man presents in the emergency department with very severe pain. His temperature is 102.3°F. His testes appear swollen and are tender to palpation. Urinalysis reveals 50 white blood cells, 0 red blood cells. Which of the following is the next step in management?

a. Antibiotics
b. Culture and sensitivity
c. Inguinal lymph node biopsy
d. Testicular ultrasound
e. Prostate biopsy

Answer: **A.** The most likely diagnosis is orchitis/epididymitis, so starting antibiotics is the best next step in management.

Testicular Torsion

Testicular torsion is a urologic emergency. It classically presents as severe, sudden-onset testicular pain without fever or pyuria. The testis is swollen, exquisitely tender, "high riding," and with a "horizontal lie."

The sensory and motor components of the cremasteric reflex are at L1/L2. Their absence is suggestive of testicular torsion.

Diagnose with **Doppler ultrasound**. Treat with **immediate surgical intervention with bilateral orchiopexy.**

Urologic Obstruction

The combination of **obstruction and infection** of the urinary tract is another urologic emergency. It can lead to destruction of the kidney in a few hours and, potentially, to death from sepsis.

Treatment is immediate decompression of the urinary tract above the obstruction and IV antibiotics. The most important intervention is a **ureteral stent or percutaneous nephrostomy**; defer more elaborate instrumentations for a later, safer date.

Congenital Urologic Diseases

Following are the urologic diseases that may require surgery:

- The most common reason for a newborn boy not to urinate during the first day of life is posterior urethral valves.
  - Catheterize to empty the bladder.
  - Diagnose with voiding cystourethrogram.
- A child who has hematuria from trivial trauma has an undiagnosed congenital anomaly until proven otherwise.
- A child with a urinary tract infection has an undiagnosed congenital anomaly until proven otherwise (e.g., vesicoureteral reflux).
  - Order a voiding cystogram to look for the reflux.
  - If found, give long-term antibiotics until the child "grows out of the problem."
- Suspect low implantation of a ureter in girls who void appropriately but are also found to be constantly wet from urinating into the vagina.
- Ureteropelvic junction (UPJ) obstruction is only symptomatic when diuresis occurs. UPJ presents classically in a teenager who drinks large volumes of beer and develops colicky flank pain.

Hydrocele

Hydrocele is a painless, swollen fluid-filled sac along the spermatic cords within the scrotum that transilluminates upon inspection. It is a remnant of tunica vaginalis.

Hydrocele usually resolves within the first 12 months of life, and it does not need to be reassessed unless present after 1 year. For most hydroceles, watchful waiting is the appropriate management. If the hydrocele does persist >12 months, surgery is recommended to reduce the risk of future inguinal hernias.

Varicocele

Varicocele is a varicose vein in the scrotal veins causing swelling and increased pressure of the pampiniform plexus. The most common complaint is dull ache and heaviness in the scrotum.

> Varicocele is the most common cause of scrotal enlargement in adult males.

The best initial diagnostic is a proper physical exam coinciding with a **"bag of worms" sensation**. The most accurate test is **ultrasound of scrotal sac**, which will show dilatation of the vessels of the pampiniform plexus to >2 mm.

- Asymptomatic patients are monitored with yearly examination.
- Surgical ligation or embolization is reserved for those with pain, infertility, or delayed growth of the testes.
- Always ultrasound the other testicle. Varicocele is a bilateral disease; if you see it on one side, it is likely indolent on the other side.

> Cryptorchidism is associated with an increased risk of malignancy, regardless of surgical intervention.

Cryptorchidism

Cryptorchidism is the congenital absence of one testicle in the scrotal sac. The "missing" testicle is usually found within the inguinal canal; in 90% of cases it can be palpated in the inguinal canal. After age 4 months, orchiopexy of congenitally undescended testes is recommended as soon as possible, and the surgery should definitely be complete before age 2.

Urethral Abnormalities

In **hypospadias**, the urethral opening is ectopically located on the **ventral side of the penis** proximal to the tip of the glans penis. Surgical correction is treatment of choice. Do not circumcise; circumcision can add to the difficulties of surgically correcting the hypospadias.

In **epispadias**, the opening to the urethra is found on the **dorsal surface**. Epispadias is highly associated with urinary incontinence and concomitant bladder exstrophy. Surgical correction is required.

Priapism

Priapism is a prolonged penile erection (>4–6 hours) in the absence of sexual stimulation. It is a **urologic emergency**. There are 2 types of priapism:

- Ischemic (low-flow) priapism (more common) is caused by decreased venous flow.
- Nonischemic (high-flow) priapism is caused by a fistula between the cavernosal artery and corporal tissue. It is often associated with trauma to the perineum.

Common causes of priapism are medication (oral phosphodiesterase-5 inhibitors, trazodone), sickle cell disease, and leukemia.

Diagnosis is with a clinical exam. To determine ischemic versus nonischemic, aspirate blood from the corpora cavernosa for blood gas analysis.

- Ischemic: sample is black, analysis shows hypoxemia, hypercarbia, and acidemia
- Nonischemic: sample is red, analysis shows normal levels of oxygen, carbon dioxide, and pH

Treatment intracavernosal injection of a vasoconstrictor (e.g., phenylephrine) and cavernosal blood aspiration for ischemic priapism, and conservative monitoring for nonischemic priapism.

Fournier's Gangrene

Fournier's gangrene is a necrotizing fasciitis consisting of a mixed aerobic/anaerobic infection of the perineum and scrotum. Patients typically present with severe pain that generally starts on the anterior abdominal wall and migrates into the gluteal muscles, scrotum, and penis.

Physical exam will show blisters/bullae, crepitus, and subcutaneous gas, as well as systemic findings such as fever, tachycardia, and hypotension.

CT scan is the most accurate test and will show air along the fascial planes or deeper tissue involvement. Treatment of necrotizing fasciitis consists of surgical exploration with debridement of necrotic tissue, and antibiotic therapy.

Male incontinence is divided into 4 specific areas:

- **Urge incontinence** is involuntary leakage of urine with significant urgency. Urgency is the complaint of a sudden and compelling desire to pass urine that is difficult to defer.
- **Stress incontinence** is involuntary leakage with exertion, sneezing, and/or coughing.
- **Mixed incontinence** is involuntary leakage associated with both urgency and also with exertion sneezing, and/or coughing.
- **Post-void dribbling** is a term used to describe dribbling of urine retained in the urethra after the bladder has emptied.

Therapies include lifestyle advice (particularly weight loss and dietary changes), bladder training biofeedback, and pelvic floor muscle exercises.

Antimuscarinic drugs and beta-adrenergic agonists are the main pharmacologic agents available for urgency incontinence, and alpha blockers are used for men with urgency incontinence associated with benign prostatic hyperplasia (BPH).

In men with stress incontinence who do not respond to lifestyle interventions like pelvic floor muscle exercise, the next step in management is to add duloxetine.

Abdominal Wall Hernias

A hernia is a protrusion, bulge, or projection of an organ or part of an organ through the body wall that normally contains it, such as the abdominal wall. Although abdominal wall hernia can go unnoticed, patients will usually report a bulge that may or may not be associated with symptoms of heaviness and localized pain.

Hernia can present with complications related to incarceration and strangulation of contents in the hernia sac, leading to sepsis. Large ventral hernia may present with skin ulceration due to pressure necrosis.

Type	Characteristics
Indirect inguinal hernia (**most common type of hernia in both men and women**)	Protrudes via the internal inguinal ring, lateral to the inferior epigastric vessels
Direct inguinal hernia	Protrudes medial to the inferior epigastric vessels within Hesselbach triangle
Femoral hernia	Protrudes through the femoral ring, which is inferior to the inguinal ligament, medial to the femoral vein, and lateral to the lacunar ligament
Umbilical hernia	Results from failure of the umbilical ring to close spontaneously
Epigastric hernias	Results from defects in the abdominal midline between the umbilicus and the xiphoid process

The best initial test for all hernias is a **thorough history and physical examination**. When the diagnosis is not clear or the most accurate test is needed, select **CT scan or MRI**.

The definitive treatment of all hernias, regardless of origin or type, is **surgical repair**. Patients who develop bowel or strangulation obstruction should undergo urgent surgical repair within 4–6 hours of presentation and receive broad-spectrum antibiotics to prevent bowel loss.

Vascular Surgery

A 48-year-old laborer complains of coldness and tingling in his left hand as well as pain in the forearm when he does strenuous work. Recently he's complained of dizziness, with blurred vision and trouble keeping steady during these episodes. Which of the following is the most important management?

a. Aspirin
b. Clopidogrel
c. Warfarin
d. Bypass surgery
e. Carotid endarterectomy

Answer: **D.** Bypass surgery is needed for **subclavian steal syndrome**.

Subclavian Steal Syndrome

Although this condition is rare in practice, it is a classic board vignette. An arteriosclerotic stenotic plaque at the origin of the subclavian allows enough blood supply to reach the arm for normal activity but not enough to meet the increased demands of an exercised arm, resulting in blood being "stolen" from the vertebral artery. When the arm is raised, increasing oxygen demand, the vessels in the arm dilate to increase perfusion. This dilation acts as a vacuum to blood in the head, neck, and shoulder, leading to syncopal episodes. Classic symptoms are the following:

- Posterior neurological signs: Visual symptoms, equilibrium problems
- Claudication in the arm during arm exercises

Diagnose with an **angiography.**

Treatment is **bypass surgery.**

Aortic Aneurysm

A 66-year-old man has vague, poorly described epigastric and upper back discomfort. He is found on physical examination to have a pulsatile mass, which is very tender to palpation. Ultrasound reveals a 6-cm abdominal aneurysm. What is the next step in management?

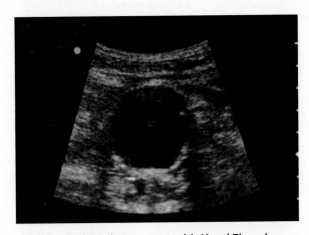

Abdominal Aortic Aneurysm with Mural Thrombus

a. ACE inhibitor
b. Urgent surgery
c. Elective repair
d. Repeat abdominal ultrasound in 6 months
e. CT angiogram of the chest

Answer: **B.** Urgent surgery within the next day is the most appropriate management in a patient with asymptomatic abdominal aortic aneurysm. Signs (hypotension) and symptoms (excruciating abdominal pain radiating to the back) suggest leaking or ruptured aneurysm and necessitate emergency surgery.

> Abdominal aortic aneurysm (AAA): one-time screening by ultrasonography in men age 65–75 who have ever smoked

Size and symptoms are key to the management of abdominal aortic aneurysm.

- Aortic diameter of 3.0–4.4 cm: image at yearly intervals
- Aortic diameter 4.5–5.4 cm: image at 3-month intervals
- Surgery is considered based on specific criteria (diameter $\geq$5.5 cm or rapid expansion of $\geq$1 cm/year). **All symptomatic AAAs get surgery!**

More urgent surgery is needed in the following cases:

- A tender abdominal aortic aneurysm will rupture within a day or two and, thus, requires urgent repair.
- Excruciating back pain in a patient with a large abdominal aortic aneurysm means that the aneurysm is already leaking, necessitating emergency surgery.

> **Basic Science Correlate**
>
> The abdominal aorta has 3 layers: intima, media, and adventitia.

A 65-year-old man presents with severe sharp chest and back pain down the spine that started 1 hour ago. His blood pressure is 219/115 mm Hg. Chest x-ray is shown. EKG and cardiac enzymes are nonrevealing. Which of the following is the most important intervention that would have prevented this presentation?

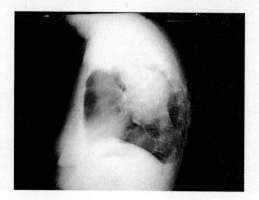

a. Aspirin prophylaxis.
b. Blood pressure control.
c. Cessation of smoking.
d. Low-fat diet.
e. Serial CT scans.

Answer: **B.** Blood pressure control is the most important strategy to prevent progression of thoracic aortic aneurysms.

Risk factors for thoracic aortic aneurysm include:

- Chronic hypertension
- Hyperlipidemia
- Smoking
- Marfan syndrome
- Untreated tertiary syphilis

The most important modifiable risk to prevent worsening of existing aneurysms is **uncontrolled hypertension.**

- **Asymptomatic lesions: blood pressure management** is most important factor to control.
- **Symptomatic lesions,** including active dissection (look for chest pain and sudden-onset "tearing" pain in the back), require **surgical intervention.**

Arteriosclerotic Occlusive Disease of the Lower Extremities

The classic presentation of this condition is pain in the legs on exercise that is relieved by rest (intermittent claudication).

If the claudication does not interfere significantly with the patient's lifestyle, no workup is indicated. The only management indicated is:

- Cessation of smoking and
- The use of cilostazol and aspirin
- Exercise/frequent ambulation

Basic Science Correlate

Cilostazol is a selective inhibitor of phosphodiesterase 3 (PDE3).

If the pain is more severe, diagnosis is with the following:

- Doppler studies looking for a pressure gradient (ankle-brachial index [ABI] <0.90)
- Arteriogram to identify stenosis

If the case describes disabling symptoms (affects work or activities of daily living) or if there is impending ischemia to the extremity, then surgery is indicated. This involves the following:

- Angioplasty and stenting for stenotic segments
- More extensive disease requires bypass grafts or sequential stents.

Pain at rest indicates end-stage disease (the patient complains of calf pain at night with disturbed sleep).

PART 6

Pediatrics

Contributing author Niket Sonpal, MD

The Newborn

At delivery, give the following:

- Erythromycin ophthalmic ointment to protect against *Neisseria gonorrhoeae ophthalmia neonatorum*
- IM vitamin K (1 mg) to prevent hemorrhagic disease

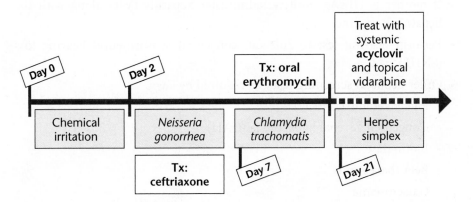

Basic Science Correlate

- Erythromycin is a bacteriostatic drug. Bacteriostatic drugs inhibit reproduction of the bacteria by blocking ribosomal formation of proteins.
- Penicillins are bactericidal. Bactericidal antibiotics kill bacteria by cell wall inhibition.

> **Basic Science Correlate**
>
> Factors II, VII, IX, and X are vitamin K–dependent clotting factors. Proteins C and S are vitamin K–dependent anticoagulants. Vitamin K adds a carboxyl group onto the glutamic acid on these factors. Protein C inhibits factor V.

Hemorrhagic Disease of Newborn

This condition occurs after 24 hours of life if vitamin K is not administered at delivery. Look for an apparently healthy neonate who suddenly presents with increased bleeding from umbilicus, GI tract, IV sites, or circumcision. The birth process causes significant trauma, so in these cases look for both intracranial bleeding (presenting with seizures) and internal bleeding.

Vitamin K is needed to produce coagulation factors II, VII, IX, X, protein C, and protein S. Babies have low vitamin K at birth because it does not cross the placenta, is not abundant in breast milk, and is not yet produced by the neonate undeveloped gut flora.

Before discharge, do the following:

- Administer hepatitis B vaccine if mother is HBsAg negative.
- If mother is HBsAg positive, administer hepatitis IVIG along with the hepatitis B vaccine.
- Perform hearing test to rule out congenital sensorineural hearing loss (SNHL).
- Order neonatal screening tests, as required by law:
  - Phenylketonuria (PKU)
  - Congenital adrenal hyperplasia (CAH)
  - Biotinidase
  - Beta-thalassemia
  - Galactosemia
  - Hypothyroidism
  - Homocystinuria

Apgar Score

The Apgar score is a measure of the need and effectiveness of resuscitation. The Apgar score does not predict outcome, but a persistently low Apgar (0–3) is associated with high mortality.

- The **1-minute** score gives an idea of what was going on **during labor and delivery.**
- The **5-minute** score gives an idea of **response to therapy** (resuscitation).

Apgar Category	0 points	1 point	2 points
Activity	Absent	Arms/legs flexed	Active movement
Pulse	Absent	<100 beats/min	>100 beats/min
Grimace	Flaccid	Some flexion	Active
Color	Cyanotic	Body pink, extremities blue	Completely pink
Respirations	Absent	Slow, irregular	Crying

Most neonates achieve a score of only 9 at 1 minute and 9 at 5 minutes because their color is usually pink with cyanosis in the extremities.

Abnormalities in the Newborn

The table lists both benign findings in the newborn and disorders with their management.

Figure	Finding/Description	Diagnosis	Association	Further Management
	Blue/gray macules on presacral back/posterior thighs	Congenital dermal melanocytosis	Usually fade in first few years	Rule out child abuse.
	Firm, yellow-white papules/pustules with erythematous base, which peak on second day of life	Erythema toxicum		Self-limited
	Permanent, unilateral vascular malformation on head and neck	Port wine stain (nevus flammeus)	Sturge-Weber syndrome (AV malformation that results in) seizures, mental retardation, and glaucoma)	Pulsed laser therapy For Sturge-Weber, evaluate for glaucoma and give anticonvulsives.

(continued next page)

Figure	Finding/ Description	Diagnosis	Association	Further Management
	Red, sharply demarcated, raised lesions appearing in first 2 months, rapidly expanding, then involuting by age 5–9 years.	Hemangioma	Consider underlying organ involvement with deep hemangiomas. (If it involves the larynx, it can cause obstruction.) May cause high output cardiac failure when large.	Treat with propranolol and/or pulsed laser if large or interferes with organ function.
	Preauricular tags/ pits	Preauricular tags/ pits	Hearing loss Genitourinary abnormalities	Hearing test Ultrasound of kidneys
	Defect in the iris	Coloboma of the iris	Other eye abnormalities CHARGE syndrome (**C**oloboma, **H**eart defects, **A**tresia of the nasal choanae, growth **R**etardation, **G**enitourinary abnormalities, and **E**ar abnormalities)	Screen for CHARGE syndrome.
	Absence of the iris	Aniridia	Wilms tumor	Screen for Wilms tumor with abdominal ultrasound Q3 months until age 8.
	Mass lateral to midline	Branchial cleft cyst	Remnant of embryonic development associated with infections	Infected cysts: Give antibiotics Surgical removal if large

(continued next page)

Figure	Finding/ Description	Diagnosis	Association	Further Management
	Mass in midline that moves with swallowing or tongue protrusion	Thyroglossal duct cyst (*see BSC after table*)	Associated with infections May have thyroid ectopia	Surgical removal Thyroid scans and thyroid function test preoperatively
	Congenital weakness where vessels of the fetal and infant umbilical cord exited through the rectus abdominis muscle	Umbilical hernia	Congenital hypothyroidism	Screen with TSH. May close spontaneously.
	Scrotal swelling, transillumination	Hydrocele	Inguinal hernia	Differentiate from inguinal hernia.
	Unilateral absence of testes in scrotal sac	Undescended testes	Associated with malignancy if >1 year of age	No treatment until 1 year of age (1) Orchiopexy is the definitive treatment (2) Hormone injections (β-hCG or testosterone)

Basic Science Correlate

A thyroglossal duct cyst may be formed anywhere along the thyroglossal tract, which is formed from the descent of the primordial thyroid gland at the base of the tongue. The duct usually atrophies, but a cyst may form.

Basic Science Correlate

In embryology, the intestines are formed outside the abdomen and extend into the umbilical cord until 10 weeks. At that time, they migrate into the abdomen.

You are called to see a 9.5-pound newborn boy who is jittery 30 minutes after birth. The pregnancy was complicated by prolonged delivery with shoulder dystocia. Physical exam reveals a large, plethoric infant who is tremulous. A pansystolic murmur is heard. Which of the following is the most appropriate diagnostic test?

a. Bilirubin level.
b. Blood glucose.
c. Galactose level.
d. Serum calcium level.
e. Serum TSH.

Answer: **B.** Blood glucose is the best initial diagnostic exam to evaluate in infants that present large for gestation, plethora, and jitteriness. This child is most likely born an **infant of a diabetic mother (IODM).**

Look for **macrosomia** (all organs except the brain are enlarged), **history of birth trauma, and cardiac abnormalities** (cardiomegaly). The case may not give a history of diabetes in the mother. Treat with **glucose and small, frequent meals.**

Infant of a Diabetic Mother (IODM)

Lab abnormalities are the following:

- Hypoglycemia (after birth)
- Hypocalcemia
- Hypomagnesemia
- Hyperbilirubinemia
- Polycythemia

IODM is associated with the following:

- Cardiac abnormalities (ASD, VSD, truncus arteriosus)
- Small left colon syndrome (abdominal distension)
- Increased risk of developing diabetes and childhood obesity

Infants of diabetic mothers become hypoglycemic after delivery because of excess insulin. In utero, they acclimate to a high-glucose environment by producing more insulin, becoming hyperinsulinemic. At birth, upon leaving this high-glucose environment, IODMs' high insulin level makes them hypoglycemic.

IODM is also associated with macrosomia. Neonates with fetal macrosomia are those above the 90th percentile of weight for gestational age or more than 4,000 g at birth.

Respiratory Distress in the Newborn

Keep the following in mind for all cases of respiratory distress in the newborn:

- Chest x-ray (**best initial test**)
- Other diagnostic studies:
  - ABG
  - Blood cultures (sepsis)
  - Blood glucose (hypoglycemia)
  - CBC (anemia or polycythemia)
  - Cranial ultrasound (intracranial hemorrhage)
- Treatment is as follows:
  - Oxygen (keep SaO_2 >95%)
  - Give nasal CPAP to prevent barotrauma and bronchopulmonary dysplasia if the neonate's oxygen requirement is high.
  - Consider empiric antibiotics for suspected sepsis.

CCS Tip: When oxygen therapy does not improve hypoxemia in a case of newborn respiratory distress evaluate the patient for cardiac causes of hypoxia (i.e., congenital heart defects).

Respiratory Distress Syndrome (RDS)

Clinical features are a premature neonate with the following:

- Tachypnea
- Nasal grunting
- Intercostal retractions within hours of birth

The hallmark finding is hypoxemia. Eventually hypercarbia and respiratory acidosis develop.

> Pneumonia and RDS look identical on chest x-ray. If in doubt, give antibiotics.

Diagnostic testing is as follows:

- Chest x-ray (**best initial test**): ground-glass appearance, atelectasis, air bronchograms
- Lecithin-sphingomyelin (L/S) ratio on amniotic fluid prior to birth (**best predictive test**)

Treatment starts with oxygen and nasal CPAP. Exogenous surfactant administration has been proven to decrease mortality.

> Lucinactant is the first synthetic peptide-containing surfactant approved for treatment of neonatal RDS.

Basic Science Correlate

Mechanism of Surfactant

- Surfactant prevents collapse of the alveoli by decreasing surface tension.
- Surfactant is produced by Type II pneumocytes, which start to develop around 24 weeks gestation. However, not enough surfactant is secreted until 35 weeks gestation.

Postnatal corticosteroids do not help RDS and are not indicated.

Do the following for primary prevention:

- Antenatal betamethasone: most effective if >24 hours before delivery and <34 weeks gestation
- Avoid prematurity: give tocolytics
- Give corticosteroids immediately to any fetus in danger of preterm delivery <34 weeks

Possible complications:

- Retinopathy of prematurity (hypoxemia)
- Bronchopulmonary dysplasia (prolonged high-concentration oxygen): prevent with CPAP
- Intraventricular hemorrhage

Transient Tachypnea of the Newborn (TTN)

This presents as tachypnea after a term birth of infant delivered by cesarean section or rapid second stage of labor, likely related to retained lung fluid. The condition usually resolves in 24–48 hours.

Basic Science Correlate

TTN is caused by retained lung fluid. That is, fluid present in the lungs in utero does not get squeezed out in passage through the birth canal. Increased fluid in the lungs causes increased airway resistance and decreased lung compliance.

Testing includes a chest x-ray to look for the following:

- Air trapping
- Fluid in fissures
- Perihilar streaking

Treatment is oxygen (minimal requirements needed), which results in rapid improvement within hours to days.

Meconium Aspiration Syndrome (MAS)

This presents as severe respiratory distress and hypoxemia in a term neonate with hypoxia or fetal distress in utero. (Meconium passed may be aspirated in utero or with the first postnatal breath.)

> **Basic Science Correlate**
>
> Meconium is the first stool a baby passes. It is sticky, like tar, and is composed of epithelial cells, lanugo, mucus, bile, and amniotic fluid. Fetuses in distress often pass meconium before birth. Meconium aspiration causes:
> - Blockage of alveoli
> - Decreased gas exchange
> - Irritation of airway, causing inflammation then pneumonia

Perform a chest x-ray to look for the following:

- Patchy infiltrates
- Increased AP diameter (barrel chest)
- Flattening of diaphragm

Treatment is as follows:

- Positive pressure ventilation
- High-frequency ventilation
- Nitric oxide therapy
- Extracorporeal membrane oxygenation

Prevention of meconium aspiration starts with prevention of fetal distress. After birth, suctioning offers no benefit and may cause harm.

Possible complications:

- Pulmonary artery hypertension
- Air leak (pneumothorax, pneumomediastinum)
- Aspiration pneumonitis

Upper Gastrointestinal Malformation

A newborn is born by normal vaginal delivery without complication. There is no respiratory distress. Upon his first feed, he is noted to have prominent drooling; he gags and develops respiratory distress. Chest x-ray reveals an infiltrate in the lung. Which of the following will confirm the diagnosis?

a. Arterial blood gas
b. Blood cultures
c. CT scan of chest
d. Nasogastric tube placement
e. Gastrografin enema

> VACTERL abnormalities are the following:
> - **V**ertebral defects
> - **A**nal atresia
> - **C**ardiac abnormalities
> - **T**racheoesophageal fistula with **E**sophageal atresia
> - **R**adial and **R**enal anomalies
> - **L**imb syndrome

Answer: **D.** This patient has a tracheoesophageal fistula (TEF). Classically, there is choking and gagging with the first feeding and then respiratory distress develops due to aspiration pneumonia. The feeding tube will be coiled in the chest. Don't forget to look for other abnormalities associated with VACTERL syndrome.

Basic Science Correlate

TEF is an embryological malformation: Division of the cranial part of the foregut into the respiratory and esophageal parts is incomplete. This occurs at week 4 of development.

> Differential diagnosis of double-bubble seen on x-ray includes duodenal atresia, annular pancreas, malrotation, and volvulus.

A premature infant is born by normal vaginal delivery without complication. There is no respiratory distress. Upon her first feed, she begins vomiting gastric and bilious material. Chest x-ray is shown. What is the most likely diagnosis?

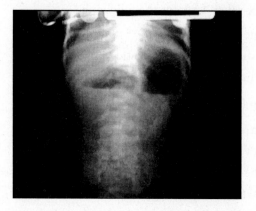

Answer: The most likely diagnosis is duodenal atresia. Half of infants with this condition are born prematurely, and the condition is associated with Down syndrome. Look for polyhydramnios in the prenatal exam. Treatment involves nasogastric decompression and surgical correction. You must search for other abnormalities (VACTERL association) with x-ray of the spine, abdominal ultrasound, and echocardiogram.

Basic Science Correlate

During duodenal development, the lumen is completely occluded by epithelium, then is re-formed. Failure to re-form a lumen = Duodenal atresia.

Annular Pancreas

In this condition, the pancreas surrounds the second part of the duodenum in a ring-like formation, potentially causing obstruction.

Symptoms include polyhydramnios, low birth weight, and feeding intolerance.

Diagnostic testing is abdominal x-ray (**best initial test**) showing double bubble sign and abdominal CT (**most accurate test**).

> ### Basic Science Correlate
>
> Annular pancreas forms when the ventral bud does not rotate with the duodenum during the 7th week of gestation. This causes encasing of the duodenum.

Jaundice in the Newborn

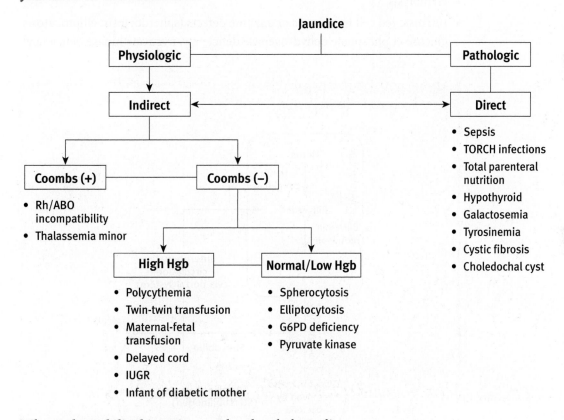

When is **hyperbilirubinemia** considered pathological?

- When it appears on day 1 of life and continues for 2 weeks
- When bilirubin rises >5 mg/dL/day
- When bilirubin >12 mg/dL in term infant
- When direct bilirubin >2 mg/dL at any time

Diagnostic testing is as follows if jaundice presents in the first 24 hours:

- Total and direct bilirubin
- Blood type of infant and mother: look for ABO or Rh incompatibility
- Direct Coombs test
- CBC, reticulocyte count, and blood smear: assess for hemolysis
- Urinalysis and urine culture if elevated direct bilirubin: assess for sepsis

If there is prolonged jaundice (>2 weeks) and no elevation of conjugated bilirubin, consider the following:

- UTI or other infection
- Bilirubin conjugation abnormalities (e.g., Gilbert, Crigler-Najjar syndromes)
- Hemolysis
- Intrinsic red cell membrane or enzyme defects (spherocytosis, elliptocytosis, glucose-6-phosphate dehydrogenase deficiency, pyruvate kinase deficiency)

Basic Science Correlate

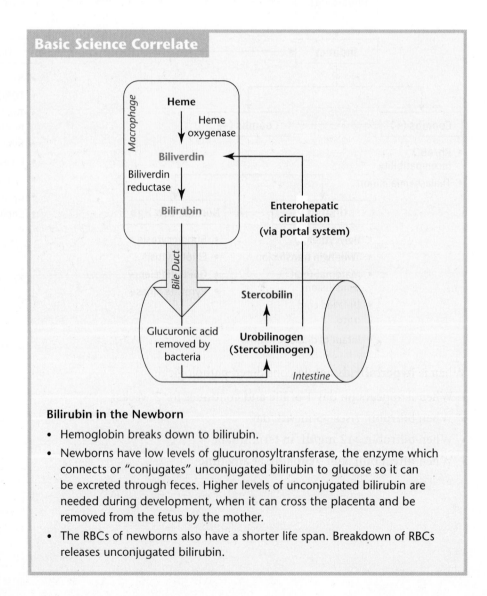

Bilirubin in the Newborn

- Hemoglobin breaks down to bilirubin.
- Newborns have low levels of glucuronosyltransferase, the enzyme which connects or "conjugates" unconjugated bilirubin to glucose so it can be excreted through feces. Higher levels of unconjugated bilirubin are needed during development, when it can cross the placenta and be removed from the fetus by the mother.
- The RBCs of newborns also have a shorter life span. Breakdown of RBCs releases unconjugated bilirubin.

Where there is prolonged jaundice (>2 weeks) AND elevation of conjugated bilirubin, consider cholestasis:

- Liver function tests (**best initial test**)
- Ultrasound and liver biopsy (**most specific tests**)

The most feared complication of jaundice results from elevated indirect (unconjugated) bilirubin, which can cross the blood brain barrier, deposit in the basal ganglia and brainstem nuclei, and cause kernicterus. Look out for hypotonia, seizures, opisthotonos, delayed motor skills, choreoathetosis, and sensorineural hearing loss. Management is immediate exchange transfusion.

Treatment is as follows:

- Phototherapy when bilirubin >10–12 mg/dL (normally decreases by 2 mg/dL every 4–6 hours)
- Exchange transfusion if bilirubin encephalopathy ever suspected or phototherapy fails to reduce total bilirubin

---

Basic Science Correlate

Phototherapy isomerizes bilirubin, making it water-soluble.

TORCH Infections Summary

Many of the TORCH infections have similar presentations, but there are notable distinguishing features.

Infection	Classic Feature(s)	Diagnostic Workup
General features	Intrauterine growth retardation, hepatosplenomegaly, jaundice, mental retardation	Elevated total cord blood IgM
Toxoplasmosis	Hydrocephalus with generalized intracranial calcifications and chorioretinitis	Positive toxoplasma IgM (after 5 days of life) and/or IgA (after 10 days of life) considered diagnostic of congenital toxoplasmosis
Rubella	• Cataracts, deafness, and heart defects • Blueberry muffin spots (extramedullary hematopoiesis)	Rubella virus RNA by PCR
CMV	• Microcephaly with periventricular calcifications • Petechiae with thrombocytopenia, sensorineural hearing loss • Blueberry-type rash	Urine or saliva CMV culture; if negative, consider CMV PCR
Herpes	First week: Pneumonia/shock Second week: Skin vesicles, keratoconjunctivitis Third to fourth week: Acute meningoencephalitis	HSV PCR (**most accurate test**)
Syphilis	Osteochondritis and periostitis; desquamating skin rash of palms and soles, snuffles (mucopurulent rhinitis); hepatomegaly (**most common finding**)	• VDRL screening (**best initial test**) • IgM-FTA-ABS (**most accurate test**)
Varicella	• Neonatal: pneumonia • Congenital: limb hypoplasia, cutaneous scars, seizures, mental retardation	• IgM serology (**best initial test**) • PCR of amniotic fluid (**most accurate test**)

Substance Abuse and Neonatal Withdrawal

Neonatal withdrawal presents with restlessness/tremors/jitters; high-pitched crying; poor feeding/irritability; seizures; fever; tachypnea; diarrhea/vomiting; and nasal stuffiness/sneezing.

The timing of withdrawal:

- Heroin, cocaine, amphetamine, and alcohol withdrawal presents within **first 48 hours** of life
- Methadone withdrawal presents within **first 96 hours** (up to 2 weeks); methadone associated with higher risk of seizures

Infants of mothers with substance use disorders are at higher risk for the following complications:

- Low birth weight
- Intrauterine growth restriction (IUGR)
- Congenital anomalies (alcohol, cocaine)
- Sudden infant death syndrome (SIDS)

Also, watch out for complications of the mother's condition, such as:

- Sexually transmitted diseases
- Toxemia
- Breech
- Abruption
- Intraventricular hemorrhage (cocaine use)

Treatment is parental support and education, optimizing the environment for mother-infant interaction, and pharmacotherapy when necessary.

Do not give naloxone to an infant born from a mother with known narcotics use. It may precipitate sudden withdrawal, including seizures.

Teratogenesis and Effect of Drugs on the Neonate

Drug	Effect	Drug	Effect
Anesthetics	Respiratory, CNS depression	Isotretinoin	Facial and ear anomalies, congenital heart disease
Barbiturates	Respiratory, CNS depression	Phenytoin	Hypoplastic nails, typical facies, IUGR
Magnesium sulfate	Respiratory depression	Diethylstilbestrol (DES)	Vaginal adenocarcinoma
Phenobarbital	Vitamin K deficiency	Tetracycline	Enamel hypoplasia, discolored teeth
Sulfonamides	Displaces bilirubin from albumin	Lithium	Ebstein anomaly
NSAIDs	Premature closure of ductus arteriosus	Warfarin	Facial dysmorphism and chondrodysplasia (bone stippling)
ACE inhibitors	Craniofacial abnormalities	Valproate/carbamazepine	Mental retardation, neural tube defects

Genetics/Dysmorphology

Condition	Classic Feature(s)	Diagnostic Workup/Disease Associations
Trisomy 21: Down syndrome Risk associated with advanced maternal age (>35 years)	Upward slanting palpebral fissures; speckling of iris (Brushfield spots); inner epicanthal folds; small stature; late fontanel closure; mental retardation; hypoplasia of the middle phalanx of the fifth finger; high arched palate microcephaly	• Hearing exam • Echocardiogram: Endocardiac cushion defect > VSD > PDA, ASD; MVP (Cardiac abnormalities are a major cause of early mortality.) • Gastrointestinal: TEF, duodenal atresia • TSH: Hypothyroidism • With advancing age, have a high probability of developing acute lymphocytic leukemia and early-onset Alzheimer disease
Trisomy 18: Edwards syndrome	Low-set, malformed ears; microcephaly; micrognathia; clenched hand—index over third, fifth over fourth; rocker-bottom feet and hammer toe; omphalocele; structural heart defect (most common is VSD)	• Echocardiogram: VSD, ASD, PDA • Renal ultrasound: Polycystic kidneys, ectopic or double ureter • Most patients do not survive first year
Trisomy 13: Patau syndrome	Defect of midface, eye, and forebrain development: Holoprosencephaly, microcephaly, microphthalmia, cleft lip/palate	• Echocardiogram: VSD, PDA, ASD • Renal ultrasound: Polycystic kidneys • Single umbilical artery
Aniridia-Wilms tumor association (WAGR syndrome)	**W**ilms **A**niridia **G**U anomalies Mental **R**etardation	• When you see an infant with aniridia, do a complete workup for WAGR syndrome.
Klinefelter syndrome (XXY) 1:500 males	Low IQ, behavioral problems, slim with long limbs, gynecomastia	• Testosterone levels: Hypogonadism and hypogenitalism • Replace testosterone at age 11–12.
Turner syndrome (XO) Sporadic; no association with maternal age	Small-stature female, gonadal dysgenesis, low IQ, congenital lymphedema, webbed posterior neck, broad chest, wide-spaced nipples	• Renal ultrasound: Horseshoe kidney, double renal pelvis • Cardiac: Bicuspid aortic valve, coarctation of the aorta • Thyroid function: Primary hypothyroidism, Hashimoto thyroiditis • Can give estrogen, growth hormone, and anabolic steroid replacement.
Fragile X syndrome Fragile site on long arm of X Molecular diagnosis—variable number of repeat CGG	Macrocephaly in early childhood, large ears, large testes Most common cause of mental retardation in boys	• Attention deficit hyperactivity syndrome
Beckwith-Wiedemann syndrome IGF-2 disrupted at 11p15.5	Multiorgan enlargement: Macrosomia, macroglossia, pancreatic beta cell hyperplasia (hypoglycemia), large kidneys, neonatal polycythemia	• Increased risk of abdominal tumors • Obtain ultrasounds and serum AFP every 6 months through age 6 to look for Wilms tumor and hepatoblastoma.
Prader-Willi syndrome Deletion of 15q11q13, which is paternally derived	Obesity, mental retardation, binge eating, small genitalia	• Decreased life expectancy related to morbid obesity

(continued next page)

Condition	Classic Feature(s)	Diagnostic Workup/Disease Associations
Angelman syndrome (happy puppet syndrome) Deletion of 15q11q13, which is maternally derived	Mental retardation, inappropriate laughter, absent speech or <6 words, ataxia and jerky arm movements resembling a puppet gait, recurrent seizures	• 80% develop epilepsy
Robin sequence (Pierre Robin) Associated with fetal alcohol syndrome, Edwards syndrome	Mandibular hypoplasia, cleft palate	• Monitor airway: Obstruction possible over first 4 weeks of life.

> **Basic Science Correlate**
>
> Trisomy is most commonly caused by nondisjunction during meiosis.

Marfan Syndrome

Marfan syndrome is an autosomal dominant mutation of the FBN1 gene on chromosome 15. It encodes for fibrillin protein, which makes up a major part of bones connective tissue, and blood vessels.

Physical exam reveals a tall and thin patient with long extremities (arm span exceeds height), arachnodactyly, pectus excavatum deformity, and hypermobile joints.

Diagnosis of Marfan is made clinically, but genetic testing is the **most accurate test**.

Aortic root dissection is also very common in Marfan.

- Do TTE at the time of diagnosis and 6 months later to establish if the aortic root is stable.
- If dilation is seen, surgical intervention may be required.

Ophthalmologic evaluation is also recommended annually to screen for ectopia lentis.

Treatment is supportive.

Ehlers-Danlos Syndromes (EDS)

The syndromes result from a mutation in one of over a dozen genes.

EDS are associated with:

- Extremely elastic, smooth skin that is fragile and bruises easily
- Wide, atrophic scars (flat or depressed scars)
- Joint hypermobility

- Molluscoid pseudotumors (calcified hematomas over pressure points such as the elbow)
- Spheroids (fat-containing cysts on forearms and shins) (common)
- Hypotonia and delayed motor development

Diagnosis may be confirmed with genetic testing or skin biopsy.

There is no known cure. Treatment is supportive and palliative. Physical therapy and bracing may help strengthen muscles and support joints.

Osteogenesis Imperfecta (OI)

Osteogenesis imperfecta is a group of disorders whose main features are fragile osteopenic bones with recurrent fractures.

- Recurrent fractures and osteopenia (hallmark features)
- Joint laxity (common)
- Blue sclerae, hearing loss, and progressive skeletal deformity (some forms of OI)

The most common form of OI is inherited in autosomal dominant encoding of the alpha-1 and alpha-2 chains of type I collagen (COL1A1 and COL1A2).

There is no definitive, readily available diagnostic test for OI. Diagnosis is based on the history, signs and symptoms, and physical exam, along with a detailed family history.

Growth, Nutrition, and Development

Developmental Milestones

The absence of milestone behavior (or persistence of it beyond a given time frame) signifies CNS dysfunction. Exam questions typically describe a child's skills and ask for the corresponding age.

Age	Milestone
Newborn reflexes	**Moro, grasp, rooting, tonic neck, and placing reflexes**: appear at birth and disappear at 4–6 months
	Parachute reflex (extension of arms when fall simulated): present at 6–8 months and persists
2 months	Lifts head and chest when prone, tracks past midline, alert to sound and "coo," recognizes parent, and has social smile
4 months	Rolls front to back and back to front, grasps a rattle, orients to voice and can laugh
6 months	Can sit unassisted and transfer objects between hands, can babble, has some stranger anxiety
9 months	Has pincer grasp, creeps and crawls, knows own name
12 months	Cruises, says 1 or more words, plays ball

(continued next page)

Age	Milestone
15 months	Builds 3-cube tower, walks alone, makes lines and scribbles
18 months	Builds 4-cube tower, walks down stairs, says 10 words, feeds self
24 months	Builds 7-cube tower, runs well, goes up and down stairs, jumps with 2 feet, threads shoelaces, handles spoon, says 2–3 sentences
36 months	Walks down stairs alternating feet, rides tricycle, knows age and sex, understands taking turns
48 months	Hops on 1 foot, throws ball overhead, tells stories, participates in group play

Newborn reflexes include:

- Sucking: baby automatically will suck on a nipple-like object
- Grasping reflex
- Babinski: toe extension
- Rooting: if cheek is touched, baby turns toward that side
- Moro: arms spread symmetrically when baby is startled
- Stepping: walking-like leg motion when toes touch the ground
- Superman: when baby is held, arms extend forward like "Superman"

Pediatric Growth

Birth weight normally doubles at 4 months and triples by 1 year. The most common cause of failure to thrive in all age groups is psychosocial deprivation.

Any child who has crossed 2 major growth percentiles must be worked up. All cases of underfeeding must be reported to child protective services.

- Best indicator for acute malnutrition: weight/height <5th percentile
- Best indicator for under- and overweight: BMI

Skeletal maturity is related to sexual maturity, and less related to chronologic age. Height percentile at age 2 normally correlates with the final adult height percentile.

> Patients with genetic short stature or constitutional delay of growth appear to have a normal birth weight and normal growth velocity, but when plotted on the normal growth curve, it will appear below and parallel to the curve.

Description of Growth Pattern	Differential Diagnosis	Workup
Decreased weight gain greater than decreased length/height	• Undernutrition • Inadequate digestion • Malabsorption (infection, celiac disease, cystic fibrosis, disaccharide deficiency, protein-losing enteropathy)	• Assess caloric intake • Perform stool studies for fat • Perform sweat chloride test
Normal weight gain and decreased length/height	• Growth hormone (GH) or thyroid hormone deficiency • Excessive cortisol secretion • Skeletal dysplasias	• GH deficiency: insulin-like growth factor 1 (IGF-1) and IGF-binding protein 3 (IGF-BP3) • Thyroid hormone: TSH, free T4, free T3 • Cushing: 24-hour urinary cortisol or free cortisol • Bone age (x-ray of hand and wrist): skeletal dysplasia, i.e., no delay in bone age and disproportionate bone length on exam
Decreased weight gain equal to decreased length/height	• **Systemic illness**: heart failure; inflammation, e.g., IBD; renal insufficiency; hepatic insufficiency • Genetic short stature • Constitutional delay in growth and development	**Inflammatory markers**: CRP, ESR, CBC with diff **Organ dysfunction**: • LFT, creatinine, BUN • Electrolytes **Bone age**: • Genetic short stature: bone age is close to chronological age; puberty occurs at the normal time • Constitutional delay of growth: bone age is delayed and puberty occurs later than usual

Basic Science Correlate

- IgM is secreted during early stages of humoral immunity. It is the first antibody secreted.
- IgG causes sustained immunity to pathogens. It is the only immunoglobulin that crosses the placenta.
- IgE binds to allergens and secretes histamine.
- IgA is found in mucosal areas (intestines, saliva, tears, breast milk). It is secreted during breastfeeding.

Monomer
IgD, IgE, IgG

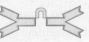
Dimer
IgA

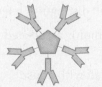
Pentamer
IgM

Behavioral Disorders

A 4-year-old boy has problems with bedwetting. The mother says that during the day, he has no problems but is usually wet 6 out of 7 mornings. He does not report dysuria or frequency and has not had increased thirst. The mother also says that he is a deep sleeper. Which of the following is the most appropriate next step in management?

a. Give anticholinergics
b. Give desmopressin
c. Give prophylactic antibiotics
d. Perform renal ultrasound
e. Reassure mother that bedwetting is normal

Answer: **E.** Bedwetting age <5 (before bladder control is anticipated) is normal.

Enuresis

Enuresis is the involuntary voiding of urine, occurring at least 2×/week for at least 3 months in children age >5 years (when bladder control is anticipated).

- **Nocturnal enuresis** (nighttime wetting) is more common in boys who are usually continent, occurring within 2 years of daytime continence; treatment is behavior therapy.
- **Diurnal enuresis** (daytime wetting) is more common in girls and is associated with a higher rate of urinary tract infection (UTI); most commonly caused by diabetes insipidus, UTI, seizure, constipation, and abuse.

Urinalysis is the **best initial test**. If signs of infection are present, do a urine culture.

For recurrent UTI, do a bladder/renal ultrasound (postvoid residual, anatomical abnormalities) or voiding cystourethrogram.

Treatment is behavioral and motivational therapy (cures 70% of patients), e.g., limit liquids and use a bed alarm. Never punish the child.

If behavioral therapy fails, consider desmopressin to decrease the volume of urine produced.

Encopresis

Encopresis is the unintentional or involuntary passage of feces in inappropriate settings, such as into clothing or onto the floor, in children age >4 (the age by which most children control bowel movements).

Abdominal x-ray (**best initial test**) will distinguish retentive from nonretentive.

- **Retentive encopresis** (most common): associated with constipation and overflow incontinence
- **Nonretentive encopresis**: associated with abuse

Do not miss uncommon causes such as Hirschsprung disease, anal fissure, ulcerative colitis, and spinal cord abnormalities.

Treatment is as follows.

- **Retentive** encopresis: disimpaction, stool softeners, and behavior intervention
- **Nonretentive** encopresis: behavior modification alone

Attention-Deficit/Hyperactivity Disorder

Attention-deficit/hyperactivity disorder (ADHD) is the most commonly diagnosed mental and behavior disorder in children and teens. Children with ADHD are hyperactive and have a problem controlling their impulses both at home and at school.

Under DSM-5 criteria, diagnosis of ADHD requires the following conditions.

- Patients age <17 must have at least 6 symptoms of hyperactivity and impulsivity or at least 6 symptoms of inattention
- Patients age ≥17 must have at least 5 symptoms of hyperactivity and impulsivity or at least 5 symptoms of inattention

Symptoms must:

- Occur in more than one setting and occur often
- Start age <12 and last >6 months
- Impair the patient's function (i.e., at school)
- Be excessive for the child's developmental status

Sample Inattention Symptoms	Sample Hyperactivity Symptoms	Sample Impulsivity Symptoms
• Distraction • Inability to follow directions • Inability to complete a task • Daydreaming • Inability to stay organized • Carelessness (making mistakes)	• Fidgeting • Excessive talking • Constant physical motion • Inability to sit still	• Blurting out answers • Inability to wait their turn

Treatment of ADHD is behavioral modification, medication, and/or educational intervention—alone or in combination. Behavioral modification includes:

- Maintaining the same daily schedule
- Using checklists and star charts for tasks
- Keeping distractions to a minimum
- Rewarding positive actions

Further treatment with medication is highly patient-specific, with dosage based on the patient's response and side effects. Stimulants (methylphenidate) are first-line.

- Elimination diets and essential fatty acid supplementation are not currently recommended as adjunct treatments for ADHD.
- Since ADHD drug treatment is so patient-specific, it is hard to test on the exam.

Immunizations

For **premature infants or low-birth-weight babies**, immunize at the chronological age. Do not delay immunizations and do not dose-adjust.

For **immunocompromised patients**, do not give live vaccines.

- The following are not contraindications to immunization:
    - A reaction to a previous DPT of temperature <40.6°C (<105.0°F), redness, soreness, and swelling
    - Mild, acute illness in an otherwise well child
    - Family history of seizures or SIDS
- MMR: Documented egg allergy is not a contraindication. Also, MMR does not cause autism or inflammatory bowel disease.
- Yellow fever vaccine: Egg allergy does contraindicate.
- Influenza vaccine: Egg allergy is no longer a contraindication. Patients age ≥6 months with a known egg allergy should receive trivalent inactivated influenza vaccine (TIV) followed by 30 minutes of observation in a facility prepared to recognize and treat anaphylaxis. Patients with a history of severe anaphylaxis to eggs should be referred to an allergy specialist to receive TIV.
- Hepatitis B vaccine does not cause demyelinating neurologic disorders.
- Meningococcal vaccination is not related to development of Guillain-Barré.

Active Immunizations after Exposure

Measles	• 0–6 months: Ig • 6–12 months: Ig plus vaccine • >12 months: vaccine only within 72 hours of exposure • Pregnant or immunocompromised: Ig only
Varicella	• Susceptible children and household contacts: VZIG and vaccine • Susceptible pregnant women, newborns whose mothers had chickenpox within 5 days before delivery to 48 hours after delivery: VZIG
Hepatitis	• Hepatitis B: Ig plus vaccine; given at birth, age 1 month, and 6 months • Hepatitis A: age >2 only, Ig plus vaccine
Mumps and rubella	• No postexposure protection available

Specific Routine Vaccinations

Hepatitis B	• **If mother is HBsAg negative**: first dose at birth; a total of 3 doses by 18 months • **If mother is HBsAg positive**: first dose of hepatitis B vaccine (HBV) plus hepatitis B Ig at 2 different sites within 12 hours of birth; a total of 3 doses by 6 months
DTaP	• Total of 5 doses is recommended before school entry (last dose age 4–6 years) • Pertussis booster vaccine is also given during adolescence, regardless of immunization. • Td is given at 11–12 years, then every 10 years
HiB conjugated vaccine	• Does not cover nontypeable *Haemophilus* • Not given age >5 • Invasive disease does not confirm immunity; patients still require vaccine if age <5
Varicella	• Associated with the development of herpes zoster after immunization
HPV	• Quadrivalent vaccine that should be administered to **all adults age 13–45**
Meningococcal conjugate vaccine	• Given at age 11–12 or at age 15 • Indicated for all college freshmen living in dormitories • Menomune (MPSV4) indicated in children age **2–10** • Type B vaccine (Trumenba) given at age 16–23

Child Abuse/Non-Accidental Trauma (NAT)

Testing includes:

- Lab studies: PT, PTT, platelets, bleeding time, CBC
- Skeletal survey
- If severe injuries (even with no neurological signs): head CT scan ± MRI; ophthalmologic examination
- If abdominal trauma: urine and stool for blood; liver and pancreatic enzymes; abdominal CT
- Urine toxicology screen, especially if there is altered mental status

> Don't forget dilated eye exam by an ophthalmologist in cases of suspected infant abuse.

Treatment is, first, to address medical and/or surgical issues. Then report any child suspected of being abused or neglected to child protective services (CPS). Initial action includes a phone report; in most states, a written report is then required within 48 hours.

Indications for hospitalization include:

- Medical condition requires it
- Diagnosis is unclear
- There is no alternative safe place

If parents refuse hospitalization or treatment, get an emergency court order.

The following must be explained to the parent: why an inflicted injury is suspected abuse; that you are legally obligated to report it; that you have made a referral to protect the child; and that a CPS worker and law enforcement officer will be involved.

Childhood Malignancy

Type	X-Ray Appearance	Most Accurate Diagnostic Test	Therapy
Ewing sarcoma	Onion-skin pattern due to lytic lesions causing laminar periosteal elevation	Analysis for a translocation t(11;22) via bone biopsy	Multidrug chemotherapy as well as local disease; control with surgery and radiation
Osteogenic sarcoma	Sclerotic destruction causing a "sunburst" appearance	CT scan of the leg	Chemotherapy and ablative surgery
Osteoid osteoma	Round central lucency with a sclerotic margin	CT scan or MRI of the affected leg	NSAIDs for pain; the condition will resolve spontaneously

Respiratory Diseases

Condition	Classic Presentation	Diagnosis	Steps in Management	Complication(s)/ Prognosis
Laryngotracheitis (Croup) Parainfluenza virus type 1 is the most common cause of acute laryngotracheitis.	Child age 3 months to 5 years with URTI symptoms (symptoms worse at night): rhinorrhea, sore throat, hoarseness, deep barking cough, inspiratory stridor, tachypnea	Diagnosis made clinically; however, neck x-ray positive for steeple sign can be diagnostic	1. Humidified oxygen 2. Nebulized epinephrine and corticosteroids. Antitussives, decongestants, sedatives, or antibiotics are not used in the management of croup.	Spontaneous resolution in 1 week Always suspect diagnosis of epiglottitis
Epiglottitis *H. influenzae* type B (now less common) *S. pyogenes, S. pneumoniae, S. aureus, Mycoplasma* **Notes:** *H. influenza* is a gram-negative coccobacillus. *S. pneumonia* is a gram-positive, alpha-hemolytic bacterium. *S. pyogenes* is a gram-positive coccus that causes group A streptococcal infection.	Sudden onset, muffled voice, drooling, dysphagia, high fever, and inspiratory stridor; patient prefers to sit in tripod position; patient has toxic appearance	A medical emergency; go straight to management based on clinical diagnosis. Perform diagnostic workup after stabilization: • Neck x-ray (thumb-print sign) • Blood cultures • Nasopharyngoscopy in the OR • Epiglottic swab culture	1. Transfer to hospital/OR 2. Consult ENT and anesthesia 3. Intubate 4. Give antibiotics (ceftriaxone) and vancomycin 5. Give rifampin prophylaxis to household contacts if *H. influenzae* positive	Airway obstruction and death
Bacterial tracheitis *S. aureus* **Notes:** *S. aureus* is a gram-positive coccus that occurs in clusters.	Brassy cough, high fever, respiratory distress, but no drooling or dysphagia; child <3; usually occurs after viral URTI	Clinical plus laryngoscopy: • Chest x-ray shows subglottic narrowing plus ragged tracheal air column • Blood cultures • Throat cultures	Antistaphylococcal antibiotics; may require intubation if severe	Airway obstruction

Clues to less common disorders:

- Diphtheritic croup (extremely rare in North America) presents with a gray-white pharyngeal membrane; may cover soft palate; bleeds easily. Don't forget that diphtheria is a notifiable disease.
- Foreign body aspiration presents with sudden choking/coughing without warning.
- Retropharyngeal abscess presents with drooling and difficulty swallowing.
- Extrinsic compression (vascular ring) or intraluminal obstruction (masses). Look for a patient with continued symptoms and who does not improve with treatment.
- Angioedema is due to a sudden allergic reaction (a trigger will be given in the case). Treat with steroids and epinephrine. If severe, intubate for airway protection. Angioedema is mediated by bradykinin. This peptide increases the permeability of the vasculature, leading to the accumulation of fluid.
- Pertussis presents with severe cough after 1–2 weeks plus characteristic whoop and spells of cough (paroxysms). Look for a child with incomplete immunization history.

> Differentiate epiglottitis from croup by the absence of a barking cough.

A toddler presents to the ED with sudden onset respiratory distress. The mother reports that earlier, the child was without symptoms, playing with toys in the living room with her siblings. On physical examination the patient is drooling and in moderate respiratory distress. There are decreased breath sounds on the right with intercostal retractions. Which of the following is the most appropriate next step in management?

a. Antibiotics
b. Bronchoscopy
c. Chest x-ray
d. Cricothyroidotomy
e. Throat cultures

Answer: **B.** Bronchoscopy is indicated both to visualize a suspected foreign body and for foreign body retrieval. if there is significant respiratory distress and hypoxemia, emergency cricothyroidotomy may be indicated. Foreign bodies are found most commonly in children <4.

Recurrent infections in a young child should always raise the suspicion of previously undiagnosed aspiration. Get a chest x-ray to look for postobstruction atelectasis or visualization of the foreign body.

Inflammation of the Small Airways

Bronchiolitis

The pathophysiology of bronchiolitis is respiratory syncytial virus (RSV) (50%); parainfluenza; adenovirus; and other viruses.

Bronchioles are the smallest parts of the airway (≤1 mm) and terminate at alveoli. They have ciliated cuboidal epithelium over a layer of smooth muscle. Bronchioles change in diameter and can reduce or increase airflow.

> The most common sites of foreign body aspiration are the **larynx** (age >1) and **trachea or right mainstem bronchus** (age <1).

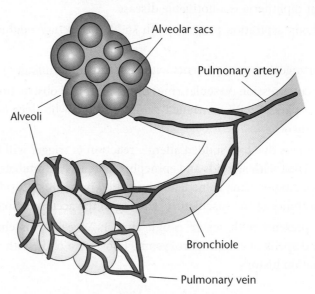

Anatomy of the Respiratory System

Bronchiolitis results in inflammation, which results in ball-valve obstruction, which results in air trapping and overinflation.

The classic presentation is in a child age <2 (most severe age 1–2 months) with the following symptoms in fall and winter months:

- Mild URI
- Fever
- Paroxysmal wheezy cough
- Dyspnea
- Tachypnea
- Apnea (in young infants)
- On exam, wheezing and prolonged expirations

Diagnosis is clinical. Diagnostic tests include:

- Chest x-ray (**best initial test**) will show hyperinflation with patchy atelectasis (may look like early pneumonia)
- Viral antigen testing (IFA or ELISA) of nasopharyngeal secretions (**most specific test**)

Treatment is supportive only. Hospitalize if severe tachypnea (>60/minute), pyrexia, and intercostal retractions are present. Steroids are not indicated.

> Ribavirin has not been shown to have clinical benefit and is generally not recommended.

General prevention methods include hand-washing, avoiding secondhand smoke, and avoiding sick contacts. For high-risk patients only (i.e., those with bronchopulmonary dysplasia and those born preterm), consider hyperimmune RSV IVIG or monoclonal antibody to RSV F protein (palivizumab).

Pneumonia

Classic presentations:

- **Viral** (most common cause **age <5**), most often RSV
  - URI symptoms
  - Low-grade fever
  - Tachypnea (most consistent finding)
- **Bacterial** (most common cause **age >5**), most often *S. pneumoniae, M. pneumoniae,* or *C. pneumoniae* (not trachomatis)

Diagnostic testing includes:

- Chest x-ray:
  - Viral: hyperinflation with bilateral interstitial infiltrates and peribronchial cuffing
  - Pneumococcal: confluent lobar consolidation
  - Mycoplasma/chlamydia: unilateral lower-lobe interstitial pneumonia; looks worse than presentation
- CBC with differential:
  - Viral usually <20,000
  - Bacterial 15,000–40,000
- Respiratory viral panel PCR: IgM titers for mycoplasma
- Blood cultures

Treatment is as follows:

- Outpatient (mild cases): amoxicillin (alternatives are cefuroxime and amoxicillin/clavulanic acid)
- Hospitalized:
  - 1–6 months: ceftriaxone or cefotaxime
  - ≥6 months: ampicillin, ceftriaxone, or cefotaxime
  - If severe and requires ICU: vancomycin and ceftriaxone + azithromycin
- *Chlamydia* or *Mycoplasma*: azithromycin

Cystic Fibrosis (CF)

CF is an autosomal, recessively inherited disease caused by a mutation in the CFTR gene. The body regulates sweat and mucus by channeling water and chloride through a specific protein. The CFTR gene controls expression of this protein. In CF, the malfunctioning protein does not allow the chloride to flow through, and the blocked channel causes a buildup of thick mucus.

The most common initial presentation is meconium ileus. Other signs and symptoms that warrant workup for CF are the following:

- Failure to thrive from malabsorption (steatorrhea due to pancreatic exocrine insufficiency, vitamin A, D, E, and K deficiency)
- Rectal prolapse: most often in infants with steatorrhea, malnutrition, and cough
- Persistent cough in first year of life with copious purulent mucus production

> Meconium ileus occurs in 10% of patients. Look for abdominal distention at birth, failure to pass meconium, and bilious vomiting.

Other associated conditions are undescended testes, infertility (absent vas deferens), and allergic bronchopulmonary aspergillosis.

Diagnostic testing is as follows:

- Two elevated sweat chloride concentrations (>60 mEq/L) obtained on separate days (**best initial and most specific test**)
- Genetic testing is highly accurate but does not detect all chromosome-7 mutations; use it to detect carrier status and for prenatal diagnosis
- Newborn screening: determine immunoreactive trypsinogen in blood spots and then confirm with sweat or DNA testing
- Chest x-ray useful to monitor course of disease and acute exacerbations
- PFTs are not done until age 5 or 6 to evaluate disease progression (obstructive → restrictive)

Treatment is as follows:

- Supportive care: aerosol treatment, albuterol/saline, chest physical therapy with postural drainage, and pancrelipase (aids digestion with pancreatic dysfunction)
- Ivacaftor: first approved CF treatment to restore the function of a mutant CF protein; has been shown to decrease sweat chloride levels, improve FEV_1, decrease pulmonary symptoms and exacerbations, and improve weight gain; recommended for all patients age ≥6 who carry at least one copy of the G551D mutation

The most common organisms that cause infection in CF are *Staphylococcus aureus*, *Haemophilus influenzae*, and *Pseudomonas aeruginosa*.

The following treatment has been shown to improve survival:

- Ibuprofen reduces inflammatory lung response, slows patient's decline
- Azithromycin slows rate of decline in FEV_1 in patients age <13
- Antibiotics during exacerbations delay progression of lung disease

Never delay antibiotic therapy (even if fever and tachypnea are absent):

- Mild disease: macrolide, TMP-SMX, or ciprofloxacin
- Documented infection with *Pseudomonas or S. aureus*: piperacillin plus tobramycin or ceftazidime (given aggressively)
- Resistant pathogens: inhaled tobramycin

Other important management considerations:

- Give all routine vaccinations plus pneumococcal and yearly flu vaccines.
- Steroids improve PFTs in the short term, but there is no persistent benefit when steroids are stopped.
- Expectorants (guaifenesin or iodides) are not effective in the removal of respiratory secretions.

> G551D mutation is present in 5% of CF patients and interferes with activation of CFTR chloride channel.
>
> All CF patients should undergo genotyping to determine whether they carry the G551D mutation.

A 3-year-old white child presents with rectal prolapse. She is noted to be in the less-than-5th percentile for weight and height. The parents also note that she has a foul-smelling bulky stool each day that "floats." They also state that the child has developed a repetitive cough over the last few months. What is the first step in workup?

a. Genetic testing
b. Pulmonary function tests (PFTs)
c. Rectal biopsy
d. Sweat chloride
e. Stool studies

Answer: **D.** Sweat chloride is the best initial test to diagnose CF.

Cardiology

Congenital Heart Disease (CHD)

The most common symptom of acyanotic defects is congestive heart failure. The most common acyanotic lesions are these:

- Ventricular septal defect
- Atrial septal defect
- Atrioventricular canal
- Pulmonary stenosis
- Patent ductus arteriosus
- Aortic stenosis
- Coarctation of the aorta

In infants with cyanotic defects, the primary concern is hypoxia. The most common defects associated with cyanosis are tetralogy of Fallot and transposition of the great arteries (TGA).

Because functional closure of the ductus arteriosus may be delayed in CHD:

- CHDs that rely on the ductus will present within 1 month
- Infants with left-to-right shunting lesions will present at age 2–6 months

Consider CHD in any child presenting with the following:

- Shock, tachypnea, cyanosis (especially if fever is absent): cyanosis and hypoxemia classically do not respond to oxygen as is seen in pulmonary conditions
- Infants: feeding difficulty, sweating while feeding, rapid respirations, easy fatigue
- Older children: dyspnea on exertion, shortness of breath, failure to thrive
- Abnormalities on exam:
  - Upper extremity hypertension or decreased lower extremity blood pressure
  - Decreased femoral pulses (obstructive lesions of left side of the heart)
  - Facial edema, hepatomegaly
  - Heart sounds: pansystolic murmur, grade 3/6 murmurs, PMI at upper left sternal border, harsh murmur, early midsystolic click, abnormal S2

> Do not be reassured by normal antenatal ultrasounds; most CHD cases are diagnosed after delivery.

The presence or absence of a heart murmur is not used to suggest CHD.

CCS Tip: Because sepsis and CHD present very similarly, begin antibiotic therapy at the same time as workup for CHD.

Diagnostic testing is as follows:

- Chest x-ray and EKG (**best initial tests**) show increased pulmonary vascular markings
  - Transposition of the great arteries (TGA)
  - Hypoplastic left heart syndrome
  - Truncus arteriosus
- Echocardiography (**most specific test**)

> On the Step 3 exam, when is a murmur innocent?
> - When the question includes fever, infection, or anxiety
> - When it is *only* systolic (never diastolic)
> - When it is grade <2/6

High-Yield Congenital Heart Defects	
Heart Defect	
Acyanotic lesions	**Comments**
Ventricular septal defect	• Harsh holosystolic murmur over lower left sternal border ± thrill; loud pulmonic S2 • Almost 50% of cases have spontaneous closure within first 6 months • Surgical repair if failure to thrive, pulmonary hypertension, or right-to-left shunt >2:1

Atrial septal defect	• Loud S1, wide fixed splitting of S2, systolic ejection murmur along left upper sternal border
	  - Majority are asymptomatic
	  - Secundum type most common
	  - Most close by age 4
	• Primary and sinus types require surgery
	• Most common type: patent foramen ovale
	• A patent foramen ovale needs to be closed if a paradoxical embolus has gone through it
	• Late complications: mitral valve prolapse, dysrhythmias, and pulmonary hypertension

Atrioventricular canal	• Combination of the primum type of atrial septal defect, ventricular septal defect, and common atrioventricular valve • Presentation similar to ventricular septal defect • Perform surgery in infancy *before* pulmonary hypertension develops
Pulmonary stenosis	• May be asymptomatic or may result in severe congestive heart failure • Give prostaglandin E1 infusion at birth • Attempt balloon valvuloplasty.
Patent ductus arteriosus	• Girls > boys (2:1), babies where maternal rubella infection was present, and premature infants • Wide pulse pressure, bounding arterial pulses, and characteristic sound of "machinery" (to-and-fro murmur) • NSAID-induced closure helpful in premature infants • Term infants often require surgical closure
Aortic stenosis	• Early systolic ejection click at apex of left sternal border • Valve replacement and anticoagulation may be required

(continued next page)

High-Yield Congenital Heart Defects	
Heart Defect	
Acyanotic lesions	**Comments**
Coarctation of the aorta	• Of all cases, 98% occur at origin of left subclavian artery • Blood pressure higher in arms than legs, bounding pulses in arms and decreased pulses in legs • Ductus dependent: give PGE1 infusion to maintain ductus patent (ensures lower extremity blood flow) • Surgery repair after stabilization
Cyanotic lesions	
Tetralogy of Fallot	• Most common CHD beyond infancy • Defects include ventricular septal defect, right ventricular hypertrophy, right outflow obstruction, and overriding aorta • Substernal right ventricular impulse, systolic thrill along the left sternal border • Intermittent hyperpnea, irritability, cyanosis with decreased intensity of murmur • Treatment: give oxygen, beta blocker, PGE1 infusion for cyanosis present at birth • Surgical repair at 4–12 months
Transposition of the great arteries	• Most common cyanotic lesion presenting in immediate newborn period • Common in infants of diabetic mothers • S2 usually single and loud; murmurs usually absent • Ductus-dependent: give PGE1 to keep ductus open • Definitive surgical switch of aorta and pulmonary artery needed as soon as possible

Summary of Cyanotic Heart Defects				
	Right to Left Shunt Present?	**PDA Dependent?**	**VSD Present?**	**Surgery Is Treatment?**
Tetralogy of Fallot	Yes		Yes	Yes
Transposition of great vessels	Yes	Yes		Yes
Hypoplastic LH	Yes	Yes		Yes
Truncus arteriosus	Yes		Yes	Yes
Total anomalous pulmonary venous return	Yes			Yes

Basic Science Correlate

Ventricular septal defect results from incomplete formation of the interventricular septum, leaving an incomplete closure of the interventricular foramen.

The **ductus arteriosus** connects the pulmonary artery and descending aorta during development. It allows the blood to bypass the lungs, since the fetus is not receiving any oxygen from them in utero.

Aortic stenosis occurs when the leaflets of the valves fuse together. It can be congenital or acquired over time.

Tricuspid Valve Atresia

Tricuspid valve atresia presents with severe cyanosis in a newborn. The lack of communication between the right heart chamber results in hypoplastic RV and pulmonary outflow tract, which results in underdevelopment of pulmonary valve and/or artery. They must have an associated PFO, ASD, or VSD for survival, which will allow for mixing of oxygenated and deoxygenated blood.

- Chest x-ray shows decreased pulmonary flow
- EKG shows left axis deviation small or absent R waves in precordial leads, and LVH

Treatment is PGE1 to keep the PDA open (until aortopulmonary shunt can be performed). Atrial balloon septostomy may be needed to make the ASD larger. Consider staged surgical correction.

Ebstein's Anomaly

Ebstein's anomaly is associated with maternal lithium use in pregnancy. The child will have downward displacement of tricuspid valve into the right ventricle.

Physical examination will show a holosystolic murmur of tricuspid regurgitation over most of the anterior left chest.

EKG will show tall P waves and right axis deviation.

Antibiotic Prophylaxis and Prevention of Endocarditis
- Antibiotic administration **prior to GU or GI procedures** is no longer recommended, even in high-risk patients.
- Antibiotic administration **prior to dental procedures** is no longer recommended except with the following:
  - Prosthetic valves
  - Previous endocarditis
  - Congenital heart disease (unrepaired or repaired with persistent defect)
  - Cardiac transplantation patients with cardiac valve abnormalities

---

Hypertension

Defining Hypertension		
	Age 1–13 Years	**Age 13 Years and Older**
Normal BP	Systolic and diastolic BP <90th percentile	Systolic BP <120 mm Hg and diastolic BP <80 mm Hg
Elevated BP	Systolic and diastolic BP ≥90th percentile to <95th percentile, or 120/80 mm Hg to <95th percentile (whichever is lower)	Systolic BP 120–129 mm Hg and diastolic BP <80 mm Hg
Stage 1 HTN	Systolic and diastolic BP ≥95th percentile to <95th percentile + 12 mm Hg, or 130/80 mm Hg to 139/89 mm Hg (whichever is lower)	130/80 mm Hg to 139/89 mm Hg
Stage 2 HTN	Systolic and diastolic BP ≥95th percentile + 12 mm Hg, or ≥140/90 mm Hg (whichever is lower)	≥140/90 mm Hg

Always work up for secondary hypertension under the following circumstances:

- Newborns: umbilical artery catheters → renal artery/vein thrombosis
- Early childhood: renal parenchymal disease, coarctation, endocrine, medications
- Adolescents:
  - Essential hypertension is associated with obesity
  - Evaluate for renal and renovascular hypertension
  - Renovascular hypertension may be caused by UTI (secondary to an obstructive lesion), acute glomerulonephritis, Henoch-Schönlein purpura with nephritis, hemolytic uremic syndrome, acute tubular necrosis, renal trauma, leukemic infiltrates, mass lesions, or renal artery stenosis

Consider renal causes of hypertension in every pediatric patient presenting with hypertension.

Diagnostic testing is as follows:

- Screening tests
  - CBC
  - Urinalysis, urine culture
  - Electrolytes, glucose
  - BUN, creatinine
  - Calcium
  - Uric acid
  - Lipid panel with essential hypertension and positive family history
- Echocardiogram for chronicity (left ventricular hypertrophy)
- Kidney evaluation
  - Renal ultrasound
  - Voiding cystourethrogram if there is a history of repeated UTI (especially <5 years)
  - 24-hour urine collection for protein excretion and creatinine clearance
  - Plasma renin activity (**best test for renovascular and renal disorders**)
- Endocrine causes
  - Urine and serum catecholamines, if pheochromocytoma is suspected
  - Thyroid and adrenal hormone levels
- Drug screening (in adolescents), if drug abuse is suspected

Treatment starts with lifestyle change, if the patient is obese (weight control, aerobic exercise, diet with no added salt, and monitoring of blood pressure). If there is no response, give antihypertensives:

- Diuretic or beta blocker
- Add a CCB and ACE inhibitor (good in high-renin hypertension secondary to renovascular or renal disease or high-renin essential hypertension)

Gastroenterology

Diarrhea

Acute Diarrhea

- Most common cause of acute diarrhea in infancy is rotavirus; immunization against rotavirus is given 3 times before age 6 months
- Most common causes of bloody diarrhea are *Campylobacter*, amoeba (*E. histolytica*), *Shigella*, *E. coli*, and *Salmonella*

Following are characteristics of selected microbes causing acute diarrhea:

- *Rotavirus*: double-stranded DNA virus
- *Shigella*: gram-negative, non-spore-forming rod
- *Campylobacter*: gram-negative spiral that is motile with flagella
- *Salmonella*: gram-negative rod that is motile
- *Clostridium difficile*: gram-positive, spore-forming bacteria
- *Giardia*: anaerobic protozoan with flagella
- *Cryptosporidium*: protozoan that mostly affects immunocompromised patients

In children with diarrhea, take a history and physical. Stool exam (**best initial test**) is done for the following:

- Leukocytes, blood, and cultures
- *Clostridium difficile* toxin if a recent history of antibiotics
- Ova and parasites

Treatment is hydration and fluid and electrolyte replacement. Do not use antidiarrheals in children.

Antibiotics are rarely used (even in bacterial diarrhea), except for the following cases:

- *Campylobacter*: self-limiting; erythromycin speeds recovery and reduces carrier state so recommended for patients with severe disease or dysentery
- *Salmonella*: only age <3 months, are toxic, who have disseminated disease, or who have *S. typhi*
- *C. difficile*: metronidazole or PO vancomycin and discontinuation of other antibiotics
- *E. histolytica* or *Giardia*: metronidazole
- *Cryptosporidium*: antiparasitics (watch for malnutrition in pediatric patients)

Hemolytic uremic syndrome (HUS) (most common cause of ARF in young children) is a complication of acute invasive (bloody) diarrhea. It is most commonly caused by *E. coli* O157:H7 (also *Shigella, Salmonella, Campylobacter*).

- Young children present 5–10 days after infection with pallor (microangiopathic hemolytic anemia), weakness, oliguria, and acute renal insufficiency or acute renal failure.
- Look for anemia, helmet cells, burr cells, fragmented cells, elevated WBCs, negative Coombs, low platelets (<100,000/mm^3), low-grade microscopic hematuria, and proteinuria.

Treatment of acute diarrhea is supportive care, treatment of hypertension, aggressive nutrition, and early dialysis. Begin complement therapy as follows:

- Eculizumab (first-line therapy in children with microangiopathic hemolytic anemia, thrombocytopenia, and renal failure in the absence of bloody diarrhea, which is suggestive of Shiga toxin–mediated HUS)
- Never give antibiotics in suspected cases of *E. coli* O157:H7, as risk of developing HUS increases
- Over 90% of patients survive the acute stage; a small number develop end-stage renal disease
- After HUS, monitor blood pressure for 5 years and renal function with BUN/creatinine for 2–3 years

Chronic Diarrhea

Chronic, nonspecific diarrhea presents with normal weight, height, and nutritional status with no fat in stool. History usually includes excessive intake of fruit juice or carbonated fluids or low fat intake. If there is weight loss and stool with high fat, screen for malabsorption syndromes.

Malabsorption

Malabsorption may appear from birth or after introduction of new foods.

Diagnostic testing includes:

- Fat malabsorption:
  - Sudan black stain (**best initial test**)
  - 72-hour stool for fecal fat (**best confirmatory test and gold standard for steatorrhea**)
- Protein malabsorption cannot be evaluated directly
  - Spot stool alpha-1 antitrypsin level (**best initial test**)
- Vitamins/minerals: measure serum Fe, folate, Ca, Zn, and Mg and vitamins B12, D, and A

- Pancreatic insufficiency presents with prominent steatorrhea. Get a sweat chloride test to rule in/out cystic fibrosis.
- Giardiasis is the only infection that causes chronic malabsorption. If giardiasis is suspected, order a duodenal aspirate/biopsy or immunoassay.
- Malrotation can present with malabsorption and incomplete bowel obstruction.

Celiac Disease

Celiac disease presents with the following within the first 2 years:

- Chronic diarrhea
- Failure to thrive
- Growth retardation
- Anorexia
- Iron deficiency anemia
- Dermatitis herpetiformis

Symptoms occur with exposure to gluten, rye, wheat, and barley. Intolerance is lifelong.

Celiac patients have an increased lifetime risk of osteoporosis and GI malignancies (most commonly enteropathy-associated T-cell lymphoma).

The **best initial diagnostic test** is anti-tissue transglutaminase (tTG) antibodies. Additional tests include endomysial and deamidated gliadin peptide antibodies.

Histology on biopsy (**most accurate test**) will show blunting of villi.

Treatment is a strict gluten-free diet.

Gastroesophageal Reflux Disease (GERD)

A 4-month-old girl presents with several weeks of chronic wheeze and apneic episodes 20–30 minutes after feeds. She has been spitting up after feeds since birth. She has presented to the office on several prior occasions with the same complaint despite adjustments in feed technique and formula consistency. She is at the 5th percentile for weight. Which of the following is the most appropriate intervention?

a. Erythromycin
b. Fundoplication
c. Metoclopramide
d. Omeprazole
e. Ranitidine

Answer: **E.** GERD results from incompetent esophageal sphincter tone early in life. Symptoms typically resolve by 12–24 months. Diagnosis is clinical. However, the best initial test is esophageal pH monitoring. Endoscopy is used to evaluate for erosive gastritis or other complications. The best initial treatment is a change in feeding technique and thickened feeds. H2-receptors are considered first line in children because of their safety profile, but PPIs are more effective in suppressing gastric acid production.

Pyloric Stenosis

A 4-week-old boy presents with recurrent vomiting after feeds. Vomitus is nonbilious in nature. Laboratory findings include chloride 88 mEq, potassium 3.1 mEq, sodium 146 mEq, and pH 7.48. What is the best initial test in the workup of this infant?

a. Abdominal x-ray
b. Barium enema
c. CT scan of the abdomen
d. Esophageal pH monitoring
e. Ultrasound

Answer: **E.** The case will describe a male with nonbilious projectile vomiting typically in first 6 weeks of life. There is hypochloremic and metabolic alkalosis, and a firm, mobile, 1-inch mass is often palpated in the epigastrium. The best initial test is ultrasound of the abdomen. Treatment is pyloromyotomy. Abdominal x-ray is less useful in identifying pyloric stenosis and is not the test of choice in cases where clinical suspicion is high. CT scan is not indicated to prevent exposure to radiation when a more appropriate test is available.

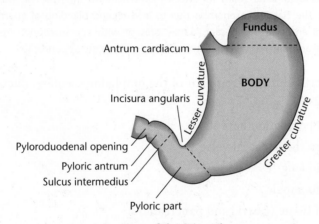

Anatomy of the Stomach

Pyloric stenosis is caused by a hypertrophied pylorus. The hypertrophied pylorus obstructs the outlet, so nothing passes to the duodenum and projectile vomiting ensues. The vomitus *does not* contain bile. (Food must be able to get to the duodenum in order to come in contact with bile.)

The absence or presence of bile in vomitus is the key difference between duodenal atresia (bile) and pyloric stenosis (no bile). Hypochloremic metabolic alkalosis is pathognomonic of pyloric stenosis. Vomiting causes loss of the gastric acid (i.e., hydrochloric acid). The low chloride level prevents the kidneys from excreting bicarbonate, leading to alkalosis.

> **Hypertrophy:** enlarged cells, but the same number of cells
>
> **Hyperplasia:** normal cell size, but more cells

Malrotation and Volvulus

Look for an infant with bilious emesis and recurrent abdominal pain with vomiting. Always suspect volvulus when the patient has an acute small-bowel obstruction without a history of bowel surgery.

The **best initial test** is ultrasound (inversion of superior mesenteric artery and vein and duodenal obstruction) or barium enema (cecum is not in the right lower quadrant). Abdominal x-ray is not helpful; it is helpful only in duodenal destruction, where it shows a "double-bubble" sign.

Treatment is surgical.

Hematochezia

A 2-year-old boy is brought to the office because his mother has noticed bleeding in his diaper for 1 week. The child has had no complaints. Physical examination is unremarkable. Which of the following is the best initial test?

a. Guaiac exam
b. Push enteroscopy
c. Red blood cell tagged scan
d. Tc-99m pertechnetate scan
e. Upper endoscopy

Answer: **D.** The Tc-99m pertechnetate scan (also known as the Meckel radionuclide scan) is the diagnostic exam for Meckel diverticulum. Intermittent, painless rectal bleeding is the classic presentation due to acid-related bleeding of aberrant mucosa (remnant of embryonic yolk sac). It may present with intussusception (remnant may become a lead point) or diverticulitis, or it looks like acute appendicitis.

Meckel diverticulum is a remnant of the omphalomesenteric duct. It follows the rule of 2s:

- 2% of the population have it
- 2 feet from the ileocecal valve
- 2 inches in length
- 2:1 male to female
- 2 types of tissue (gastric and pancreatic)
- Occurs in first 2 years of life

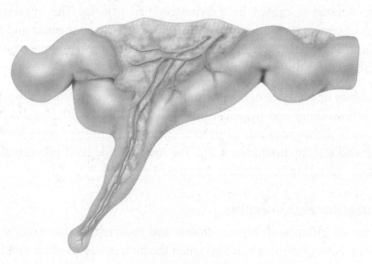

Meckel Diverticulum

Esophageal Atresia

The esophagus ends blindly, and in nearly 90% of cases it communicates with the trachea through a fistula known as a tracheoesophageal fistula (TEF).

The child will have a typical "vomiting with first feeding" or choking/coughing and cyanosis due to the TEF.

The **best initial test** is a water-soluble contrast esophagram. The **most accurate test** is CT scan. Treatment is surgical repair.

Choanal Atresia

The infant is born with a membrane between the nostrils and pharyngeal space that prevents breathing during feeding.

- Associated with CHARGE syndrome
- Child turns blue when feeding and then pink when crying

This recurrent sequence of events is clinically diagnostic. Confirmatory testing is CT scan.

Treatment is surgical intervention to perforate the membrane and reconnect the pharynx to the nostrils.

> CHARGE syndrome is a set of congenital defects seen in conjunction:
> **C:** coloboma of the eye, CNS anomalies
> **H:** heart defects
> **A:** atresia of the choanae
> **R:** retardation of growth and/or development
> **G:** genital and/or urinary defects (hypogonadism)
> **E:** ear anomalies and/or deafness

Nephrology and Urology

Urinary Tract Infection

Urinary tract infection (UTI) is seen in boys age ≤1 and girls age >2. Most girls develop their first UTI by age 5 (peaks are during infancy and toilet training). The most common agent is gram-negative rods.

The **best initial test** is urinalysis, and the **most accurate test** is urine culture.

Treatment is as follows:

- Cystitis (dysuria): amoxicillin, trimethoprim-sulfamethoxazole
- Pyelonephritis (fever, flank pain): IV ceftriaxone or ampicillin plus gentamicin

Do not give the following:

- Sulfonamides or nitrofurantoin to infants age <1 month (give ceftriaxone)
- Tetracyclines to children age <7
- Quinolones to children age <16

Children are at great risk of kidney damage, including kidney scars, poor kidney growth, poor kidney function, and high blood pressure, especially if an underlying urinary tract abnormality exists.

Vesicoureteral Reflux (VUR)

VUR is abnormal movement of urine from the bladder into the ureters/kidneys. Urine usually travels from the kidneys through the ureters, then into the bladder. In this condition, urine flow is reversed.

VUR predisposes the child to pyelonephritis, which leads to scarring and possible reflux nephropathy (hypertension, proteinuria, renal insufficiency to end-stage renal disease, impaired kidney growth).

Primary VUR (most common) results from incompetent or inadequate closure of the ureterovesical junction, which contains a segment of the ureter within the bladder wall (intravesical ureter).

Testing is a voiding cystourethrogram (VCUG) and renal scan. If scarring is present, follow creatinine periodically.

Treatment is antibiotic prophylaxis. Consider surgery for any breakthrough UTI, new scars, and failure to resolve.

> A 2-year-old girl presents with a urinary tract infection (UTI). She has had multiple UTIs since birth but has never had follow-up studies to evaluate these infections. Physical examination is remarkable for an ill-appearing child who has a temperature of 40°C (104°F) and is vomiting. Voiding cystourethrogram reveals abnormal urinary backflow from the bladder. Which of the following is the most important step to prevent permanent damage?
>
> a. ACE inhibitors
> b. Trimethoprim-sulfamethoxazole
> c. NSAIDs
> d. Regular creatinine measurement
> e. Surgical reconstruction
>
> Answer: **B**. Antibiotic prophylaxis (trimethoprim-sulfamethoxazole or nitrofurantoin) is used for the first year following diagnosis for any grade of VUR, particularly in younger infants, to prevent kidney scarring from recurrent infections.

Obstructive Uropathy

The first presentation of obstructive uropathy is often infection or sepsis. The most common causes are the following:

- **Boys:** posterior urethral valves (**most common cause of bladder obstruction**): look for walnut-shaped mass (bladder) above pubic symphysis and weak urinary stream
- **Newborns:** hydronephrosis and polycystic kidney disease (**most common causes of a palpable abdominal mass**)

The **best initial diagnostic tests** are VCUG and renal ultrasound.

Acute Poststreptococcal Glomerulonephritis

Acute poststreptococcal glomerulonephritis (APGN) presents age 5–12, usually 1–2 weeks after strep pharyngitis or 3–6 weeks after skin infection (impetigo). The **classic triad** of symptoms is edema, hypertension, and hematuria.

Diagnostic testing includes:

- Urinalysis: dysmorphic RBCs, RBC casts, protein, polymorphonuclear cells
- Low C3 (returns to normal in 6–8 weeks)
- Need positive throat culture or increasing antibody titer to streptococcal antigens
- Most specific test: anti-DNase B antigen

Treatment is penicillin (erythromycin if penicillin-allergic) and supportive care (sodium restriction, diuresis, fluid and electrolyte management).

- Give antihypertensives only in acute management if patient has hypertension with poststreptococcal glomerulonephritis
- Do not give steroids

There is complete recovery in >95% of patients.

> A 10-year-old boy presents with lower extremity swelling. He has had a sore throat for 2 weeks and fever. His mother has noticed very dark, brownish-red urine over the past couple of days. He has no known allergies. On physical examination, his blood pressure is 185/100 mm Hg. Which of the following is indicated for management?
>
> a. ACE inhibitors
> b. Diuretics
> c. Erythromycin
> d. Oral prednisone
> e. Penicillin
>
> Answer: **E.** The most appropriate therapy for **APGN** is antibiotics to eradicate the underlying infection. Penicillin is the drug of choice. Erythromycin is used on patients who are penicillin-allergic.

Proteinuria

- Transient, from fever, exercise, dehydration, or cold exposure
- Orthostatic (most common form of persistent proteinuria in school-aged children and adolescents): look for history of normal proteinuria in supine position but greatly increased proteinuria in upright position. Rule this out *before* any other evaluation is done.
- Glomerular or tubular disorders: suspect a glomerular disorder with proteinuria >1 g/24 hours or if there is hypertension, hematuria, or renal dysfunction

Minimal Change Disease

Minimal change disease (nephrotic syndrome) is common age 2–6, often arising after a minor infections. It presents with the following:

- Proteinuria (>40 mg/m^2/hour) (creatinine usually normal)
- Hypoalbuminemia (<2.5 g/dL)
- Edema (initially around eyes and lower extremities)
- Hyperlipidemia
- Normal C3 and C4

Complications include:

- Infection (spontaneous bacterial peritonitis most common): you must immunize against *Pneumococcus* and *Varicella*
- Increased risk of thromboembolism due to increased prothrombotic factors and decreased fibrinolytic factors

Treatment is supportive care (sodium and fluid restriction) and oral prednisone. For steroid dependency or resistance, give cyclophosphamide, cyclosporine, and high-dose pulsed methylprednisolone.

> A 3-year-old child presents to the physician with puffy eyes. The mother reports diarrhea 2 weeks ago. On physical examination there is no erythema or evidence of trauma, insect bite, cellulitis conjunctival injection, or discharge. Urinalysis reveals 3+ proteinuria. Laboratory profile is significant for albumin 2.1 mg/dL, creatinine 0.9; and normal C3 and C4. What is the next step in management?
>
> a. Outpatient prednisone
> b. Hospitalize and observe
> c. Heparin
> d. High-dose methylprednisone
> e. Intravenous antibiotics
>
> Answer: **A.** Outpatient prednisone is the first step for mild cases of minimal change disease. Continue daily for 4–6 weeks, then taper to alternate days for 2–3 months without initial biopsy.

Endocrinology and Rheumatology

Rickets

Rickets is a disorder arising from insufficient intake of vitamin D, calcium, or phosphate. It leads to softening and weakening of the bones and makes the child more susceptible to fractures. Children age 6–24 months are at highest risk because their bones are rapidly growing.

Rickets has 3 main etiologies:

- Vitamin D–deficient rickets is caused by a lack of enough vitamin D in the child's diet.
- Vitamin D–dependent rickets arises from an inability to convert 25-OH to $1,25(OH)_2$; the infant is therefore dependent on vitamin D supplementation.
- X-linked hypophosphatemic rickets stems from a kidney defect compromising its ability to retain phosphate. Adequate bone mineralization cannot take place without phosphate, so bones are weak.

Type	Calcium	Phosphate	$1,25(OH)_2$ Vit D	25(OH) Vit D
Vitamin D-deficient	Increased	Decreased	Normal	Decreased
Vitamin D-dependent	Normal	Normal	Normal	Normal
X-linked Hypophosphatemia	Normal	Decreased	Decreased	Normal

The child will present with a waddling gait due to tibial/femoral bowing, along with ulnar/radial bowing.

Treatment is supplemental dietary phosphate, calcium, and vitamin D in the form of ergocalciferol or $1,25(OH)_2$ (also known as *calcitriol*). Monitor blood vitamin D annually.

Pediatric Hip Disorders				
Disease	**Age**	**Presentation**	**Diagnosis**	**Treatment**
Congenital hip dysplasia	Infancy	Usually found on screening during the first few newborn exams	Ortolani and Barlow maneuvers "Click" or "clunk" in the hip can be heard	Pavlik harness
Legg-Calve-Perthes disease (avascular necrosis of the femoral head)	Age 2–8 years	Painful limp	X-ray shows joint effusions and widening	Rest and NSAIDs, followed by surgery on both hips
Slipped capital femoral epiphysis (SCFE)	Adolescence	Painful limp and externally rotated leg in an obese adolescent	X-ray shows widening of the joint space	Internal fixation with pinning

Kawasaki Disease

Kawasaki disease is an acute vasculitis of medium-sized arteries and the leading cause of acquired heart disease in the United States and Japan. It is most common among age <5.

The condition presents with fever for ≥5 days, plus 4 of the following symptoms:

- Bilateral bulbar conjunctivitis without exudate
- Intraoral erythema, strawberry tongue, dry and cracked lips
- Erythema and swelling of hands and feet; desquamation of fingertips 1–3 weeks after onset
- Nonvesicular rash
- Nonsuppurative cervical lymphadenitis, diameter >1.5 cm and usually unilateral

Diagnostic testing includes:

- Increased ESR, C-reactive protein (CRP) at 4–8 weeks
- Platelets increase in weeks 2–3 (often > 1 million)
- Cardiac findings: early myocarditis; pericarditis; coronary artery aneurysms in 2nd to 3rd week

Treatment is intravenous immunoglobulin (IVIG) and high-dose aspirin as soon as possible, based on clinical diagnosis.

- 2D echocardiogram and EKG: get baseline at diagnosis; repeat at 2–3 weeks and at 6–8 weeks
- Add anticoagulant (warfarin) for high-risk thrombosis (e.g., when platelet count is very high)

Steroids have no benefit. Only IVIG has been shown to reduce the incidence of cardiovascular complications. There is a 1–2% mortality due to coronary artery thrombosis secondary to coronary artery aneurysms.

An 18-month-old presents with a fever for 1 week and a rash on his hands with desquamation that developed today. On examination he is noted to have conjunctival injection, erythematous tongue, cracked lips, and edema of the hands. He has palpable and painful lymph nodes in the neck. What is the next step in management?

a. Anticoagulation
b. Echocardiogram
c. IVIG
d. Methylprednisolone
e. Prednisone

Answer: **C.** For Kawasaki disease, IVIG and high-dose aspirin should be started immediately to prevent coronary artery involvement (reduces risk from 25% to <5%). Echocardiogram should be performed at diagnosis for baseline measurement; however, coronary artery abnormalities occur in the second or third week.

Hematology

Anemia

In term infants, normal hemoglobin nadir occurs at 12 weeks at 9–11 mg/dL. The anemia results from a progressive drop in RBC production (due to erythropoietin suppression at birth) until tissue oxygen needs are greater than at delivery. No treatment is needed.

In preterm infants, response is exaggerated and earlier. Hemoglobin nadir occurs at 3–6 weeks at 7–9 mg/dL. Some patients may require transfusion.

Iron-Deficiency Anemia

A normal newborn has sufficient stores of iron to meet requirements for 4–6 months, but iron stores and absorption are variable.

Breast milk has less iron than most formulas but has higher bioavailability. Iron in breast milk is more readily absorbed in the proximal intestine.

Decreased dietary iron will cause anemia at 9–24 months.

Treatment is oral ferrous salts. Continue iron replacement for 8 weeks after blood value normalizes to replete bone marrow iron stores. Limit cow's milk.

Lead Poisoning

Consider lead poisoning when the case describes hyperactivity, aggression, and learning disability (may be mistaken for ADHD). Other clues include impaired growth, constipation, and mental lethargy.

Diagnostic testing includes:

- Blood lead testing at 12 and 24 months in high-risk children (**best initial test**): level ≤5 mcg/dL is acceptable
- Labs: microcytic, hypochromic anemia, increased free erythrocyte porphyrins (FEP), and basophilic stippling
- X-ray of long bones (dense lead lines)

Treatment is referral to the department of health when blood lead level >15 mcg/dL, and chelation when blood lead level >45 mcg/dL.

Neurology

Seizures

In the newborn intensive care unit, an infant is noted to be "jittery" and has repetitive sucking movements, tongue thrusting, and brief apneic spells. Blood counts and chemistries are within normal limits. What is the initial workup of this patient?

Answer: Seizures classically present with subtle repetitive movements, such as chewing, tongue thrusting, apnea, staring, blinking, or desaturations. Classic tonic-clonic movements are uncommon. Look for ocular deviation and failure of jitteriness to subside with stimulus (e.g., passive movement of a limb). Complete diagnostic workup for seizures is listed.

Diagnostic testing includes:

- EEG: may be normal
- CBC, electrolytes, calcium, magnesium, glucose (hypoglycemia is a common cause of seizures in infants of diabetic mothers)
- Amino acid assay and urine organic acids to detect inborn errors of metabolism and pyridoxine deficiency
- To look for infectious causes, perform the following:
  - TORCH infection studies: total cord blood IgM for screening
  - Blood and urine cultures
  - Lumbar puncture if meningitis is suspected
- Ultrasound of head in preterms to look for intraventricular hemorrhage; intracranial hemorrhage causes seizures typically 2–7 days after birth

Treatment is to correct the underlying cause, including electrolyte abnormalities. For acute seizure, use lorazepam or diazepam (rectally). For chronic seizure, it depends on the type; with absence seizures, use ethosuximide.

> **Basic Science Correlate**
>
> Benzodiazepines bind the alpha-1 receptor site of the GABA receptor.
>
>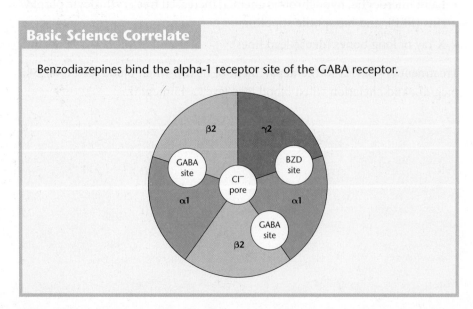

You are asked to see a previously well 13-month-old boy who is brought in after a generalized tonic-clonic seizure 1 hour ago. The seizure lasted several minutes. The mother remembers that a similar episode occurred when she was a child. On examination vitals are BP 100/52 mm Hg, HR 110, temp 101.4°F, RR 32. She wishes to know if her child has epilepsy. What is the most appropriate response?

a. No increased risk of epilepsy

b. Slightly increased risk of epilepsy

c. High risk of epilepsy developing in the next year

d. Patient has epilepsy but medications will be withheld until second episode of seizure

e. Patient has epilepsy and will require anti-seizure medications

Answer: **A.** This patient presents with simple febrile seizure—generalized tonic-clonic seizure <10 min duration occurring with rapid onset high fever (when >39°C [102°F]) in child age 9 months to 5 years. There is usually a positive family history. Management includes evaluation for meningitis and controlling fever. DO NOT order EEG or neuro-imaging.

The risk of epilepsy is increased in a case presenting as febrile seizure under any of the following conditions:

- Atypical seizure: >15 minutes, more than 1×/day, and focal findings
- Family history of epilepsy and initial seizure age <9 months
- Abnormal development
- Preexisting neurologic disorder

Seizure Disorder

Epilepsy is present when at least 2 unprovoked seizures occur more than 24 hours apart.

Early treatment with antiseizure medication reduces the risk of subsequent seizures and improves time to remission. Antiseizure medications may be stopped after the patient has been seizure-free for 2 years.

Seizure Disorder	Classic Features	EEG Findings	Treatment
Absence seizures	• Frequent seizures with cessation of motor activity or speech, blank facial expression, and flickering of eyelids • More common in girls, rare in children age <4 • Rarely lasts >30 seconds • No aura or postictal state	• 3-second spike and generalized wave discharge	• First line: ethosuximide (alternative: valproic acid)
Juvenile myoclonic epilepsy (JME)	• Jerky movement occurring in the morning • Onset around adolescence	• Irregular spike-and-wave pattern	• First line: valproic acid

(continued next page)

Seizure Disorder	Classic Features	EEG Findings	Treatment
West syndrome (infantile spasms)	• Infantile spasms during year 1 of life • Clusters of mixed flexor and extensor spasms of trunk and extremities, persisting for minutes with brief intervals between each spasm • Of children with West syndrome, 75% have an underlying CNS disorder (Down syndrome most common)	• Hypsarrhythmia (very high-voltage slow waves, irregularly interspersed with spikes and sharp waves)	• First line: ACTH, prednisone, vigabatrin, pyridoxine (vitamin B6)
Partial seizure	• Simple: tonic or clonic movements involving most of the face, neck, and extremities and lasting 10–20 seconds • No postictal period • Generalized: includes impaired consciousness	• Spike and sharp waves or multifocal spikes	• First line: carbamazepine and valproic acid
Generalized seizure	• Aura, loss of consciousness, eyes roll back, tonic contraction, apnea then clonic rhythmic contractions alternating with relaxation of all muscle groups • Tongue biting, loss of bladder control • Prominent postictal state	• Anterior temporal lobe shows sharp waves or focal spikes	• Generalized tonic clonic: carbamazepine or valproic acid • Generalized myoclonic: topiramate

Duchenne and Becker Muscular Dystrophies

The dystrophinopathies are inherited as X-linked recessive traits leading to progressive muscle weakness:

- Duchenne muscular dystrophy (DMD) (more common) is a frameshift or deletion of the dystrophin gene, which results in complete loss of dystrophin.
- Becker muscular dystrophy (BMD) is a non-frameshift mutation that results in partial function of dystrophin.

DMD has earlier onset and more severe symptoms. Mean age of death is age 25–30 due to cardiopulmonary arrest.

BMD is seen later in life and has a less severe course.

Both diseases present with progressive muscle weakness, commonly seen in the proximal muscles and lower extremity. Gower sign signifies weakness of the proximal lower extremity muscles: The patient uses the upper extremity to stand.

Molecular genetic testing is the **most accurate diagnostic test**. Labs show elevated creatine kinase, and muscle biopsy will reveal degeneration, regeneration, isolated "opaque" hypertrophic fibers, and significant replacement of muscle with fat and connective tissue.

Treatment is as follows:

- **DMD**: glucocorticoids are mainstay of treatment for patients age ≥4 whose motor skills have plateaued or are declining
- **BMD**: physical therapy and supportive care aimed at improving quality of life; no specific therapy reverses this condition

---

DMD Treatment

Those with a confirmed mutation of the dystrophin gene that is amenable to exon 51 binding are candidates for **eteplirsen**, a synthetic strand of nucleic acid that binds to exon 51 of the messenger RNA, which encodes for dystrophin. It allows for production of a partially functional dystrophin protein, as in BMD.

The success rate of eteplirsen in DMD is only 13%.

Infectious Disease

Fever without a Focus in the Young Child

Fever without a focus of infection is an acute febrile illness seen in children age <36 months, defined as rectal temperature at least 38.0°C (100.4°F) with no localizing signs and symptoms.

Give empiric antibiotics under the following conditions:

- Documented rectal temperature >38.0°C/100.4°F
- WBC >15,000, neutrophils >1,500 with band forms
- Neonate: hospitalize, pan-culture (blood, urine, CSF), and give prophylactic antibiotics to cover for group B *Streptococcus*, *E. coli*, and *Listeria*
- Infant (most common organism *Streptococcus pneumoniae*)
  - Well appearing: single-dose IM ceftriaxone and follow up in 24 hours
  - Toxic appearing: empiric IV antibiotics

Neonatal Sepsis

A 3-week-old infant is brought into the clinic with irritability, weight loss of 3 lb over the past week, and "grunting." Physical examination reveals temperature of 102.5°F. There is a bulging anterior fontanel, delayed capillary refill. What is the next step in management?

Answer: The next step in management is to transfer the patient to the ED and initiate a full sepsis workup. This includes CBC with differential; blood culture; CSF culture; urinalysis/urine culture; and chest x-ray before antibiotics are given.

Basic Science Correlate

Gram-positive bacteria stain purple due to their *thick* peptidoglycan layer.
Gram-negative bacteria stain red due to the *thin* peptidoglycan layer.

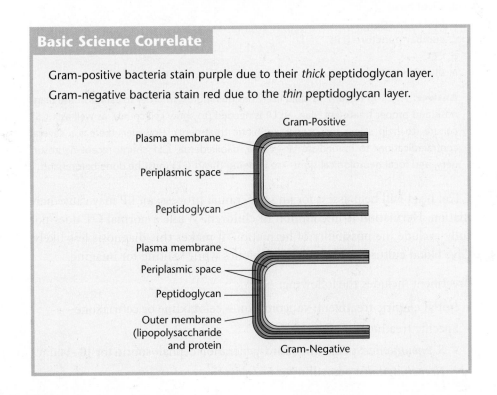

Gram-Positive
- Plasma membrane
- Periplasmic space
- Peptidoglycan

Gram-Negative
- Plasma membrane
- Periplasmic space
- Peptidoglycan
- Outer membrane (lipopolysaccharide and protein

In cases of **early-onset sepsis** (within first 24 hours), pneumonia is the most common cause. The most common organisms involved are:

- Group B *Streptococcus* (beta-hemolytic, gram-positive)
- *E. coli* (gram-negative, rod shaped)
- *Haemophilus influenzae* (gram-negative coccobacilli)
- *Listeria monocytogenes* (gram-positive, motile with flagella)

In cases of **late-onset sepsis** (after first 24 hours), meningitis and bacteremia are the most common causes. The most common organisms are:

- *Staphylococcus aureus* (gram-positive cocci)
- *E. coli*
- *Klebsiella* (gram-negative, oxidase-negative rod)
- *Pseudomonas* (gram-negative aerobic bacteria)

Empiric treatment of neonatal sepsis is ampicillin and gentamicin until 48- to 72-hour cultures are negative. If meningitis is possible, add cefotaxime. If child is younger than age <28 days, add acyclovir.

Meningitis

A 10-year-old boy with no past medical history presents to the office for headache, neck stiffness, nausea, and vomiting for the past 12 hours. He had an upper respiratory infection last week that was treated with amoxicillin. Vital signs are stable. Physical exam is significant for papilledema. Which of the following is next step in management?

a. CT of head
b. MRI of head
c. Lumbar puncture (LP)
d. CBC
e. Blood cultures

Answer: A. CT of head. This child likely has meningitis. In order to establish the diagnosis and proper treatment plan, an LP is needed (to show cell count), as well as a CSF culture (to help select the proper antibiotic treatment). However, there are several contraindications to immediate LP—coma, papilledema, CSF shunt, recent neurosurgery, and focal neurological signs—so imaging (head CT) must be done beforehand.

CT of head will help assess for an intracranial process; an LP may cause herniation. Herniation is uncommon in children. While a normal CT does not fully exclude the possibility of herniation, it makes this diagnosis less likely. Give blood cultures and empiric antibiotics while waiting for imaging.

Treatment includes the following:

- Initial empiric treatment: vancomycin + cefotaxime or ceftriaxone
- Specific treatment:
  - *S. pneumoniae*: penicillin or 3rd-generation cephalosporin for 10–14 days
  - *N. meningitidis*: penicillin for 5–7 days

- HiB: ampicillin for 7–10 days plus IV dexamethasone
- Pretreated and no organism identified: third-generation cephalosporin for 7–10 days
- Gram-negative (*E. coli*): third-generation cephalosporin for 3 weeks

Complications of meningitis include hearing loss (most common) especially with pneumococcus; neurologic dysfunction, thrombosis, or mental retardation especially if therapy is delayed; subdural effusion (seizures and persistent fever) especially with HiB; and meningococcus (septic shock, DIC, acidosis, adrenal hemorrhage, renal/heart failure).

Meningitis can be prevented with chemoprophylaxis with rifampin for *N. meningitidis* and HiB but not for *S. pneumoniae*. Regardless, give prophylaxis to all close contacts.

Catscratch Disease

Catscratch disease is infectious disease caused by the bacterium *Bartonella henselae* that develops 1–2 weeks after a cat scratch or bite. On the Step 3 exam, it will commonly be from a kitten.

Symptoms include swollen lymph nodes near the site of the scratch/bite; headache; and low-grade fever.

Physical exam reveals lymphadenopathy and a pustule at the site of inoculation.

Diagnosis is most often confirmed with a positive serologic test for *B. henselae*. The **most accurate test** is PCR.

Treat with azithromycin.

Lysosomal and Glycogen Storage Diseases

Lysosomal Storage Diseases					
Type	**Defective/Deficient Enzyme**	**Organ Affected**	**Clinical Manifestation**	**Diagnosis**	**Treatment**
I - Von Gierke	Glucose-6-phosphatase	Liver and kidney	Ketotic hypoglycemia, hepatomegaly	Liver biopsy, and DNA testing	Cornstarch, allopurinol, granulocyte-colony stimulating factor (G-CSF)
II - Pompe	Lysosomal acid maltase deficiency	All organs	Hypotonia (floppy baby) Hypertrophic cardiomyopathy	Muscle or liver enzyme assay, DNA testing	Enzyme replacement
IV -Andersen	Glycogen branching enzyme deficiency	Muscle	Cirrhosis of the liver and liver failure by age 2	Liver biopsy, DNA testing	Liver transplant
V - McArdle	Muscle phosphorylase deficiency	Muscle	Fatigability and limited physical activity	Muscle enzyme assay, DNA testing	Sucrose prior to strenuous activity

Glycogen Storage Diseases				
	Deficient/ Defective Enzyme	**Inheritance Pattern**	**Accumulated Substance**	**Clinical Findings**
Tay-Sachs disease	Hexosaminidase A	Autosomal recessive disease Chromosome 15q	Ganglioside	Cherry red macula Mental retardation and developmental delay; death by age 2 years Seizures Lysosomes with onionskin–whorled membranes
Gaucher disease	β-glucocerebrosidase Most common of all	Chromosome 1 Autosomal recessive disease	Glucocerebroside	Hepatosplenomegaly Aseptic necrosis of femur Lytic lesions Gaucher cell: macrophages that look like crumpled paper due to fibrillary cytoplasm
Krabbe disease	Galactocerebrosidase	Autosomal recessive	Galactocerebroside	Optic atrophy Developmental delay
Fabry disease	Alpha galactosidase A	X-linked recessive	Ceramide trihexoside	Peripheral neuropathy (burning pain) of hands/feet
Niemann-Pick disease	Sphingomyelinase	Autosomal recessive disease Chromosome 11p	Sphingomyelin	Cherry red macula Neurodegeneration Hepatosplenomegaly Foam cells—foamy vacuolated macrophages in the marrow
Metachromatic leukodystrophy	Arylsulfatase A	Autosomal recessive disease	Cerebroside sulfate	Demyelination with ataxia and dementia

Infections

The following pediatric infections are commonly seen on the Step 3 exam.

Causative Organism	Disease	Rash	Progression
Streptococcus pyogenes	Scarlet fever	Erythematous, sandpaper-like with numerous papules	Groin/axilla → trunk and extremities, sparing palms and soles. Rash is followed by desquamation.
Staphylococcus aureus	Toxic shock syndrome	Sunburn-like (diffuse, erythematous, macular) with desquamation on palms and soles	Trunk and neck → extremities
Rickettsia rickettsii	Rocky Mountain spotted fever	Blanching, erythematous macules → petechial	Wrists/ankles → trunk. Rash then appears in later stage disease on the palms and soles.
Treponema pallidum	Secondary syphilis	Copper-colored maculopapular, including palms and soles	Diffuse rash and condyloma lata, alopecia
Borrelia burgdorferi	Lyme disease	Erythema chronicum migrans (expanding target-shaped red rash)	Expanding circle
Coxsackievirus type A	Hand, foot, and mouth	Vesicular	Palms and soles only
Rubella virus	German measles (rubella)	Maculopapular	Head → body. Lasts 3 days.
Rubeola virus	Measles	Maculopapular	Head → entire body. Becomes confluent as it spreads downward. Cough, coryza, conjunctivitis, and Koplik spots
Mumps virus	Mumps	None	No rash progression but does cause parotitis, orchitis
VZV	Chickenpox	Asynchronous	Trunk → face/extremities
HHV-6	Roseola infantum	Blanching, maculopapular, occurs after fever	Neck/trunk → face/extremities
Parvovirus B19	Erythema infectiosum	"Slapped cheek"	Face → body

PART 7

Obstetrics

Contributing author Victoria Hastings, DO, MPH, MS

The Uncomplicated Pregnancy

Diagnosing Pregnancy

Pregnancy is suggested in a patient with amenorrhea, enlargement of the uterus, and a (+) urinary β-hCG. Pregnancy is confirmed with the following:

- **Presence of a gestational sac:** Seen by transvaginal ultrasound at 4–5 weeks; corresponds to a serum β-hCG level of about 1,500 mIU/mL
- **Presence of yolk sac:** Visualized within the gestational sac at 4–6 weeks
- Fetal heart motion: Seen by ultrasound at 5–6 weeks

CCS Tip: Order pregnancy counseling (e.g., "Avoid alcohol and tobacco.") in newly diagnosed pregnant patients via the ORDER icon. Type in, "Counsel patient, pregnancy."

> Intrauterine pregnancy is normally seen on the following:
>
> - **Vaginal sonogram** at 5 weeks gestation when serum β-hCG >1,500 mIU
> - **Abdominal sonogram** at 6 weeks gestation when β-hCG >6,500 mIU

Routine Prenatal Screening Tests

Gravidity means the number of pregnancies. **Parity** means the number of births. For parity, use the mnemonic **TPAL**:

- Term (>37 weeks)
- Preterm (20–36+6 weeks)
- Abortions (<20 weeks)
- Living children

First Trimester

A 21-year-old primigravida, para 0 (G1 P0) presents for her first prenatal visit at 11 weeks' gestation, which is confirmed by obstetric sonogram. She has no risk factors. What screening tests should be performed?

Answer: **See chart below.**

Screening	Test	Diagnostic Significance	Next Step in Management
FIRST TRIMESTER ROUTINE TESTS			
Anemia, blood disorders	CBC	• Anemia = Hb <11 g/dL in the first and third trimesters and <10.5 g/dL in the second trimester. The most reliable indicator of true anemia is MCV. • Most common cause of anemia is iron deficiency. (See BSC below) • WBC >16,000/mm³ is abnormal.	• ↓ hemoglobin ↓ MCV: Give iron. Test for thalassemia if anemia does not improve. • ↓ hemoglobin ↑ MCV • ↑RDW: Give folate. • Thrombocytopenia • (<150,000/ mm³): Correlate clinically for ITP.
Blood type, Rh, and antibody	Type and screen Direct and indirect Coombs	• Rh negative mothers may become sensitized (anti-D Ab) → risk of erythroblastosis fetalis in the next pregnancy. • Indirect Coombs test (or atypical antibody test [AAT]) detects atypical RBC Abs.	• Give RhoGAM to Rh negative mothers at 28 weeks *after* first rescreening for absence of anti-D antibodies. • Give RhoGAM in Rh negative mothers after any procedure (CVS, amniocentesis) and after delivery.
Genitourinary screening	Cervical PAP smear	• Detects cervical dysplasia or malignancy.	• See Gynecology section for management.
	Urinalysis/ Urine culture	• UA: Screen for underlying renal disease and infection. • UCx: Screen for asymptomatic bacteriuria (ASB).	• Always treat ASB in pregnancy to prevent pyelonephritis (30% risk when untreated). • Rx: Cephalosporins, amoxicillin • Need test of cure in pregnant women
Immunization status	Rubella antibody	• (–) Rubella IgG Abs means ↑ risk of primary rubella infection.	• Do *not* give rubella immunization in pregnancy. • Immunize seronegative patients *after* delivery.
	Hepatitis B surface antigen	• (+) HBsAg: Indicates risk for vertical transmission of HBV	• (+) HBsAg: Order HBVe antigen. • (+) HBeAg signifies a highly infectious state.
Infection: Syphilis	VDRL or RPR	• Confirm (+) VDRL/RPR with treponemal-specific tests (MHATP or FTA). Alternatively, may start with treponemal specific tests (EIA/CIA) followed by VDRL/RPR ("reverse algorithm screening").	• (+) confirmatory test: Treat with intramuscular penicillin. • Penicillin allergic: Desensitize and then treat with penicillin.
Infection: HIV	Fourth-generation HIV-1/HIV-2 immunoassay	• If (+), perform HIV-1/HIV-2 antibody differentiation immunoassay. • If the fourth-generation test is positive and the confirmatory HIV-1/HIV-2 antibody differentiation immunoassay is indeterminate or negative, get plasma HIV RNA level.	• All babies born to HIV (+) women will be HIV antibody (+) (passive transport of maternal Abs). (+) Abs do not indicate infection in infant. • Antiretrovirals (triple therapy) are recommended in pregnancy. • Give zidovudine in labor.
Infection: Chlamydia/ Gonorrhea	Cervical culture	• Gram stain • Chlamydia and gonorrhea culture (see BSC below) • Also treat *Trichomonas vaginalis* (can cause premature labor).	• (+) Chlamydia/gonorrhea • PO azithromycin + IM ceftriaxone (treatment of choice) • (+) Bacterial vaginitis PO or vaginal metronidazole or clindamycin • (+) *Trichomonas vaginalis* PO metronidazole for mother and partner

(continued next page)

Screening	Test	Diagnostic Significance	Next Step in Management
FIRST TRIMESTER ROUTINE TESTS			
Tuberculosis	Quantiferon gold (QFT) (preferred) or PPD	• Test for exposure to TB in high risk mothers. • (+) PPD test is induration, not erythema.	• (−) QFT or PPD: No further follow-up is needed. • (+) QFT or PPD: Order chest x-ray to rule out active disease. • Treatment for positive screen: 　- (+) QFT or PPD/(−) CXR: INH and B6 for 9 months if treatment was initiated prior to pregnancy. If not, may defer Tx until after delivery. 　- (+) QFT or PPD/(+) CXR (+) sputum: Begin triple therapy antituberculosis Rx if sputum stain positive. Obtain sputum for culture. 　- Avoid streptomycin in pregnancy because of the risk of ototoxicity in the fetus.
Trisomy 21: Early testing	β-hCG Pregnancy-associated plasma protein A (PAPP-A) Fetal nuchal translucency OR fetal cell-free DNA	• **Offered to all pregnant women** regardless of maternal age or other risk factors.	• (+) screening test is confirmed with chorionic villus sampling or amniocentesis.

Abs = antibodies; CIA = chemiluminescence; EIA = treponemal enzyme immunoassay; FTA: fluorescent treponemal antibody absorption; Hb = hemoglobin; IM = intramuscular; MHATP: microhemagglutination assay for antibodies to *T. pallidum*; PO = oral

---

Basic Science Correlate

Anemia in pregnancy is caused by increased levels of hepcidin, which inhibits iron transport. Pregnancy increases iron demand, but hepcidin prevents absorption.

Basic Science Correlate

Chlamydia trachomatis is an obligate intracellular parasite: It needs a host cell to survive.

Neisseria gonorrhea is a gram-negative diplococcus that grows on chocolate agar. Nuclear acid amplification test (NAAT) is the test of choice.

MS-AFP increases with gestational age and is expressed in multiples of the median (MoM).

- Elevated: >2.5 MoM
- Normal: <2.5 MoM

Inhibin A is made by the placenta during pregnancy and normally remains constant during 15th–18th week of pregnancy. Inhibin A levels are increased in the blood of mothers of fetuses with Down syndrome.

Second Trimester

A 23-year-old woman (G3 P1 Abortion 1) is seen at 17 weeks gestation. She recently underwent a triple marker screen with the maternal serum alpha fetoprotein (normal <2.2 MoM). Her test showed an elevation in maternal serum alpha fetoprotein. On examination her uterus is at the umbilicus. What is the next step in management?

a. Amniocentesis
b. Chorionic villus sampling
c. Inhibin A
d. Recommendation of termination of pregnancy
e. Ultrasound

Answer: **E.** The most common cause of an abnormal MS-AFP is gestational dating error. The first step is to get an obstetric ultrasound to confirm the gestational age. A first trimester ultrasound is the most accurate way to date a pregnancy.

Screening	Test	Diagnostic Significance	Next Step in Management
SECOND TRIMESTER OPTIONAL TESTS			

Quadruple Marker Screen (testing window is 15–20 weeks gestation)	1. MS-AFP
	2. β-hCG
	3. Estriol
	4. Inhibin A (↑ sens to 80%)
		• MS-AFP alone: only 20% sensitivity → ↑ to 70% sensitivity with triple screen
		• **↑ MS-AFP:**
		  - NTD, ventral wall defect, twin pregnancy, placental bleeding, renal disease, sacrococcygeal teratoma
		• **↓ MS-AFP:**
		  - **Trisomy 21 (Down syndrome)**
		    ○ ↓ MS-AFP
		    ○ ↓ Estriol
		    ○ ↑ β-hCG
		    ○ ↑ Inhibin A
		  - **Trisomy 18 (Edward Syndrome)**
		    ○ ↓ MS-AFP
		    ○ ↓ Estriol
		    ○ ↓ β-hCG
		    ○ ↓ Inhibin A
			1. Abnormal MS-AFP:
			First step in management:
			• Ultrasound to confirm dating
			• If dating error, repeat MS-AFP
			• A normal repeat MS-AFP is reassuring
			Accurate gestational dating is needed for interpretation of results.
			2. Dates confirmed by ultrasound:
			Next step in management:
			For ↑ MS-AFP: amniocentesis for AF-AFP level and acetylcholinesterase activity
			For ↓ MS-AFP: amniocentesis for karyotyping
			Elevated amniotic fluid-acetylcholinesterase activity is specific to open NTD.

Third Trimester

A 38-year-old woman (G2 P1) is at 27 weeks' gestation. She weighs 227 pounds. She has gained 30 pounds during her pregnancy but reports that most of this is "fluid retention." She was diagnosed with gestational diabetes during her last pregnancy. Which of the following is the next step in management?

a. Begin insulin therapy.
b. Begin glipizide therapy.
c. Obtain 1-hr 50 g OGTT.
d. Obtain 3-hr 75 g OGTT.
e. Obtain 3-hr 100 g OGTT.

Answer: **C.** The first step in evaluating for gestational diabetes is with the 1 hr *50 g OGTT in weeks 24–28*. When this is positive, the patient must then undergo the confirmatory *3 h 100 g OGTT*.

Screening	Test	Diagnostic Significance	Next Step in Management
THIRD TRIMESTER ROUTINE TESTS			
Diabetes	1 hr 50 g OGTT given between weeks 24–28.	Abnormal result: 1 hr blood glucose >130–140 mg/dL	(+) screening: perform 3-hr 100 g OGTT (the definitive test for glucose intolerance in pregnancy). Requires overnight fast. Positive if 2 or more elevated values.
Anemia	CBC Measured at weeks 24–28.	• Hemoglobin <11 g/dl = anemia. • The most common cause is iron deficiency (even if not present in 1st trimester).	Give iron supplementation for iron deficiency.
Atypical antibodies	Indirect Coombs test	Performed in Rh-negative women to look for atypical antibodies (anti-D Ab) before giving RhoGAM.	RhoGAM is not indicated in Rh negative women who have developed anti-D antibodies.
GBS screening	Vaginal and rectal culture for group B streptococci at 35–37 weeks (ideally performed after 36 weeks)	• (+) GBS is a high risk for sepsis in newborn. • Treat with intrapartum IV antibiotics.	Intrapartum antibiotic • IV penicillin G • IV clindamycin or erythromycin in penicillin-allergic patient if sensitivities available • IV vancomycin if sensitivities not available

GBS = Group B Streptococcus; IV = intravenous; OGTT = oral glucose tolerance test

Gestational diabetes does not present with typical symptoms of diabetes. The vast majority of patients are diagnosed on OGTT screening.

The confirmatory test for diabetes in pregnancy is the **3 hr 100 g OGTT.**

- Abnormal plasma glucose measurements
  - >95 mg/dL fasting
  - >180 mg/dL at 1 hr
  - >155 mg/dL at 2 hr
  - >140 mg/dL at 3 hr
- If one postglucose load measurement is abnormal, the diagnosis is impaired glucose tolerance. If ≥2 postglucose load measurements are abnormal, the diagnosis is gestational diabetes.
- The 1 hr 50 g OGTT is a **sensitive** test; it must catch all patients that may have the disease.
- The 3 hr 100 g OGTT is a **specific** test; it must catch all the people that actually have the disease.

Give Rh(D) immunoglobulin in Rh negative mothers in the following settings:

- At 28 weeks
- Within 72 hours of delivery
- After miscarriage or abortion
- During amniocentesis or CVS
- With heavy vaginal bleeding

> **Basic Science Correlate**
>
> $$\text{Sensitivity} = \frac{\text{true positives}}{\text{true positives} + \text{false negatives}}$$
>
> $$\text{Specificity} = \frac{\text{true negatives}}{\text{true negatives} + \text{false positives}}$$

Advanced Maternal Age

Perhaps surprisingly, pregnant women who will be older than age 35 upon giving birth are considered to have advanced maternal age. "Advanced maternal age" means that patients are at increased risk for:

- Spontaneous abortion
- Chromosomal abnormalities (e.g., Down syndrome)
- Birth defects
- Ectopic pregnancy

These patients are also at increased risk for complications (e.g., hypertension, diabetes) during the pregnancy.

Three tests can help detect fetal chromosomal abnormalities in women of advanced maternal age: cell-free DNA (cfDNA), chorionic villus sampling, and amniocentesis.

- **cfDNA testing** (noninvasive, not diagnostic, i.e., screening test) is now offered to all women, regardless of age, to assess for aneuploidy. It is performed on a sample of maternal blood, in which apoptotic fetal cells and placental cells circulate. Although the sample contains DNA from both mother and fetus, the test can distinguish the fetal cell-free DNA from the mother's DNA.
  - Used to determine the karyotype of fetus
  - Can be done as early as 10 weeks
  - Risks of the test: none
- **Chorionic villus sampling** (invasive, diagnostic) is done at 10–14 weeks' gestation. Under ultrasound guidance, a sample of the placenta (chorionic villi) is removed and tested for chromosomal abnormalities.
  - Indications for the test are advanced maternal age; abnormal cfDNA test; parents who are carriers of chromosomal disorders; mother with a sex-linked disorder; previous child with chromosomal disorder
  - Risks of the test include fetal loss; maternal bleeding; infection; rupture of membranes
- **Amniocentesis** (invasive, diagnostic) can determine the fetal karyotype at 15–17 weeks.
  - A needle introduced transabdominally through the uterus aspirates a sample of amniotic fluid that is sent for testing

- Used to determine the karyotype of fetus and can be done throughout the pregnancy for various other reasons (e.g., determining fetal lung maturity later in pregnancy)
- Risks of the test include fetal loss; maternal bleeding; infection; rupture of membranes; fluid leakage; or direct/indirect injury to fetus

---

Basic Science Correlate

Formation of chorionic villi begins in week 2 of gestation. Chorionic villi are composed of the syncytiotrophoblast and cytotrophoblast and form fingerlike projections.

Third Trimester Bleeding

CCS Tip: Initial steps in management of late pregnancy bleeding:

- Perform initial management:
    - Get the patient's vitals
    - Place external fetal monitor
    - Start IV fluids with normal saline
- Order lab tests:
    - CBC
    - DIC workup (platelets, PT, PTT, fibrinogen, and D-dimer)
    - Type and cross-match
    - Obstetric ultrasound to rule out placenta previa
- Perform further steps in management:
    - Give blood transfusion for large volume loss
    - Place Foley catheter and measure urine output
    - Perform vaginal exam to rule out lacerations
    - Schedule delivery if maternal or fetal instability

Never perform a digital vaginal exam in a patient with late vaginal bleeding—placenta previa must be ruled out first.

Abruptio Placenta

Placental abruption (abruptio placenta) is a cause of third-trimester bleeding. It is an **obstetrical emergency** with a high fetal and maternal morbidity. It is distinguished by painful vaginal bleeding secondary to the premature separation of the placenta from the uterine walls. There is an association with DIC.

Frank placental abruption is where the vaginal bleeding is observed. Concealed placental abruption is where the blood accumulates behind the placenta.

Risk factors:

- Abdominal trauma (auto accidents)
- Maternal cocaine use
- Polyhydramnios
- Chronic hypertension
- Preeclampsia/eclampsia
- Maternal smoking

Diagnosis is made via the clinical picture. Look for a woman in her third trimester with severe abdominal pain, sudden vaginal bleeding, and uterine contractions. Testing might include transabdominal ultrasound and fibrinogen level.

Treatment depends on the severity and state of both mother and fetus. If either one is unstable, C-section delivery is the answer (the other options are complicated and thus won't be tested on the exam). Always test for DIC in these patients.

A 28-year-old woman at 31 weeks' gestation with her first child wakes in the middle of the night to find that she has vaginal bleeding. She is not experiencing any pain or fluid leakage. What is the next step in management?

a. Transvaginal ultrasound
b. Transabdominal ultrasound
c. Delivery immediately
d. Cervical exam
e. Nitrazine test

Answer: **B.** Transabdominal ultrasound is indicated as a screening test for this patient, who most likely has placenta previa. A transvaginal ultrasound could then be done as a confirmatory test. Delivery before a diagnosis would be indicated only if mother or baby was unstable, which was not indicated in the question. Cervical exam should be deferred until placenta previa is ruled out. Nitrazine testing would be done to assess for the presence of amniotic fluid, indicating possible rupture of membranes; this patient has no fluid leakage.

Placenta Previa

Placenta previa is implantation of the placenta that extends over the internal cervical os. Consider this diagnosis in all patients with painless third trimester vaginal bleeding.

Risk factors:

- Previous placenta previa
- Previous C-section
- Previous multiple-gestation pregnancy
- Previous abortion
- Advanced maternal age
- Maternal smoking or cocaine use

The **best initial test** is trans*abdominal* ultrasound to detect the placenta previa; it is done first to avoid the risks of entering the vagina.

Do not do a cervical exam in painless vaginal bleeding! In a cervical exam the fingers must enter the internal cervical os to assess cervical opening width/softness and fetal head position. In complete previa, the fingers will strike the placenta and separate it from the uterine wall—worsening the patient's condition and, if severe, causing fetal loss.

The **most specific test** is trans*vaginal* ultrasound is done if diagnosis is uncertain or positive for previa. Done correctly, transvaginal ultrasound does not put the patient at risk for bleeding, because the optimal view of the placenta previa keeps the transvaginal probe 2–3 cm from the cervix.

Treatment begins with ultrasound monitoring. Start at 32 weeks in an asymptomatic patient (no bleeding episodes).

> Placenta previa = **painless** vaginal bleeding
>
> Abruptio placenta = **painful** vaginal bleeding

- At 32 weeks, if the placenta is >2 cm away from the os, the patient may deliver vaginally; if <2 cm, repeat ultrasound at 36 weeks.
- At 36 weeks, a placenta that is >2 cm away from the os permits vaginal delivery.

In a patient with an acute episode of painless vaginal bleeding where the fetus or mother is at risk (nonreassuring stress test, mother in shock) and not responding to resuscitative measures, immediate delivery via C-section is needed.

Placenta Accreta

Placenta accreta is one of the 3 types of adherent placentas:

- Placenta **accreta:** placental villi **attach** to myometrium
- Placenta **increta:** placental villi **invade** the myometrium
- Placenta **percreta:** placental villi **penetrate** to or through the uterine serosa (possible to adhere to bladder or intestines)

Risk factors:

- Placenta previa after C-section (**most important** risk factor)
- C-section
- Uterine surgeries
- Advanced maternal age
- History of fertility treatments (in vitro)

Diagnosis is often made on routine ultrasound. Otherwise, the first symptom is significant bleeding after manual separation of the uterus or inability to remove the placenta from the uterus. In a patient with placental percreta with invasion to bladder, the initial symptom is hematuria during pregnancy.

Treatment is a peripartum hysterectomy if severe and the hemorrhage cannot be controlled.

Vasa Previa

Vasa previa is life-threatening for the fetus. It occurs when velamentous cord insertion results in umbilical vessels crossing the placental membranes over the cervix. When membranes rupture, the fetal vessels are torn, and blood loss is from the fetal circulation. Fetal exsanguination and death occur rapidly. The classic triad is as follows:

1. Rupture of membranes
2. Painless vaginal bleeding
3. Fetal bradycardia

The **first step in management** is always emergency cesarean section.

If the question describes an antenatal Doppler sonogram showing a vessel crossing the membranes over the internal cervical os, do not perform amniotomy. Amniotomy may rupture the fetal vessels and cause fetal death.

Uterine Rupture

Uterine rupture is the diagnosis when there is a history of a uterine scar with sudden-onset abdominal pain and vaginal bleeding associated with a loss of electronic fetal heart rate, uterine contractions, and recession of the fetal head.

A summary of third-trimester bleeding appears below.

	Abruptio Placenta	Placenta Previa	Vasa Previa	Uterine Rupture
Pain	Yes	No	No	Yes
Risk factors	• Previous abruption • Hypertension • Trauma • Cocaine abuse	• Previous previa • Multiparity • Structural abnormalities (e.g., fibroids) • Advanced maternal age	• Velamentous insertion of the umbilical cord • Accessory lobes • Multiple gestation	• Previous classic uterine incision • Myomectomy (fibroids) • Excessive oxytocin • Grand multiparity
Diagnosis: sonogram	Placenta in normal position ± retroplacental hematoma	Placenta implanted over the internal cervical os	Vessel crossing the membranes over the internal cervical os	N/A
Management	1. C-section: best choice for placenta previa or if patient/fetus is deteriorating (emergent) 2. Vaginal delivery if ≥36 weeks or continued bleeding in a stable patient 3. Admit and observe if bleeding has stopped, vitals and fetal heart rate (FHR) stable, or <34 weeks		Immediate C-section	Immediate surgery and delivery
Complication	Disseminated intravascular coagulation	Placenta accreta/increta/percreta → hysterectomy	Fetal exsanguination	Hysterectomy for uncontrolled bleeding

Fetal Complications

Perinatal Infections

Group B β-Hemolytic Streptococci (GBS)

A 28-year-old woman presents at 36 weeks' gestation with rupture of membranes. On examination she is found to have 7 cm cervical dilatation. She received all of her prenatal care, and her only complication was a course of antibiotics for asymptomatic bacteriuria. GBS screening was negative. Her first baby was hospitalized for 10 days after delivery for GBS pneumonia and sepsis. What is the most appropriate management?

a. Intrapartum IV penicillin
b. Intramuscular azithromycin
c. Rescreen for group B streptococci
d. Schedule cesarean section
e. No intervention needed

Answer: **A.** Intrapartum IV penicillin is indicated because the patient's previous birth was complicated with neonatal GBS sepsis.

With GBS, 30% of women have asymptomatic vaginal colonization.

Vertical transmission results in pneumonia and sepsis in the neonate within hours to days of birth. There is a 50% mortality rate with neonatal infection.

Treatment for GBS is intrapartum IV penicillin. With penicillin allergy, use IV erythromycin or clindamycin if sensitivities are available (if not available, use vancomycin).

Use antibiotics in the following situations:

- GBS (+) urine culture at any time during pregnancy
  - Presence of high-risk factors: preterm delivery
  - Membrane rupture >18 hours
  - Maternal fever
  - Previous baby with GBS sepsis

Do not use antibiotics in the following situations:

- Planned C-section without rupture of membranes (even if culture is [+])
- Culture (+) on a previous pregnancy, but culture (–) in the current pregnancy

Toxoplasmosis

Toxoplasmosis is present in undercooked meat and cat feces (after the cat has eaten an affected rodent). Toxoplasmosis can live in the environment for >1 year.

Infection with *Toxoplasma gondii* parasite is the most common diagnosis when the case describes a patient handling cat feces or litter boxes, drinking raw goat milk, eating raw meat, or possibly gardening.

> GBS-related meningitis occurs after the first week and is a hospital-acquired infection that is unrelated to vertical transmission.

> IgG antibodies in the mother indicate past exposure and are protective. IgM antibodies suggest recent exposure and risk of exposure to the fetus.

Vertical transmission only occurs with primary infection of the mother. The most serious infections occur during the first trimester.

The classic triad of congenital toxoplasmosis includes:

- Chorioretinitis
- Intracranial calcifications
- Hydrocephalus

Suspect primary infection of toxoplasmosis when the question gives a history of a mild mononucleosis-like syndrome and presence of a cat in the household. Intrauterine growth retardation may be seen on ultrasound. Testing includes *Toxoplasma* IgG and IgM levels.

The most important management is prevention: pregnant women should be told to not handle cat feces, raw goat milk, and undercooked meat during pregnancy.

Treatment of serologically confirmed fetal/neonatal infection via amniocentesis is pyrimethamine and sulfadiazine.

Varicella

Transplacental infection results from primary varicella infection in the mother (25–40% infection rate). The greatest risk to the fetus is if a rash appears in the mother between 5 days antepartum and 2 days postpartum.

Neonatal infection presents with "zigzag" skin lesions, limb hypoplasia, microcephaly, microphthalmia, chorioretinitis, and cataracts.

Prevention includes vaccination (live-attenuated varicella virus to nonpregnant women) and postexposure prophylaxis: VariZIG (purified human immunoglobulin with high levels of antivaricella antibodies) within 10 days of exposure. Note that VariZIG does not prevent infection but only attenuates the clinical effects of the virus.

Treatment is as follows:

- Maternal varicella (uncomplicated): oral acyclovir to mother plus VariZIG to mother and neonate
- Congenital varicella: VariZIG and IV acyclovir to neonate

Basic Science Correlate

Varicella is in the family *Herpesviridae*, **human herpesvirus type 3**. Primary infection causes varicella. After clinical symptoms disappear, the virus lies dormant in the dorsal root ganglia.

Later in life it may reactivate, causing shingles. Herpesvirus commonly reactivates in immunocompromised patients.

Rubella

A 24-year-old child-care worker is 29 weeks pregnant and is currently working. One of the children she cares for was diagnosed with rubella last week. Rubella antigen testing is performed and her IgG titer is negative. What is the next step in management?

a. Anti-rubella antibodies
b. Betamethasone
c. Rubella vaccine now
d. Rubella vaccine after delivery
e. Ultrasound of the fetus

Answer: **D.** There is no postexposure prophylaxis available, and immunization during pregnancy is contraindicated (live vaccine). The only correct management is to await normal delivery and give vaccination to the mother after delivery.

Vertical transmission of rubella virus (the causative virus of German measles) occurs with primary infection during pregnancy (70–90%).

Neonates with congenital rubella present with congenital deafness (most common sequelae), congenital heart disease (e.g., patent ductus arteriosus, or PDA), cataracts, mental retardation, hepatosplenomegaly, thrombocytopenia, and "blueberry muffin" rash. Adverse effects occur with primary infection in the first 10 weeks of gestation.

Basic Science Correlate
Rubella is a single-stranded RNA virus of the family *Togaviridae*.

Prevention includes a first-trimester screening and cautioning the mother to avoid infected individuals. Do not immunize pregnant women; immunize seronegative women only after delivery.

No post-exposure prophylaxis is available.

> Congenital CMV syndrome is the most common congenital viral syndrome in the United States.

Cytomegalovirus

Cytomegalovirus (CMV) is spread by infected body fluid secretions. It is the most common cause of sensorineural deafness in children.

Basic Science Correlate
CMV is another member of the family *Herpesviridae*, **HHV-5**.

The greatest risk for vertical transmission occurs with primary infection (infection rate is 50%).

Most mothers develop asymptomatic infections or describe mild, mononucleosis-like symptoms. About 10% of infants with congenital CMV infection are symptomatic at birth.

Manifestations include intrauterine growth restriction, prematurity, microcephaly, jaundice, petechiae, hepatosplenomegaly, periventricular calcifications, chorioretinitis, and pneumonitis.

Diagnostic testing includes CMV IgM and IgG levels from the mother:

- IgG (+)/IgM (−) indicates past exposure and no risk for primary infection
- IgG (+)/IgM (+) or IgG (−)/IgM (+) indicates recent infection

Prevention includes following universal precautions with all body fluids. Avoid transfusion with CMV-positive blood.

Treatment is as follows:

- Antiviral therapy with ganciclovir or foscarnet to prevent viral shedding and hearing loss (but does not cure the infection)
- CMV hyperimmune globulin to potentially reduce the risk of congenital infection in pregnant women with primary CMV infection

Herpes Simplex Virus (HSV)

A 21-year-old multipara is admitted to the birthing unit at 39 weeks gestation in active labor at 6 cm dilation. Membranes are intact. She has a history of genital herpes preceding the pregnancy. Her last outbreak was 8 weeks ago. She now complains of pain and pruritus. On examination she has localized, painful, ulcerative lesions on the right vaginal wall. Which of the following is the next step in management?

a. IV acyclovir
b. Terbutaline
c. Obtain culture of ulcer
d. Proceed with vaginal delivery
e. Schedule cesarean section

Answer: **E.** Active genital herpes is an indication for cesarean section.

Contact with maternal genital lesions during an active HSV episode is the most common cause of transmission. Transplacental infection can also occur with primary infection during pregnancy (50% risk). The greatest risk is primary infection in the third trimester.

Suspect primary HSV infection if the case describes fever, malaise, and diffuse genital lesions during pregnancy.

Neonatal infection acquired during delivery has 50% mortality rate. Surviving infants develop meningoencephalitis, mental retardation, pneumonia, hepatosplenomegaly, jaundice, and petechiae.

Diagnostic testing is (+) HSV culture from vesicle fluid or ulcer or HSV PCR.

Treatment includes:

- C-section for women with lesions suspicious for active genital HSV at the time of labor
- Acyclovir to patient for primary infection during pregnancy
- Do not use fetal scalp electrodes for monitoring (risk of HSV transmission increases if mother has active HSV lesion)
- Advise standard precautions: avoid intercourse if partner has active lesions, oral sex in presence of oral lesions, kissing neonate in presence of oral lesions

Human Immunodeficiency Virus (HIV)

A 24-year-old HIV positive woman (G2 P1) presents in her 16th week of pregnancy. Her previous child was diagnosed HIV positive after vaginal delivery. What is the most effective method to decrease the risk of vertical transmission?

a. Avoid artificial rupture of membranes
b. Avoid breastfeeding
c. Antiretroviral triple therapy
d. Cesarean section
e. Zidovudine (ZDV) monotherapy

Answer: C. All of the strategies are recommended, but triple ART is indicated for more effective management of HIV in the mother to drive the viral load to <1,000. ZDV monotherapy is less effective than triple therapy in reducing the risk of HIV transmission to the fetus (25% to 8%). (ZDV monotherapy alone is never indicated.) Cesarean section (before rupture of membranes), avoidance of breastfeeding and intrapartum invasive procedures (artificial ROM, fetal scalp electrodes) also decrease transmission rate. Combining all of the strategies listed would reduce the transmission rate to 1%.

Basic Science Correlate

HIV is a single-stranded, positive, enveloped RNA virus, a member of the family Retroviridae, genus Lentivirus. Once the virus enters a host cell, *viral reverse transcriptase* converts the viral RNA genome into double-stranded DNA. This allows integration of the *viral DNA* into the host *cellular DNA*.

The major route of vertical transmission is contact with infected genital secretions at the time of vaginal delivery. Without treatment, the vertical transmission rate is 25–30%.

Elective cesarean is of most benefit in women with low CD4 count and high RNA viral load (>1,000). All neonates of HIV-positive women will have positive HIV tests from transplacental passive IgG passage.

> HIV-infected pregnant women should receive ART therapy regardless of HIV RNA level.

Prevention and treatment are as follows. First, continue antiretrovirals in all pregnant patients.

- Triple-drug therapy:
  - Start triple therapy immediately—regardless of CD4 and viral load—to decrease risk of transmission
  - IV intrapartum ZDV at time of delivery if viral load not fully suppressed
  - Combination ZDV-based ART for 6 weeks after delivery
- Give the infant prophylaxis against HIV, with 6 weeks of **ZDV**
- Vaginal delivery is preferred unless maternal viral load >1,000 viral copies/mL
- Advise mother not to breastfeed (breast milk transmits the virus)
- Avoid invasive procedures (e.g., artificial rupture of membranes, fetal scalp electrodes)

Syphilis

There is no immunity from prior infection with syphilis, and reinfection can occur over and over again. If an exam question describes a previously treated syphilis infection, never assume immunity.

Transplacental infection results from primary and secondary infection (60% risk of transmission). Latent or tertiary infection has the lower risk of transmission.

Early acquired (first trimester) congenital syphilis includes the following symptoms:

- Nonimmune hydrops fetalis
- Maculopapular or vesicular peripheral rash
- Anemia, thrombocytopenia, and hepatosplenomegaly
- Large and edematous placenta
- Perinatal mortality rate ~50%

Late-acquired congenital syphilis (diagnosed after age 2) includes the following symptoms:

> Always order an HIV test in any pregnant patient who has tested positive for an STD.

- Hutchinson teeth
- "Mulberry" molars
- "Saddle" nose
- "Saber" shins
- Deafness (cranial nerve 8 palsy)

Diagnostic testing is as follows:

- VDRL or RPR screening in first trimester; confirm (+) screen with FTA-ABS
- You could also reverse-screen, i.e., start with a treponemal-specific test
- In primary syphilis, a screening test will be falsely negative.
- When there is a painless genital ulcer, order darkfield microscopy to diagnose primary syphilis.

Treatment is benzathine penicillin IM × 1 for (+) mothers. With penicillin allergy, do oral desensitization followed by full dose benzathine penicillin.

A 34-year-old multigravida presents for prenatal care in the second trimester. She reports a history of substance abuse but states she has been clean for 6 months. With her second pregnancy, she experienced a preterm delivery at 34 weeks' gestation of a male neonate who died within the first day of life. At that delivery, the baby was swollen, with skin lesions, and the placenta was very large. She was treated with antibiotics but she can't remember what they were. On a routine prenatal panel with this current pregnancy, she is found to have a positive VDRL test. What is the next step in management?

a. FTA-ABS
b. Intramuscular penicillin
c. Lupus anticoagulant
d. Oral penicillin
e. RPR
f. Ultrasound

Answer: **A.** The next step after any positive screening test is the confirmatory test before starting therapy. FTA-ABS or MHA-TP is the confirmatory tests for syphilis. Once syphilis is confirmed, give intramuscular penicillin.

Hepatitis B Virus (HBV)

Neonatal infection results from primary infection in the third trimester or ingestion of infected genital secretions during vaginal delivery. Of the neonates who get infected, 80% will develop chronic hepatitis (compared with only 10% of infected adults).

A 29-year-old multigravida was found on routine prenatal laboratory testing to be positive for hepatitis B surface antigen. She is an intensive care unit nurse. She received 2 units of packed red blood cells 2 years ago after experiencing postpartum hemorrhage with her last pregnancy. Which of the following indicates the greatest risk of transmission?

a. Anti-HBc
b. Anti-HBs
c. HBe Ag
d. HBs Ag
e. IgM anti-HBc

Answer: **C.** Mothers who are (+) for HBsAg, anti-HBe antibody, and IgM anti-HBc are acutely infected. There is only a 10% vertical transmission risk. Mothers who are also (+) for **HBeAg** have an **80% risk** of transmission to fetus. Anti-HBs (antibody to surface antigen) indicates immunity to infection from previous immunization. Hepatitis B surface antibody is an IgG antibody that can cross the placenta.

Hepatitis B infection is not an indication for cesarean delivery.

- During pregnancy (e.g., amniocentesis), avoid invasive procedures.
- Once the neonate has received active immunization and HBIG, breastfeeding is not contraindicated.
- Immunizations:
  - **HBsAg-negative:** give active immunization during pregnancy
  - **Postexposure prophylaxis for the mother:** HBIG (antibodies to hepatitis B) passive immunization and vaccine

Treatment is hepatitis immunization and HBIG in the neonate. Chronic HBV can be treated with interferon or lamivudine.

Zika Virus

Zika is spread by the bite of an infected *Aedes* mosquito, and can also be sexually transmitted by exposed individuals. Zika can then be passed from mother to fetus during pregnancy, leading to birth defects such as microcephaly.

Symptoms include fever, rash, headache, joint pain, and body aches.

Diagnosis is based on a finding of Zika virus, Zika virus RNA, or antigen in any body fluid or tissue specimen, commonly serum or urine. Individuals with possible exposure and symptoms should be screened with **RNA nucleic acid testing (NAT)** and **Zika virus IgM** testing. Where there is exposure without symptoms, NAT alone is sufficient.

There is currently no available treatment. All efforts focus on prevention.

- Avoid travel to endemic areas (Caribbean, Central America) and protect against mosquito bites.
- Avoid intercourse with other individuals who may be exposed.
- Avoid pregnancy for 6 months after potential exposure of either partner.

Intrauterine Growth Restriction (IUGR)

IUGR is the diagnosis when the estimated fetal weight (EFW) is <10 percentile for gestational age. Accurate, early pregnancy dating is essential for making the diagnosis.

If accurate dates are not known, an early sonogram (<20 weeks) is the next step in management. Never change the gestational age based on a late sonogram.

	Symmetric IUGR	Asymmetric IUGR	
	Fetal Causes	Maternal Causes	Placental Causes
	Decreased growth potential	Decreased placental perfusion	
Etiology	- Aneuploidy - Infection (e.g., TORCH) - Structural anomalies (e.g., congenital heart disease, NTD, ventral wall defects)	- Hypertension - Small vessel disease (e.g., SLE) - Malnutrition - Tobacco, alcohol, street drugs	- Infarction - Abruption - Twin-twin transfusion - Velamentous cord insertion
Ultrasound	↓ *in all measurements*	↓ *abdomen measurements; normal head measurements*	
Workup	- Detailed sonogram - Karyotype - Screen for fetal infections	- Monitor with serial sonograms, nonstress test, amniotic fluid index (AFI), biophysical profile, and umbilical artery Doppler - AFI is often decreased, especially with severe uteroplacental insufficiency	

Basic Science Correlate

Symmetric IUGR is caused by *intrinsic* factors (e.g., genetic issue, fetal infection).

Asymmetric IUGR is caused by *extrinsic* factors, such as **low oxygen** and **nutrient transfer from the placenta** leading to hypoxia in the fetus. These conditions can lead to hypoglycemia (from ↓ glycogen and fat stores) and polycythemia (from ↑ erythropoietin).

Macrosomia

Macrosomia is indicated by a fetus with estimated fetal weight (EFW) >90th–95th percentile for gestational age or birth weight of 4,000–4,500 g.

Risk factors include GDM, overt diabetes, prolonged gestation, obesity, ↑ in pregnancy weight gain, multiparity, and male fetus.

Complications include:

- Maternal: Injury during birth, postpartum hemorrhage, and emergency cesarean section
- Fetus: Shoulder dystocia, birth injury, asphyxia
- Neonate: Hypoglycemia, Erb palsy

Management is **elective cesarean** (if EFW >4,500 g in diabetic mother or >5,000 g in nondiabetic mother).

Medical Complications in Pregnancy

Hypertension

Hypertension (BP ≥140/90 mm Hg) during pregnancy can be classified as chronic hypertension or gestational hypertension. Both types predispose the mother and the fetus to more serious conditions.

When hypertension is accompanied by signs and symptoms of end-organ damage or neurological sequelae, the diagnosis is preeclampsia, eclampsia, or HELLP syndrome.

With hypertension is sustained, the fetus may be growth restricted and hypoxic and is at risk for abruptio placenta.

Diagnosis is as follows:

- Chronic hypertension: a history of elevated blood pressure before pregnancy or before 20 weeks' gestation
- Gestational hypertension: when blood pressure develops after 20 weeks' gestation and returns to normal baseline by 6 weeks postpartum
- Preeclampsia: when there is proteinuria and/or presence of "warning signs"

Preeclampsia and Eclampsia

Preeclampsia without severe features is indicated with **either** of the following:

- Sustained BP elevation >**140/90 mm Hg** and proteinuria of at least 1+ (on dipstick) or >**300 mg** (on a 24-hour urine)
- Sustained BP elevation >**140/90 mm Hg** and end-organ dysfunction with or without proteinuria

Preeclampsia with severe features is indicated by preeclampsia **plus** any of the following:

- Systolic blood pressure ≥160 mm Hg or diastolic blood pressure ≥110 mm Hg
- New onset cerebral or visual disturbance (includes headache)
- Hepatic abnormality (RUQ pain and/or transaminases more than doubled)
- Thrombocytopenia (<100,000)
- Renal abnormalities
- Pulmonary edema

Primigravidas are most at risk. Other risk factors are multiple gestation, hydatidiform mole, diabetes mellitus, age extremes, chronic hypertension, and chronic renal disease.

> A 19-year-old primigravida presents at 32 weeks' gestation for routine follow-up. She denies headache, epigastric pain, or visual disturbances. She has gained 2 pounds since her last visit 2 weeks ago. On examination blood pressure is 155/95, which is persistent on repeat BP check 10 minutes later. She has only trace pedal edema. Which of the following is the next step in management?
>
> a. Methyldopa
> b. Labetalol
> c. Electrocardiogram
> d. Fetal ultrasound
> e. Urinalysis
>
> Answer: **E.** Always rule out preeclampsia in a hypertensive pregnant patient. Even if she is asymptomatic, proteinuria indicates preeclampsia and a worse prognosis.

Warning signs of maternal jeopardy:

- Hallmark symptoms: headache; epigastric pain; changes in vision
- Signs: pulmonary edema, oliguria (peripheral edema not a warning sign)
- Labs: thrombocytopenia, elevated liver enzymes

Further diagnoses:

- Chronic hypertension with superimposed preeclampsia: when there is new onset of proteinuria, end-organ dysfunction, or both after 20 weeks of gestation in a woman with chronic/preexisting hypertension
- Eclampsia: when a case describes unexplained grand mal seizures in a hypertensive and/or proteinuric pregnant woman in the last half of pregnancy; patients present with same signs and symptoms as in preeclampsia plus unexplained tonic-clonic seizures (seizures from severe diffuse cerebral vasospasm cause cerebral perfusion deficits and edema)
- HELLP syndrome: when there is hemolysis (H), elevated liver (EL) enzymes, and low platelets (LP)

Diagnostic testing is as follows:

- CBC, chem-12 panel, coagulation panel, and urinalysis with urinary protein
- Labs will show:
  - Hemoconcentration: hemoglobin, hematocrit, BUN, serum creatinine, and serum uric acid all increased
  - Proteinuria
  - In severe preeclampsia, DIC, and liver enzyme elevation

Treatment is as follows:

- Blood pressure control:
  - Do not treat unless BP >160/110 mm Hg (antihypertensives decrease uteroplacental blood flow); goal SBP is 140–150 mm Hg and DBP 90–100 mm Hg
  - Maintenance therapy: (first line) methyldopa, labetalol (alpha and beta blocker that preserves blood flow to uterus and placenta), and nifedipine (CCB)
  - IV hydralazine or labetalol
- Seizure management and prophylaxis:
  - Protect patient's airway and tongue
  - Give IV $MgSO_4$ (magnesium sulfate) bolus for seizure and infusion for continued prophylaxis.
  - Give IV $MgSO_4$ in preeclampsia with severe features to prevent seizures— stop them before they happen!
- Monitoring:
  - Serial sonograms (evaluate for intrauterine growth restriction [IUGR])
  - Serial BP monitoring
- Labor:
  - Induce labor if ≥37 weeks in preeclampsia without severe features: attempt vaginal delivery with IV oxytocin if mother and fetus are stable.
  - Aggressive, prompt delivery is the best step for preeclampsia with severe features, superimposed preeclampsia, or eclampsia at *any* gestational age.
  - Give intrapartum IV $MgSO_4$ and hydralazine and/or labetalol to manage BP

> Eclampsia = Preeclampsia + Seizures

> Seizure disorder is not a risk factor for eclampsia.

> The only definitive cure is delivery and removal of all fetal-placental tissue.

> Never give ACE inhibitors, ARBs, renin inhibitors, or thiazides during pregnancy.

Gestational thrombocytopenia (most common cause of thrombocytopenia in pregnancy)

- Mild: counts >70,000/mm^3
- Not associated with other abnormalities, and no symptoms
- Usually develops in third trimester

A 32-year-old multigravida at 36 weeks' gestation was found to have BP 160/105 mm Hg on routine prenatal visit. Previous BP readings were normal. She complained of some right-upper-quadrant abdominal pain. Urinalysis showed 3+ proteinuria. She is emergently induced for labor and delivers an 8 lb. 3 oz. boy. Two days after delivery, routine labs reveal elevated total bilirubin, lactate dehydrogenase, alanine aminotransferase, and aspartate aminotransferase. Platelet count is 85,000/mm^3. Postpartum evaluation reveals that she has no complaints of headache or visual changes. Which of the following is the most likely diagnosis?

a. Cholecystitis
b. HELLP syndrome
c. Hepatitis
d. Gestational thrombocytopenia
e. Preeclampsia

Answer: **B.** Patient has evidence of hemolysis (elevated LDH), elevated liver enzymes, and thrombocytopenia.

A 24-year-old woman in week 36 of her second pregnancy presents to the office with abdominal pain and nausea for the past 2 days. The patient states that she feels weak and tired. BP 156/92 mm Hg, HR 90 bpm, UA 1+ protein. What is the next step in the management of this patient?

a. CBC, CMP
b. UA
c. Transfer and admit for immediate delivery
d. Recheck blood pressure
e. No intervention is needed

Answer: **A.** A CBC/CMP should be done, along with 24-hour urine testing. Patients in the third trimester need close observation. While the symptoms observed here could simply result from a viral infection (in which case nothing needs to be done—the most common pitfall in these patients), you should at least have labs drawn to assess for HELLP. Urinalysis (B) is already positive for 1+ protein and would not elicit any new information. Although the patient's elevated blood pressure could indicate preeclampsia, immediate delivery (C) is not needed at this time. Blood pressure monitoring should continue (D), but blood work is the essential next step and would be the correct answer.

HELLP Syndrome

HELLP syndrome occurs in preeclamptic patients with the addition of hemolysis, elevated liver enzymes, and low platelets. It usually occurs in the third trimester, but it can occur up to 2 days after delivery.

Risk factors include:

- Previous HELLP syndrome
- Sisters and offspring of people with HELLP syndrome

Diagnosis is based on the presence of elevated liver enzymes, low platelets, and hemolysis.

H = hemolysis
E = elevated
L = liver enzymes
L = low
P = platelet count

Treatment for HELLP depends on the gestational age of the fetus. However, delivery is the only effective treatment and is curative. Immediate delivery is recommended in the following circumstances:

- >34 weeks' gestation
- Fetal distress
- Severe maternal disease
- Maternal DIC, liver infarction, renal failure
- Placental abruption

If the fetus is <34 weeks' gestation and none of the criteria are met, give a dose of corticosteroids to mature the fetal lungs.

Initiate platelet transfusion if:

- Actively bleeding patient
- Platelet count <20,000/mm^3
- C-section. Transfuse to raise platelet count >50,000/mm^3

Serious complications of HELLP:

- DIC
- Placental abruption
- Renal failure
- Pulmonary edema
- Fetal demise
- Maternal death

Cardiac Abnormalities

- Heart disorders account for 15% of maternal obstetric deaths.
- Women with high-risk disorders (e.g., pulmonary hypertension, Eisenmenger syndrome, severe valvular disorders, prior postpartum cardiomyopathy) should be advised *not* to become pregnant due to risk of sudden death.
- Cardiovascular changes in pregnancy (30–50% ↑ cardiac output) may unmask or worsen underlying cardiac conditions. These changes are maximal at 28 and 34 weeks' gestation.

Peripartum Cardiomyopathy

- Heart failure with no identifiable cause can develop between the last month of pregnancy to 5 months postpartum.
- Risk factors include multiparity, age ≥30, multiple gestations (i.e., twins or triplets, etc.), and preeclampsia.
- Mortality rate is 10% in 2 years.

Management of Specific Cardiac Conditions

- Heart failure: risk of maternal or fetal death is associated with class III or IV heart failure
  - Never use an ACE inhibitor or aldosterone antagonist in pregnancy.
  - Loop diuretics, nitrates, and β-blockers may be continued.
  - Digoxin may be used in pregnancy to improve symptoms, but it does not improve outcomes.
- Arrhythmias
  - Continue rate control as with nonpregnant patients
  - Do not give amiodarone or warfarin.
- Valvular disease
  - Regurgitant lesions are well tolerated and require no therapy.
  - Stenotic lesions have an increased risk of maternal/fetal morbidity and mortality.
  - Mitral stenosis has an increased risk of pulmonary edema and A-fib.

Hypercoagulable States

Pulmonary embolus (PE) is the third leading cause of maternal death in the United States; 50% of pregnant women who develop thromboemboli have an underlying thrombophilic disorder. Virchow triad consists of endothelial injury, vascular stasis, and hypercoagulability.

Diagnosis of venous thromboembolic events is made as follows:

- When DVT is suspected, get lower extremity Doppler
- When PE is suspected, get V/Q scan first and consider chest x-ray
- Avoid CT angiogram unless initial testing is equivocal or negative
- Do not order D-dimer in pregnancy because it will be elevated

Treatment is anticoagulation. Low molecular weight heparin (LMWH) is the drug of choice, since it does not cross the placenta.

- Warfarin is contraindicated, as it crosses the placenta, causes fetal abnormalities, and may cause death.
- Patients with a history of DVT or PE in a previous pregnancy or history of underlying thrombophilic condition should receive prophylactic LMWH throughout pregnancy, unfractionated heparin during labor and delivery, and warfarin for 6 weeks postpartum.

When is **anticoagulation** the answer?

- When there is DVT or PE in pregnancy, A-fib with underlying heart disease (but not A-fib alone); antiphospholipid syndrome; severe heart failure (EF <30%); and Eisenmenger syndrome

> Most common underlying thrombophilias:
> - Factor V Leiden mutation
> - Prothrombin gene mutation
> - Antiphospholipid syndrome
> - Hyperhomocysteinemia (MTHFR)
> - Antithrombin III deficiency

Thyroid Disorders

Hyperthyroidism in pregnancy causes fetal growth restriction and stillbirth. **Hypothyroidism** in pregnancy causes intellectual deficits in offspring and miscarriage.

Pregnancy does not change the symptoms of hyperthyroidism or hypothyroidism, nor does it change the normal values/ranges of free serum thyroxine (T4) and thyroid-stimulating hormone (TSH).

- For symptomatic hyperthyroidism, beta blockers are the drug of choice. (Do not use radioactive iodine in pregnancy.)
- For hypothyroidism, levothyroxine is the drug of choice. (Do not use triiodothyronine or desiccated thyroid as thyroid replacement in pregnancy.)
  - Hormone replacement should be continued in those with hypothyroidism during pregnancy.
  - However, on initial pregnancy diagnosis, increase the dose by 25–30%.

Graves Disease

- Propylthiouracil (PTU) is the drug of choice during the first trimester (methimazole is the second-line therapy).
  - PTU crosses the placenta and may cause goiter and hypothyroidism in the fetus, so in the second and third trimesters, use methimazole.
  - Congenital Graves disease in the fetus may be masked until 7–10 days after birth, when the drug's effect subsides.
- Maternal thyroid-stimulating immunoglobulins and thyroid-blocking Igs can cross the placenta and cause fetal tachycardia, growth restriction, and goiter.

> **Basic Science Correlate**
>
> PTU and methimazole are Class D drugs that harm the fetus by inhibiting thyroperoxidase, an enzyme needed to produce T3 and T4.

Diabetes in Pregnancy

- Target values of FBS <90 mg/dL and <120 mg/dL 2 hours after a meal.
- Gestational diabetes (GDM) is managed initially with diet and light exercise.
- If target glucose measurements are not met, pharmacologic treatment is required
- Insulin, glyburide, and metformin are acceptable treatment options.
- Insulin requires additional needle-sticks, resulting in lower compliance. However, insulin is still considered first line for treatment of gestational diabetes.
- Avoid oral hypoglycemics while breastfeeding, as they can cause hypoglycemia in neonates.
- All pregnant women with diabetes should take aspirin daily to reduce the risk of developing preeclampsia.

Diagnosis is made with the following:

- Screen for GDM with a 1-hour 50 g glucose challenge test (GCT); the test is positive when glucose ≥130–140 mg/dL.
- A positive 1-hour GCT should prompt a confirmatory 3-hour glucose tolerance test (GTT).
- **At least 2 values** must be elevated to make a diagnosis of diabetes in pregnancy. There is no consensus regarding the optimum thresholds for a positive GTT, but these values can be used as a rule of thumb.

Time since Glucose Consumption	Measured Serum Glucose
Fasting	>95 mg/dL
1 hour	>180 mg/dL
2 hours	>155 mg/dL
3 hours	>140 mg/dL

Routine Monitoring in Diabetic Patients

- If you suspect that the patient has diabetes, get an **early GCT and HbA1C**. If HbA1c elevated in first trimester:
  - Obtain targeted ultrasound at 18–20 weeks to look for structural anomalies; and
  - Obtain fetal echocardiogram at 22–24 weeks to assess for congenital heart disease.
- **MSAFP at 16–18 weeks** to assess for neural tube defects (NTD)
- Monthly sonograms to assess fetal macrosomia or IUGR
- Monthly biophysical profiles
- **Start 2×/week nonstress test (NST) and amniotic fluid index (AFI) at 32 weeks** if taking medication, macrosomia, previous stillbirth, or hypertension.
- For gestational diabetes mellitus (GDM) patients, order a **2-hour 75 g OGTT** 6–12 weeks postpartum to determine if diabetes has resolved; 35% of women with GDM will develop overt diabetes within 5–10 years after delivery.
- Caudal regression syndrome is an uncommon congenital abnormality associated with overt DM.

Congenital malformations (especially NTDs) are strongly associated with HbA1c >8.5 in the first trimester.

GDM is *not* associated with congenital anomalies, since hyperglycemia is not present in the first half of pregnancy.

Labor in Diabetic Patients

- Target delivery gestational age is **40 weeks** because of delayed fetal maturity.
- Induce labor at **39–40 weeks if** <**4,500 g** or if there is poor glycemic control. Lecithin/sphingomyelin (L/S) ratio 2.5 and the presence of phosphatidyl glycerol ensures fetal lung maturity.
- Option to schedule cesarean section if >**4,500 g** because of the risk of **shoulder dystocia.**
- Check blood glucose every 2 hours during labor, and give insulin at glucose >120 mg/dL.
- Blood glucose monitoring is no longer needed after delivery.

Liver Disease

A 31-year-old primigravida woman presents at 32 weeks' gestation with dizygotic twins of different genders. She is of Swedish descent and complains of intense skin itching. Her sister experienced similar complaints when she was pregnant and delivered her baby prematurely. No identifiable rash is noted on physical examination. She states that her urine appears dark colored. What is the diagnosis?

Answer: The diagnosis is **intrahepatic cholestasis of pregnancy**. It occurs in genetically susceptible women (of European heritage) and is associated with multiple pregnancies.

Intrahepatic Cholestasis of Pregnancy

- Symptoms: intractable nocturnal pruritus on the palms and soles of the feet without skin findings
- Diagnosis: 10- to 100-fold increase in serum bile acids
- Treatment: ursodeoxycholic acid (reduces cholesterol absorption and dissolves gallstones, but gallstones re-form when patient stops taking the medication); symptoms may be relieved by antihistamines and cholestyramine

Acute Fatty Liver of Pregnancy (AFLP)

- Symptoms: initial symptoms include nausea, vomiting, and abdominal pain; clinically, it can present similar to HELLP syndrome and can be distinguished by the addition of more severe symptoms (hypoglycemia, acute kidney injury, jaundice, ascites, and encephalopathy); can lead to multiorgan failure
- Diagnosis: ↑ bilirubin, ammonia, uric acid, creatinine, WBC, PT/PTT ↓ glucose, fibrinogen, platelets. Proteinuria present. Liver biopsy will reveal microvesicular fatty infiltration of the hepatocytes; however, liver biopsy is not performed in clinical practice.
- Treatment: prompt delivery, maternal stabilization, and monitoring

Urinary Tract Infection, Pyelonephritis, and Bacteriuria

Asymptomatic Bacteriuria	Acute Cystitis	Pyelonephritis
1. Urine culture (+) 2. No urgency, frequency, or burning present 3. No fever	1. Urine culture (+) 2. Urgency, frequency, or burning present 3. No fever	1. Urine culture (+) 2. Urgency, frequency, or burning present 3. Fever 4. CVA tenderness
Tx: *Outpatient* PO antibiotics (cephalexin or amoxicillin). Nitrofurantoin is avoided in first trimester.		**Tx:** Admit to hospital; IV hydration, IV cephalosporins or gentamicin, and tocolysis (if having contractions).
Cx: 30% of cases develop acute pyelonephritis when untreated. Pregnant women need test of cure.		**Cx:** Preterm labor and delivery Severe cases → sepsis, anemia, and pulmonary dysfunction

- All pregnant women require a test of cure with a urine culture.
- All pregnant women with pyelonephritis will require suppressive antibiotic therapy (nitrofurantoin or cephalexin) and monthly urine culture.

Termination of Pregnancy

Induced Abortion

The more advanced the gestation, the higher the rate of complications.

First-Trimester Methods

- Dilation and curettage (D&C) (most common) is performed before 13 weeks' gestation; complications include endometritis (outpatient antibiotic) and retained products of conception (repeat curettage)
- Medical abortion with oral mifepristone (progesterone antagonist) and oral misoprostol (prostaglandin E1); must be used in first 63 days of amenorrhea
  - Rarely, results in incomplete abortion which then requires D&C
  - Rarely, *Clostridium sordellii* sepsis can occur

Spontaneous Abortion/Fetal Demise

Death of an embryo/fetus is based on gestational age or weight at the time of in-utero death.

- Spontaneous abortion
  - Expulsion of an embryo/fetus <500 g or <20 weeks' gestation
  - Most common symptoms are uterine pain and vaginal bleeding
  - Most common cause is chromosomal abnormalities of the embryo or fetus
  - Risk factors are advanced maternal age, previous spontaneous abortion, and maternal smoking

- Fetal demise
  - In-utero death of a fetus after 20 weeks' gestation
  - Most common symptom is loss of fetal movements
  - Most commonly idiopathic
  - Risk factors are antiphospholipid syndrome, overt maternal diabetes, maternal trauma, severe maternal isoimmunization, and fetal infection

When there is prolonged fetal demise (>2 weeks), the most serious complication to watch for is disseminated intravascular coagulation (DIC), resulting from release of tissue thromboplastin from deteriorating fetal organs.

CCS Tip: In patients presenting with fetal demise, always rule out coagulopathy by ordering platelet count, D-dimer, fibrinogen, PT, and PTT. If DIC is identified, deliver immediately.

Ultrasound must be done to assess the type of abortion. Give RhoGAM to Rh-negative women.

Spontaneous Abortion		
Type	**Ultrasound Finding**	**Treatment**
Complete	No products of conception; cervix closed	Follow up with β-hCG
Incomplete	Some products of conception present; cervix open	Medical induction or D&C
Inevitable	Products of conception present; intrauterine bleeding; dilation of cervix	Medical induction, expectant management, or D&C
Threatened	Products of conception present; intrauterine bleeding; no dilation of cervix	Pelvic rest
Missed	Fetus is dead but remains in uterus	Medical induction or D&C
Septic	Infection of the uterus	D&C + IV levofloxacin + metronidazole

Diagnostic testing is as follows:

- Speculum exam to evaluate for cervical/vaginal sources of bleeding and presence of vaginal dilation
  - **Never the first step in management for late trimester bleeding** because of risk of bleeding in a low implanted placenta
- Ultrasound to evaluate fetal cardiac activity and ± of products of conception.

Ectopic Pregnancy

Ectopic pregnancy (1% of pregnancies, but higher if there is a history or ectopic pregnancy) occurs when a fertilized egg grows outside of the uterus. It can be very serious.

Any cause of tubal scarring or adhesions increases the risk for ectopic pregnancy: pelvic inflammatory disease (PID) (most common); history of surgery (tubal ligation/surgery); or congenital risks (diethylstilbestrol [DES] exposure).

Salping**ostomy** = open the fallopian tube

Salping**ectomy** = remove the fallopian tube

Indications for methotrexate are as follows:

- Pregnancy mass <3.5 cm diameter
- Absence of fetal heart motion
- β-hcg level <6,000 mIU
- No history of folic supplementation

Diagnosis is suspected when β-hCG >1,500 mIU and no intrauterine pregnancy is seen on vaginal sonogram.

- Absence of an adnexal mass does not rule out ectopic pregnancy.
- Presume ectopic pregnancy has ruptured when the patient is unstable (hypotension, tachycardia) and there are symptoms of peritoneal irritation (abdominal guarding or rigidity).

When β-hCG <1,500 mIU or if the location of the pregnancy cannot be visualized, you cannot rule out a normal intrauterine pregnancy.

- The next step is to repeat β-hCG and repeat the sonogram.
- In a normal viable intrauterine pregnancy, β-hCG should double in 48 hours.

Treatment is as follows:

- Immediate laparotomy/salpingectomy for ruptured ectopic pregnancy (look for an unstable patient)
- Methotrexate or laparoscopy (salpingectomy or salpingostomy) for unruptured ectopic pregnancy
- RhoGAM to Rh negative women
- Follow up β-hCG to ensure there has been complete destruction of the ectopic trophoblastic villi

> ### Basic Science Correlate
>
> Methotrexate is a folate antagonist. Folate is needed for the synthesis of thymidine (remember that nucleoside?), which is essential for the formation of DNA.

A 24-year-old woman visits the clinic with left-sided abdominal and flank pain and vaginal spotting. Her last menstrual period was 7 weeks ago. She denies fevers, nausea, or vomiting. She has one prior pregnancy with spontaneous vaginal delivery. She has used OCPs in the past but currently uses an intrauterine device for contraception. Pelvic examination reveals a slightly enlarged uterus, closed cervix. No palpable adnexal mass is identified however there is tenderness on bimanual exam. Quantitative serum β-hCG value is 2,650 mIU. What is the most likely diagnosis?

a. Ectopic pregnancy
b. Hydatidiform mole
c. Incomplete abortion
d. Missed abortion
e. Threatened abortion

Answer: **A.** The classic presentation of ectopic pregnancy is amenorrhea, vaginal bleeding, and unilateral pelvic-abdominal pain. When there is also abdominal guarding or rigidity, hypotension, and tachycardia, the diagnosis is ruptured ectopic pregnancy.

Preterm Labor

Cervical Insufficiency

A 29-year-old primigravida presents to the ED at 19 weeks' gestation with lower pelvic pressure without contractions. She reports increased clear vaginal mucus discharge. Fetal membranes are found to be bulging into the vagina, and the cervix cannot be palpated. Fetal feet can be felt through the membranes. What is the next step in management?

a. Abdominal cerclage
b. Prophylactic antibiotics
c. Tocolysis
d. Vaginal cerclage
e. Rule out chorioamnionitis

Answer: **E.** In a patient with preterm labor or preterm PROM, rule out chorioamnionitis first. Emergency cerclage is indicated when there is minimal cervical dilation in the absence of labor or abruption. This patient is already fully dilated (no palpable cervix) so cerclage is no longer an option. Prophylactic antibiotics and tocolytics are not recommended.

Risk factors for cervical insufficiency are a history of any of the following:

- Second-trimester abortion
- Cervical laceration during delivery
- Deep cervical conization
- Diethylstilbestrol (DES) exposure

Treatment is as follows:

- Elective cerclage placement at 12–14 weeks' gestation for patients with ≥3 unexplained midtrimester pregnancy losses
- Urgent cerclage only after labor and chorioamnionitis have first been ruled out
- Cerclage removal at 36–37 weeks, after fetal lung maturity

> **Cervical cerclage:**
> - Performed at 12–14 weeks
> - Suture encircles cervix to prevent cervical canal from dilation
> - Indicated electively or emergently in cervical insufficiency

Prelabor Rupture of Membranes (PROM)

This is rupture of the fetal membranes before the onset of labor. Ascending infection from the lower genital tract is the most common risk factor.

Diagnostic testing includes:

- Sterile speculum examination, revealing:
  - Posterior fornix pooling of clear amniotic fluid (AF)
  - Fluid is nitrazine-positive; AF has a more basic pH compared to physiologic vaginal discharge and will turn nitrazine paper from yellow to blue
  - Fluid is ferning-positive
- Ultrasound: oligohydramnios (AFI <5)

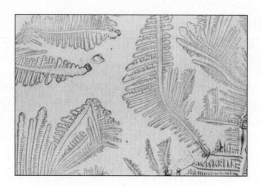

Ferning pattern of amniotic fluid

Chorioamnionitis is the feared complication. It is diagnosed clinically as:

- Maternal fever and uterine tenderness
- Confirmed PROM
- Absence of a URI or UTI

Treatment is as follows:

- If uterine contractions are present, do not give tocolysis.
- If chorioamnionitis is present:
  - Cultures
  - IV antibiotics
  - Delivery
- If infection is absent:
  - Before viability (<24 weeks): discuss benefits/risks of pregnancy termination versus expectant management
  - Preterm viability (24–33 weeks): hospitalize and give IM betamethasone if <37 weeks; obtain cervical cultures and administer prophylactic ampicillin and erythromycin for 7 days
  - Late preterm or term (>34 weeks): initiate delivery

Normal and Abnormal Labor

Stages of Labor

Labor Stage	Definition	Duration	Abnormalities
Stage 1— Latent phase	Begins: Onset of regular uterine contractions Ends: 6 cm cervical dilation	<20 hours (nullipara) <14 hours (multipara)	Prolonged latent phase: No cervical change in 20 h (nullipara)/14 h (multipara) Cause: Most common cause is analgesia Management: Rest and sedation
Stage 1— Active phase	Begins: 6 cm cervical dilation Ends: 10 cm (complete) Rapid cervical dilation	>1.2 cm/hour (nullipara) >1.5 cm/hour (multipara)	**Active phase prolongation or arrest:** • Prolongation: cervical dilation <1.2 cm/h (nullipara) / <1.5 cm/h (multipara) • Arrest: no cervical change in ≥2 h Cause: Abnormalities with passenger (fetal size or abnormal presentation), pelvis, or power (dysfunctional contractions) **Management:** • Hypotonic contractions → IV oxytocin • Adequate contractions → cesarean section
Stage 2— Descent	Begins: 10 cm (complete) Ends: delivery of baby Descent of the fetus	2 hours (nullipara) 1 hour (multipara) + 1 hour if epidural	**Second-stage arrest:** • Failure to deliver within 2 hours (nullipara) or 1 hour (multipara) • Add additional 1 hour if epidural Cause: abnormalities with passenger, pelvis, or power **Management:** • Fetal head is not engaged → cesarean • Fetal head is engaged → trial of obstetric forceps or vacuum extraction
Stage 3— Expulsion	Begins: delivery of baby Ends: delivery of placenta Delivery of placenta	<30 minutes	**Prolonged third stage:** • Failure to deliver placenta within 30 minutes Cause: consider placenta accreta/increta/percreta **Management:** • IV oxytocin • If oxytocin fails, attempt manual removal • Hysterectomy may be needed

An adequate uterine contraction:

- Occurs every 2–3 minutes
- Lasts 45–60 seconds
- At least 200 Montevideo units total intensity within 10 minutes

Umbilical Cord Prolapse

An obstetric emergency because a compressed cord has jeopardized fetal oxygenation, cord prolapse most often occurs with rupture of membranes before the head is engaged in breech or transverse lie. A fetal heart rate (FHR) rate that suggests hypoxemia (e.g., severe bradycardia, severe variable decelerations) may be the only clue. Clinically, the practitioner may palpate a pulsatile umbilical cord in the vagina.

Treatment is as follows.

- *Never* attempt to replace the cord.
- Place the patient in knee-chest position, elevate the presenting part, and give **terbutaline** to decrease force of contractions.
- Perform **immediate cesarean delivery.**

> **Basic Science Correlate**
>
> Terbutaline is a beta-adrenergic agonist that causes myometrial relaxation. It binds to the beta-2 receptors, increasing intracellular adenylyl cyclase.

Evaluating Fetal Heart Rate (FHR) Tracings

Baseline heart rate is the mean FHR during a 10-minute segment of time, excluding periodic changes. Changes in fetal heart rate and normal periodic changes of FHR are related to the following:

- Uterine hyperstimulation (commonly caused by medications)
- Fetal head compression
- Umbilical cord compression
- Placental insufficiency

Normal baseline FHR = 110–160 beats/minute.

- **Tachycardia** (>160 beats/minute) is most commonly related to medications (β-agonist: terbutaline, ritodrine).
- **Bradycardia** (<110 beats/minute) is most commonly related to medications (β-blockers or local anesthetics).

Periodic changes in heart rate include the following:

- Accelerations: Abrupt increases in FHR lasting <2 minutes that are unrelated to contractions. They always occur in response to fetal movements and are always reassuring.
- **Early decelerations:** Gradual decreases in FHR beginning and ending simultaneously with contractions. They occur in response to **fetal head compression.**

Reassuring FHR tracing:
- Baseline FHR 110–160 beats/minute
- (+) Accelerations
- (–) Decelerations
- (+) Beat-to-beat variability

Nonreassuring FHR tracing:
- Baseline FHR shows tachycardia or bradycardia
- (–) Accelerations
- (+) Variable or late decelerations
- (–) Beat-to-beat variability

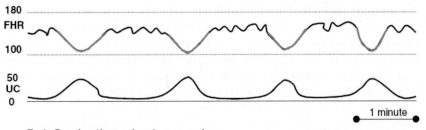

Early Decelerations – head compression

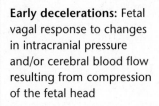

Early decelerations: Fetal vagal response to changes in intracranial pressure and/or cerebral blood flow resulting from compression of the fetal head

- **Variable decelerations:** Abrupt decreases in FHR that are unrelated to contractions. These are related to umbilical cord compression. Recurrent variable decelerations with minimal or no variability and no accelerations are nonreassuring and indicate **fetal acidosis.**

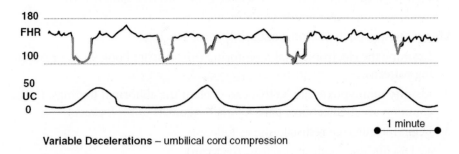

Variable Decelerations – umbilical cord compression

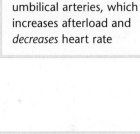

Variable decelerations: Thin-walled umbilical vein is compressed, decreasing venous return, and heart rate increases; further compression then occludes umbilical arteries, which increases afterload and *decreases* heart rate

- **Late decelerations** are *gradual* decreases in FHR that are *delayed* in relation to contractions. These are related to **uteroplacental insufficiency.** All late decelerations are nonreassuring and indicate **fetal acidosis.**

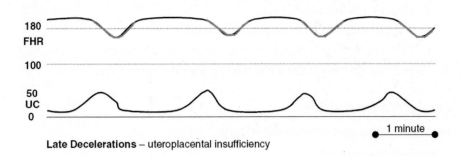

Late Decelerations – uteroplacental insufficiency

Late decelerations: Decreased placental perfusion leads to fetal hypoxemia, activating chemoreceptors to cause vasoconstriction; baroreceptors then sense this increased afterload, leading to parasympathetic reflex and drop in heart rate

- **Variability:** Beat-to-beat fetal heart rate normally has variability. Normal variability is 6–25 beats/minute. **Absence of variability** is a nonreassuring pattern.

A 31-year-old primigravida at term is in the maternity unit in active labor. She is 6 cm dilated, 100% effaced 0 station, with the fetus in cephalad position. IV oxytocin is being administered because of arrest of cervical dilation at 6 cm. Fetal membranes are intact. The nurse informs you that the external fetal monitor tracing now shows the fetal heart rate baseline at 175 beats/min with minimal variability and repetitive late decelerations. There is no vaginal bleeding. What is the most appropriate next step in management?

a. Change maternal position.
b. Discontinue oxytocin.
c. Immediate cesarean section.
d. Perform obstetric ultrasound.
e. Obtain fetal scalp pH.

Answer: **B.** Medications are a common cause of baseline fetal tachycardia or bradycardia. For management of nonreassuring fetal tracing, use a stepwise approach.

Stepwise Approach to Nonreassuring Fetal Tracings

1. Examine the electronic fetal monitoring (EFM) strip: Look for nonreassuring patterns.
2. Identify nonhypoxic causes that can explain the abnormal findings. (Most common are medications, particularly β-agonists or β-blockers.)
3. Begin intrauterine resuscitation as follows:
   a. Discontinue medications (e.g., oxytocin).
   b. Change patient's position (left lateral). This will remove pressure from the gravid uterus on the maternal inferior vena cava, improving maternal blood flow and subsequent placental blood flow.
   c. Provide high-flow oxygen.
   d. Give IV normal saline bolus.
   e. Vaginal exam to rule out prolapsed cord.
   f. Perform fetal scalp stimulation to observe for accelerations (reassuring).
4. Prepare for delivery if the EFM tracing does not normalize.

Operative Obstetrics

Forceps- or Vacuum-Assisted Delivery

When is it the answer?

- Prolonged second stage (most common indication)
- Nonreassuring EFM strip in absence of contraindications
- To avoid maternal pushing when mother has cardiac and/or pulmonary conditions that would increase her risk.

When is it *not* the answer?

- Mother has small pelvis
- Cervix is not fully dilated
- Membranes have not ruptured
- Fetal head is not engaged
- Orientation of the head is not certain

Cesarean Delivery

- Risks include the following: Increased risk of hemorrhage, infection, visceral injury (bladder, bowel, ureters), and DVTs.
- Low segment transverse incision: This is the most common procedure. It can only be performed with longitudinal lie of the fetus.
- Classic vertical incision: Can be performed with any fetal lie. Because of the increased risk of uterine rupture in subsequent pregnancies, cesarean must be initiated before labor begins.

When is it the answer?

- Cephalopelvic disproportion (CPD): With failure of progression or arrest in labor
- Fetal malpresentation
- Nonreassuring EFM strip
- Placenta previa
- Infection: Mother who is HIV-positive with a viral load >1,000 or has active vaginal herpes
- Uterine scar: Prior myomectomy (fibroid) or prior classic incision C-section

Trial of vaginal birth after cesarean (VBAC) should be attempted in patients in the absence of C-section indications when the previous cesarean was a low segment uterine incision.

Abnormal Fetal Lies

Breech

Breech presentation means the baby's buttock is the part closest to the vaginal canal. There are 3 types of breech presentation:

- **Frank breech:** The fetus has both hips flexed and knees extended so that the feet are near the fetal head.
- **Complete breech:** The fetus has both hips and knees flexed.
- **Incomplete breech:** The fetus has one or both hips not flexed.

Incidence of breech presentation decreases with gestational age. Early in pregnancy, the fetus is highly mobile and turns often. With increasing gestational age and size, there is less room for movement and less turning happens. However, some fetuses remain in the breech presentation.

Risk factors:

- Previous breech
- Uterine abnormalities
- Placental abnormalities
- Short umbilical cord
- Multiparity
- Multiple gestation

External cephalic version (ECV) is done to change a baby from breech or other non-cephalic presentation to the cephalic position. The physician pushes on the baby through the mother's abdomen to attempt to roll the baby into position.

Atony = *a tony*, or without tone.

Diagnosis of breech fetal lie is made on ultrasound.

Treatment can include C-section delivery or a trial of external cephalic version (moving the fetus to head-down position). If external cephalic version is successful, a trial of labor and vaginal delivery is possible. A vaginal breech delivery will be the wrong answer on the test.

External Cephalic Version

When is it the answer?

- Is first attempted in patients with transverse lie or breech presentation.
- The optimum time for external version is 37 weeks' gestation, and success rates are 50–60%.

Postpartum Hemorrhage

Postpartum hemorrhage is the **most common cause of maternal death worldwide**.

- Uterine atony is the most common cause of excessive postpartum bleeding worldwide. Consider in rapid or protracted labor, chorioamnionitis, medications ($MgSO_4$, halothane), and overdistended uterus. Manage with uterine massage and uterotonic agents (e.g., oxytocin, methylergonovine, or carboprost).

> **Basic Science Correlate**
>
> **Carboprost** is a prostaglandin F2 alpha analog that causes myometrial contractions. Increasing contractions causes the blood vessels to get squeezed and decreases bleeding. Hypertension is a contraindication to its use.
>
> **Misoprostol** is a prostaglandin E1 analog that also induces contractions, and can be given in hypertension.
>
> **Methylergonovine** causes vasospasm, and is contraindicated in hypertension or scleroderma patients.

- Lacerations: Management involves surgical repair.
- Retained placenta is associated with accessory placental lobe or abnormal uterine invasion. Suspect this with any missing placental cotyledons. Manage through manual removal or uterine curettage under ultrasound guidance. Placenta accreta/increta/percreta is the diagnosis when the examination shows placental villi infiltration. Placental villi may be infiltrated to the deeper layers of the endometrium (accreta), myometrium (increta), or serosa (percreta). Hysterectomy may be needed to control the bleeding.

- DIC is most commonly related to abruptio placenta. It is also associated with severe preeclampsia, amniotic fluid embolism, or prolonged retention of a dead fetus. Suspect DIC when there is generalized oozing or bleeding from IV or laceration sites in the presence of a contracted uterus.
- **Uterine inversion:** Suspect this when there is a beefy-appearing bleeding mass in the vagina and failure to palpate the uterus. Management involves uterine replacement, followed by IV oxytocin.

Postpartum Contraception

Breastfeeding is not reliable as a form of contraception. Patients should use another form. An intrauterine device (IUD) can be offered to all women immediately postpartum to improve compliance and efficacy. Most of those women will not experience expulsion.

- Combined estrogen-progestin formulations (e.g., pills, patch, vaginal ring): Reserved until 3 weeks postpartum to prevent hypercoagulable state and risk of DVT. Not used in breastfeeding women because of diminished lactation.
- Progestin contraception (e.g., mini-pill, Depo-Provera, Implanon) can safely be used during breastfeeding. They can be begun immediately after delivery. Progestin is the only contraception that can be used while breast-feeding. It works by thickening cervical mucus and thinning endometria.

> **Basic Science Correlate**
>
> Combined hormone contraception decreases secretion of FSH and LH by inhibiting midcycle secretion of gonadotropin (GnRH). FSH promotes follicular development; LH surge causes ovulation. Absence of these hormones suppresses ovulation.

Postpartum Fever

Postpartum Day	Diagnosis	Risk Factors	Clinical Findings	Management
0	Atelectasis	General anesthesia with incisional pain Cigarette smoking	Mild fever with rales Patient is unable to take deep breaths	Incentive spirometry and ambulation Chest x-rays are unnecessary
1	UTI	Multiple catheterizations and vaginal exams	High fever, CVA tenderness, (+) urinalysis, (+) urine culture (suspect pyelonephritis)	Single-agent intravenous antibiotics
2–3	Endometritis	C-section, prolonged rupture of membranes, multiple vaginal exams	Moderate-to-high fever, uterine tenderness, (−) peritoneal signs	Multiple-agent IV antibiotics (e.g., gentamycin and ampicillin); add clindamycin if C-section
4–5	Wound infection	Emergency C-section after PROM	Persistent spiking fever despite antibiotics Wound erythema, fluctuance, or drainage	IV antibiotics Wet-to-dry wound packing Closure by secondary intention
5–6	Septic thrombophlebitis	Prolonged labor	Persistent wide fever swings despite broad-spectrum antibiotics	IV heparin for 7–10 days
7–21	Infectious mastitis	Nipple trauma and cracking	Unilateral breast tenderness, erythema, and edema*	PO nafcillin Breastfeeding should be continued

*These symptoms, in the absence of fever, describe breast engorgement, which does not require antibiotics.

Postpartum Depression

Brexanolone, an analogue of allopregnanolone, is a newly approved treatment for postpartum depression. Patients see relief within 48 hours.

Diagnostic criteria are the same as for the general population; however, symptoms and onset occur during pregnancy or within the postpartum period, up to 12 months after delivery. All women should be screened for postpartum depression at the postpartum visit using the Edinburgh Postnatal Depression Scale. First-line treatment is psychotherapy, followed by the addition of SSRIs.

Breastfeeding

Breastfeeding is recommended as the exclusive feeding modality for infants' first 6 months of life and a continuing source of nutrition after solid foods are introduced. Infants who are exclusively breastfed should also receive vitamin D supplementation.

Besides promoting bonding between mother and baby, breastfeeding generates many benefits not only to the infant, but also to the mother.

	Benefits to Breastfeeding	**Contraindications to Breastfeeding**
Infant	Improved GI function	Galactosemia
	Increased immunity (passive transfer of T-cell immunity)	
	Prevention of acute illness	
	Decreased necrotizing enterocolitis in preemies	
	Decreased risk of obesity	
	Decreased risk of cancer, adult heart disease, diabetes, allergies	
	Increased IQ	
Mother	Faster recovery from childbirth, increased maternal-infant bonding	Infection: HIV, active TB, HTLV-1, herpes simplex (if lesion on breast)
	Lower incidence of stress	Drugs of abuse (except cigarettes, alcohol)
	Increased weight loss	Cytotoxic medication (e.g., methotrexate, cyclosporine)
	Prolonged postpartum anovulation (although not a reliable form of contraception)	Acute maternal disease if absent in infant (e.g., TB, sepsis)
	Decreased risk of breast cancer, ovarian cancer, type 2 diabetes	
	Economic benefits	

Note: Breastfeeding is not contraindicated in mastitis.

PART 8

Gynecology

Contributing author Victoria Hastings, DO, MPH, MS

The Breast

Nipple Discharge

Nipple discharge is a common occurrence in women and can be secondary to a variety of causes:

- Breastfeeding
  - The normal secretions of the breast are milk and colostrum.
  - Lactation occurs after delivery, and milk production can continue for 6 months after breastfeeding has stopped.
- Galactorrhea
  - This physiologic, milk-like bilateral nipple discharge is unrelated to pregnancy and breastfeeding.
  - It is caused by hyperprolactinemia.
- Medications
  - Haloperidol, risperidone, metoclopramide, and SSRIs can cause nipple discharge (commonly tested on Step 3).
- Neurogenic etiology from chronic stimulation (e.g., poor-fitting clothes)
- Malignant tumors of the breast

Diagnosis always starts with a good history and physical exam. Note the consistency of the discharge and whether it is unilateral or bilateral, to help direct the diagnostic testing.

Bilateral and multiduct discharge evaluation always begins with labs:

- TSH
- Pregnancy test
- Prolactin level
- CMP (for renal function)

> Surgical duct excision is never the answer for bilateral, milky nipple discharge. Do a workup for prolactinoma.

Treatment is as follows.

- **Unilateral/uniductal** discharge
  - Breast imaging (mammogram and ultrasound)
  - Unilateral discharge is more likely than bilateral to indicate underlying breast pathology
  - Surgical evaluation and ductal excision with biopsy (**best diagnostic tests**)
- **Bilateral** discharge
  - If prolactin levels are elevated, MRI of the brain (**best diagnostic test**)
  - Other symptoms of a prolactinoma often accompany nipple discharge: menstrual irregularities; headaches; bitemporal hemianopia (pathognomonic); and infertility

A 30-year-old woman complains of bilateral breast enlargement and tenderness, which fluctuates with her menstrual cycle. On physical examination the breast feels lumpy, and there is a painful, discrete 1.5-cm nodule. A fine-needle aspiration draws clear liquid and the cyst collapses with aspiration. Which of the following is the next step in management?

a. Clinical breast exam in 6 weeks
b. Core needle biopsy
c. Mammography
d. Repeat FNA in 6 weeks
e. Ultrasound in 6 weeks

Answer: **A.** Clinical breast exam in 6 weeks is appropriate follow-up for a cystic mass that disappears after FNA. If the mass recurs on the 6-week follow-up, FNA may be repeated, and a core biopsy can be performed.

Breast Mass

Benign Breast Disease	Malignant Breast Disease (i.e., Breast Cancer)
• Fibroadenoma	• Ductal carcinoma in situ
• Fibrocystic disease	• Lobular carcinoma in situ
• Intraductal papilloma	• Invasive ductal carcinoma
• Fat necrosis (think of this with trauma to the breast)	• Invasive lobular carcinoma
• Mastitis (inflamed, painful breast in women who are breastfeeding)	• Inflammatory breast cancer
	• Paget disease of the breast/nipple

Fibrocystic disease classically presents age 20–50 with cyclical, bilateral painful breast lump(s). Pain varies with the menstrual cycle (**clue to diagnosis**).

- A simple cyst will have sharp margins and posterior acoustic enhancement on ultrasound.
- It will collapse on FNA.

Fibroadenoma classically presents as a discrete, firm, nontender, and highly mobile breast nodule (**clue to diagnosis**). Fibroadenoma is made up of stromal and epithelial cells.

Diagnostic testing of any breast mass (including those found during pregnancy) includes:

- Clinical breast exam (never diagnose based on this alone; always do further testing)
- Ultrasound or diagnostic mammography
- FNA biopsy

For fibrocystic disease, treatment is oral contraceptive pills (OCPs), with danazol for severe pain. For fibroadenoma, no treatment is necessary, but consider surgical removal if the mass is growing.

When is the **ultrasound** the correct answer?

- First step in workup of a palpable mass that feels cystic on exam
- Imaging test for younger women with dense breasts

When is **mammography and biopsy** the correct answer?

- Cyst recurs >2× within 4–6 weeks
- Bloody fluid on aspiration
- Mass does not disappear completely upon FNA
- Bloody nipple discharge (excisional biopsy)
- Skin edema and erythema that are suggestive of inflammatory breast carcinoma (excisional biopsy)

When is **FNA or core biopsy** the correct answer?

- A palpable mass

When is **cytology** the correct answer?

- Any aspirate that is grossly bloody

When is **observation with repeat exam in 6–8 weeks** the correct answer?

- Cyst disappears on aspiration and the fluid is clear
- Needle biopsy and imaging studies are negative

> Do mammogram before biopsy. Biopsy distorts radiography.

> Core biopsy is superior to FNA. It offers more detailed histologic diagnosis and avoids inadequate samples.

A 47-year-old woman completes her annual mammogram and is asked to return for evaluation. The mammogram reveals a "cluster" of microcalcifications in the left breast. What is the next step in management?

a. Excision biopsy
b. Core needle biopsy
c. Repeat screening mammogram in 6 months
d. Repeat screening mammogram in 12 months
e. Ultrasound

Answer: **B.** Microcalcification clusters are most commonly benign; however, 15–20% represent early cancer. The next step in workup is core needle biopsy under mammographic guidance. An excisional biopsy runs the risk of taking too much tissue in the event that mammography findings were benign. Ultrasound would not add to the diagnosis, as abnormal radiologic findings are already detected on mammography. Repeat imaging after short time intervals is not appropriate, as a potential cancer diagnosis could be missed.

Breast Cancer

Preinvasive Disease

Both ductal carcinoma in situ (DCIS) and lobular carcinoma in situ (LCIS) increase the risk of invasive disease.

- If biopsy reveals **DCIS**, do surgical resection with clear margins (lumpectomy; i.e., breast conserving surgical resection) and radiation plus tamoxifen for 5 years to prevent the development of invasive disease
  - For postmenopausal women, replace tamoxifen with an aromatase inhibitor such as anastrozole
  - For women >age 35 who have 2 first-degree relatives with breast cancer, anastrazole can be used as primary prevention
- If biopsy reveals **LCIS,** give tamoxifen for 5 years; alternatively, surveillance without medical intervention
  - Classically seen in premenopausal women
  - Has low malignancy potential and is considered a small risk factor rather than a precursor

> **Tamoxifen**
> - Risks: endometrial carcinoma, thromboembolism
> - Contraindications: patient is active smoker, had previous thromboembolism, or is at high risk for thromboembolism

---

Basic Science Correlate

Tamoxifen is an estrogen receptor antagonist in the breast tissue. It acts as an endometrial agonist.

- Agonist drugs bind to and activate a receptor. Agonists cause an action.
- Antagonists are drugs with high affinity (bind to receptors well) but no efficacy (do not make the receptors work). Antagonists block an action.

Invasive Breast Disease

- Invasive ductal carcinoma (most common form of breast cancer, 85%) is unilateral. It metastasizes to bone, liver, and brain.
- Invasive lobular carcinoma (10% of breast cancers) tends to be multifocal (within the same breast), and 20% are bilateral.
- Inflammatory breast cancer (uncommon) grows rapidly and metastasizes early. Look for a red, swollen, and warm breast and pitted, edematous skin (classic *peau d'orange* appearance).
- Paget disease of the breast/nipple presents with a pruritic, erythematous, scaly nipple lesion. It is often confused with dermatosis-like eczema or psoriasis. Look for an inverted nipple or discharge.

Established risk factors for breast cancer include:

- Age ≥50
- Familial BRCA1/BRCA2 mutation carrier
- Exposure to ionizing radiation
- First childbirth age >30 or nulliparity

- History of breast cancer
- History of breast cancer in a first-degree relative
- Hormone therapy
- Obesity (BMI $\geq$30 kg per m^2)

When are **BRCA1 and BRCA2 gene testing** indicated?

- Family history of early-onset (age <50) breast cancer or family history of ovarian cancer at any age
- Breast and/or ovarian cancer in the same patient
- Family history of male breast cancer
- Ashkenazi Jewish heritage

Treatment is as follows:

- Invasive carcinoma with tumor size <5 cm: lumpectomy + radiotherapy $\pm$ adjuvant therapy $\pm$ chemotherapy
- Inflammatory, tumor size >5 cm and metastatic disease: systemic therapy
- Sentinel node biopsy is preferred over axillary node dissection.
- Always test for estrogen and progesterone receptors + HER2/neu receptor protein.

Benefit is greatest when both ER+ and PR+ receptors are present. Therapy is nearly as good when there are only ER+ estrogen receptors. Adjuvant hormonal therapy has the least benefit when only PR+ receptors are present.

- Tamoxifen competitively binds estrogen receptors; 5-year treatment leads to 50% decrease in recurrence and 25% decrease in mortality; can be used in pre- or postmenopausal patients
- Aromatase inhibitors (anastrozole, exemestane, letrozole) block peripheral production of estrogen (standard of care in HR+ postmenopausal women, i.e., more effective than tamoxifen); do not cause menopausal symptoms but do increase risk of osteoporosis
- LHRH analogs (e.g., goserelin) or ovarian ablation (surgical oophorectomy or external beam RT) is an alternative or an addition to tamoxifen in premenopausal women at high risk of recurrence.

> Breast cancer screening guidelines per the U.S. Preventive Services Task Force (USPSTF):
> - **Age 50–74:** mammogram recommended every 1–2 years
> - **Age <50:** routine screening no longer recommended; screen according to high individual risk for early onset breast cancer
> - Teaching self breast exam is no longer encouraged.
> - Clinical breast exam every 1–3 years can be considered.

A 68-year-old woman visits her physician with a solid peanut-shaped hard mass in the upper outer quadrant of the left breast. A biopsy of the lesion reveals "infiltrating ductal carcinoma." What is the next step in management?

a. Lumpectomy plus radiotherapy
b. Modified radical mastectomy
c. Modified radical mastectomy plus radiotherapy
d. Neoadjuvant chemotherapy plus lumpectomy plus radiotherapy
e. Tamoxifen and radiotherapy

Answer: **A.** Breast-conserving surgical therapy (lumpectomy) plus radiotherapy is the standard of care for invasive disease. Modified radical mastectomy gives no survival benefit and is more invasive.

When is **breast-conserving therapy not the answer?**

- Pregnancy
- Prior irradiation to the breast
- Diffuse malignancy or ≥2 sites in separate quadrants
- Positive tumor margins
- Tumor >5 cm

When is **adjuvant hormonal therapy** included in management?

- In any hormone receptor-positive (HR+) tumor, regardless of age, menopausal status, stage, or type of tumor

Benefits of Tamoxifen	Adverse Effects of Tamoxifen
• Decreased incidence of contralateral breast cancer • Increased bone density in postmenopausal women • Decreased fractures • Decreased serum cholesterol • Decreased cardiovascular mortality risk	• Exacerbates menopausal symptoms • ↑↑ risk of endometrial cancer (1% in postmenopausal women after 5 yrs therapy) • ↑↑ risk of thromboembolism All women with a history of tamoxifen use and vaginal bleeding need evaluation & endometrial biopsy if uterine bleeding is present.

When is **chemotherapy** included in management?

- Tumor size >1 cm
- Lymph node-positive disease

When are **trastuzumab and pertuzumab** included in management?

- When there is metastatic breast cancer overexpressing HER2/neu

Trastuzumab is cardiotoxic.

- Trastuzumab is a monoclonal antibody directed against the extracellular domain of the HER2/neu receptor and is used to treat and control visceral metastatic sites.

For invasive breast cancer, use the following treatment guidelines:

HR-negative, pre- or postmenopausal	HR-positive, premenopausal	HR-positive, postmenopausal
Chemotherapy ± RT alone	Chemotherapy ± RT + tamoxifen	Chemotherapy ± RT + aromatase inhibitor

Uterus

Premenarchal Vaginal Bleeding

The average age at menarche is age 12. Bleeding which occurs before that time can have several causes:

- Presence of a foreign body (most common cause)
- Sarcoma botryoides (cancer of vagina or cervix suggested by a grape-like mass arising from the vaginal lining or cervix)
- Tumor of the pituitary adrenal gland or ovary
- Sexual abuse

Perform a pelvic exam under sedation. Order CT or MRI of pituitary, abdomen, and pelvis to look for estrogen-producing tumor. If the workup is negative, the diagnosis is idiopathic precocious puberty.

Abnormal Uterine Bleeding

A 31-year-old woman complains of 6 months of heavy menses with irregular menstrual bleeding. The patient states that she started menstruating at age 13 and that she has had regular menses until the past 6 months. The pelvic examination, including a Pap smear, is normal. She has no other significant personal or family history. What is the next step in management?

a. β-hCG
b. LH, FSH levels
c. Pelvic ultrasound
d. Oral contraceptive pills
e. Progestin-only pills

Answer: **A.** Irregular bleeding in reproductive age should always be evaluated first for pregnancy. If pregnancy is ruled out, workup for anatomical causes of bleeding or anovulation can be started.

Abnormal uterine bleeding (AUB) is characterized by the mnemonic PALM-COEIN.

- PALM refers to structural causes including endometrial polyp, adenomyosis, leiomyoma, malignancy, and hyperplasia.
- COEIN refers to non-structural causes including coagulopathy, ovulatory dysfunction, endometrial dysfunction, iatrogenic, and not otherwise classified.

Management of Abnormal Uterine Bleeding

History and Physical Exam
- Pattern of bleeding and any associated symptoms
- Past medical, surgical, and gynecology history
- Patient medications
- Family history of bleeding disorders and gynecologic cancers

If acute bleeding with hemodynamic instability, send patient to ED for dilation and curettage

Laboratory Evaluation
- Urine or serum bHCG
- CBC

Laboratory Evaluation

Based on results of H&P and initial lab testing.
Consider the following
- Endometrial biopsy if age >45 or risk factors for endometrial carcinoma
- Ultrasound or hysteroscopy to assess for structural abnormalities
- Pap smear, cultures for gonorrhea and chlamydia
- Additional labs: coagulation profile, TSH, prolactin, FSH, LH, estradiols

Enlarged Uterus

An enlarged uterus may be caused by pregnancy (discussed in *Obstetrics* section), leiomyoma, adenomyosis, and malignancy (typically presents with postmenopausal bleeding).

> Rule out pregnancy before considering leiomyoma or adenomyosis.

> **Basic Science Correlate**
>
> Three layers form the uterus: endometrium (inner layer), myometrium (middle layer), and perimetrium (outer layer).
>
> The myometrium is made up of smooth muscle, composed mainly of the proteins myosin and actin.

Leiomyoma

Leiomyoma (fibroids) is a common benign tumor of the uterus seen in women of reproductive age. It arises from the smooth muscle cells of the myometrium. Symptoms include heavy/prolonged menstrual bleeding, pelvic pain, and/or infertility.

Risk factors:

- African American
- Early menarche (age <10)

Diagnosis is made by physical exam, which shows an enlarged, asymmetric, nontender uterus. If physical exam is normal but symptoms are present, diagnostic testing is transvaginal ultrasound, which has high sensitivity.

There are 3 types of leiomyoma, further distinguished by their location:

- Subserosal leiomyomas develop on the outer uterine wall.
  - Pedunculated subserosal leiomyomas grow on a stalk outside uterine wall.
- Submucosal leiomyomas develop just under the uterine lining.
  - Pedunculated submucosal leiomyomas grow on a stalk into the uterus.
- Intramural leiomyomas develop inside the uterine wall (most common type).

Treatment is medical or surgical.

- Medical: OCPs and observation
- Surgical (**definitive treatment**): abnormal uterine bleeding, infertility, or recurrent miscarriages
  - Hysterectomy, endometrial ablation, and uterine artery embolization done in women who have completed childbearing
  - Myomectomy done in women who have not completed childbearing

> Hysterectomy = removal of uterus
>
> Myomectomy = removal of the myoma

> Myomectomy puts the patient at risk for uterine rupture during pregnancy.

Adenomyosis

Adenomyosis occurs when the endometrial glands and stroma are present within the myometrium. This can cause a diffusely enlarged uterus. Symptoms include dysmenorrhea and menorrhagia. On physical exam, the uterus feels enlarged, globular, soft, symmetric, and tender.

Diagnostic testing is transvaginal ultrasound which shows an enlarged uterus with cystic areas within the myometrium. Treatment is hysterectomy.

> Asymmetric and nontender uterus = Leiomyoma

> Symmetric and tender uterus = Adenomyosis

CCS Tip: The first test to order in a patient with an enlarged uterus is β-hCG.

Postmenopausal Bleeding

The most common cause of postmenopausal bleeding is vaginal or endometrial atrophy, but the most important diagnosis to rule out is endometrial carcinoma (most common gynecologic malignancy).

The most important risk factors for endometrial carcinoma are unopposed estrogen states (obesity, nulliparity, late menopause/early menarche, chronic anovulation) and a history of tamoxifen use.

- All bleeding in postmenopausal women is suspected endometrial carcinoma until proven otherwise.
- All chronic anovulation (e.g., PCOS) in reproductive age women is a high risk for endometrial carcinoma.

Give progestins to prevent endometrial hyperplasia and cancer. Never give estrogen alone to a woman with a uterus; always combine with progestins to prevent unopposed endometrial stimulation.

> A 65-year-old obese woman complains of vaginal bleeding for 3 months. Her last menstrual period was at age 52. She has no children. She has type 2 diabetes and chronic hypertension. Physical examination is normal with a normal-sized uterus and with no vulvar, vaginal, or cervical lesions. What is the next step in management?
>
> a. Progestin therapy
> b. Estrogen and progestin therapy
> c. Endometrial biopsy
> d. Pap smear and endocervical sampling
> e. Topical estrogen cream
>
> Answer: **C.** Endometrial biopsy is the first step in management of any patient with postmenopausal bleeding.

Diagnosis	Management
Pelvic Exam	If the endometrial biopsy reveals atrophy and no cancer, no further workup is needed.
	• If the endometrial biopsy reveals adenocarcinoma, do surgery staging (total abdominal hysterectomy and bilateral salpingo-oophorectomy; pelvic and para-aortic lymphadenectomy; and peritoneal washings). • If there is lymph node metastasis, >50% myometrial invasion, positive surgical margins, or poor differentiation, add radiation. • If there is metastasis, add chemotherapy.
Hysteroscopy	Identifies endometrial or cervical polyps as source of bleeding
Ultrasonography	• Measures thickness of endometrial lining. • In postmenopausal patients, endometrial lining stripe should be <4 mm thick.

Ovaries

Ovarian enlargement may be found incidentally on physical exam or may present with symptoms. The following conditions should be considered.

Simple Cyst: Physiologic Cyst (Luteal or Follicular Cyst)

Simple cyst (most common cyst during reproductive years) is asymptomatic, unless torsion has occurred (occurs with large cysts). β-hCG is negative and ultrasound shows fluid-filled simple cystic mass.

Management is transvaginal or transabdominal ultrasound to assess initial visit. If it is asymptomatic, no further follow up is necessary.

If the cyst >10 cm diameter or there has been previous steroid contraception without resolution of the cyst, use laparoscopic removal.

Complex Cyst: Benign Cystic Teratoma (Dermoid Cysts)

Complex cyst is a benign tumor. It can contain cellular tissue from all 3 germ layers. Rarely, squamous cell carcinoma can develop. β-hCG is negative and ultrasound shows a complex mass.

> Fine needle aspiration of a complex ovarian cyst is never the correct answer on the test.

Management is laparoscopic/laparotomy removal—cystectomy (to retain ovarian function) or oophorectomy (if fertility is no longer desired).

Prepubertal or Postmenopausal Ovarian Mass

Any ovarian enlargement in prepubertal or postmenopausal women is always suspicious for an ovarian neoplasm.

> The **initial workup of an ovarian mass** involves β-hCG; ultrasound; and laparoscopy/laparotomy if complex or >7 cm.

- **Risk factors** include BRCA1 gene, positive family history; high # of lifetime ovulations, and infertility.
- **Protective factors** include conditions which lower # of lifetime ovulations: OCPs, chronic anovulation, breastfeeding, and short reproductive life.

A 31-year-old woman is taken to the ED with severe, sudden lower abdominal pain that started 3 hours ago. On examination the abdomen is tender, no rebound tenderness is present, and there is an adnexal mass in the cul-de-sac area. Ultrasound evaluation shows an 8-cm left adnexal mass. β-hCG is negative. What is the next step in management?

a. Appendectomy
b. High-dose estrogen and progestin
c. Laparoscopic evaluation of ovaries
d. Observation
e. Oophorectomy

Answer: **C.** Sudden onset of severe lower abdominal pain in the presence of an adnexal mass is presumed to be ovarian torsion. Laparoscopy and detorsioning of the ovaries are needed. If blood supply is not affected, cystectomy can be done. If there is necrosis, oophorectomy is needed. She should then receive a 4-week follow-up and yearly evaluation to ensure there is complete resolution.

Ovarian masses are characterized as shown in the table.

Type of Tumor	Clinical Presentation	Tumor Marker	Facts
Germ cell tumor	• Young women • Pain in adnexa • Complex cystic mass	• LDH • β-HCG • AFP	Most common malignant type: dysgerminoma
Epithelial tumor	• Postmenopausal women • Distended abdomen, weight loss, adnexal mass/pain	• Ca-125 • CEA	• Most common ovarian cancer • Most malignant subtype: serous
Granulosa-theca cell tumor	• Postmenopausal woman • Postmenopausal bleeding • Ovarian mass	Estrogen	Secretes estrogen and causes endometrial hyperplasia
Sertoli-Leydig tumor	Woman with masculinization (deepening of voice, more hair)	Testosterone	Secretes testosterone
Krukenberg tumor	History of gastric ulcer with worsening epigastric pain	CEA	Mucin-producing adenocarcinoma from stomach but with metastasis to ovaries

Diagnostic testing includes:

• Ultrasound to confirm ovarian mass

• Bloodwork for tumor markers

• Biopsy may be needed if metastasis or ascites present; never biopsy the ovary

Treatment is as follows:

• Salpingo-oophorectomy for premenopausal women who are not done with childbearing

• Total abdominal hysterectomy with bilateral salpingo-oophorectomy for postmenopausal women/women who are done with childbearing

Cervix

As per U.S. Preventive Services Task Force recommendations, Pap screening is not needed in the following patients:

• Women age >65 with recent normal Pap

• Women who have had total hysterectomy for benign disease

Cervical Neoplasia

The following risk factors are associated with cervical neoplasia:

• Early age of intercourse

• Multiple sexual partners

• Cigarette smoking

• Immunosuppression

Basic Science Correlate

HPV is a non-enveloped DNA virus.
- **HPV 16, 18, 31, 33, and 35:** associated with cervical cancer
- **HPV 6 and 11:** benign condyloma acuminata

Pap smear classifications:

- Indeterminate smears
  - Atypical squamous cells of undetermined significance (ASCUS)
- Abnormal smears
  - Low-grade squamous intraepithelial lesion (LSIL): HPV, mild dysplasia, or CIN 1 (cervical intraepithelial neoplasia)
  - High-grade squamous intraepithelial lesion (HSIL): moderate dysplasia, severe dysplasia, CIS, CIN 2 or 3
  - Cancer: invasive cancer

When is **screening started?**

- Age 21, regardless of the onset of sexual activity

What is the **frequency of screening?**

- If **age <30** and average risk, every 3 years with cytology only
- If **age >30** and average risk, every 3 years with cytology only or every 5 years with co-testing (cytology + HPV); HPV testing alone every 5 years can also be considered

A 35-year-old woman is referred because of a Pap smear reading of ASCUS. Her last Pap, done 1 year ago, was negative. She has been sexually active for the last 4 years, using combination oral contraceptive pills. Today, 1 year later, her Pap reveals ASCUS. Which of the following is the next step in evaluation?

a. Endocervical curettage
b. Colposcopy and biopsy
c. HPV DNA typing
d. Repeat Pap smear in 6 months
e. Repeat Pap smear in 12 months

Answer: **B.** ASCUS is often found in women with inflammation due to early HPV infection. Approximately 10–15% of patients with ASCUS have premalignant or malignant disease. Two Pap smears revealing ASCUS must be followed up with colposcopy and biopsy.

Management of ASCUS is based on age and HPV infection status.

Age 21–24	Repeat cytology in 1 year
Age ≥25	• **HPV negative:** cervical cytology alone in 1 year **or** repeat cervical cytology + HPV testing in 3 years • **HPV positive:** colposcopy

Cervical cancer screening guidelines per the USPSTF:
- Pap screening not recommended for women age >65 with recent normal Pap smear
- Pap smear not recommended for women with total hysterectomy for benign disease

Workup of an Abnormal Pap		
Step in Workup	**When is this step the answer?**	**Next Step**
Repeat Pap	First ASCUS Pap with negative HPV testing	Repeat Pap in 1 year with HPV testing; if that is again ASCUS, refer for colposcopy.
HPV DNA testing	First ASCUS Pap in women age >25	• If liquid-based cytology was used on initial Pap, use specimen for DNA testing • Colposcopy is then performed only if HPV 16 and 18 identified
Colposcopy and ectocervical biopsy	• LSIL with positive HPV • HSIL • Two ASCUS Pap smears	• Colposcopy is a magnification of the cervix (10–12x) • Abnormal lesions (e.g., mosaicism, inflammatory punctuation, white lesions, abnormal vessels) are biopsied and sent for histology
Endocervical curettage (ECC)	All nonpregnant patients with Pap smear result requiring colposcopy & biopsy.	All nonpregnant patients undergoing colposcopy for an abnormal Pap smear must undergo an ECC to rule out endocervical lesions.
Cone biopsy or Loop electrosurgical excision procedure of cervix (LEEP)	• Performed after colposcopy or ECC if Pap and biopsy findings are not consistent (suggests abnormal cells were not biopsied) • Abnormal ECC histology • Biopsy showing microinvasive carcinoma of the cervix • Biopsy showing CIN II or CIN III	**NOTE:** Deep cone biopsies can result in an incompetent cervix or cervical stenosis.

Management of Abnormal Histology		
Step in management	**When is this step the answer?**	**Details**
Observation and follow-up	• CIN 1 • CIN 2 or 3 after excision	• Follow-up with repeat Pap, colposcopy + Pap smear, or HPV DNA testing every 6 months for 2 years
Ablative modalities	• CIN 2 or 3 when patient does not want excisional procedure	• Cryotherapy • Laser vaporization • Electrofulguration
Excisional procedures	• CIN 2 or 3 • Superior to ablative modalities	• LEEP • Cold-knife conization
Hysterectomy	• Biopsy-confirmed if less than stage II • Recurrent CIN 2 or 3	

Invasive Cervical Cancer

The average age of diagnosis is age 45. Diagnostic testing is cervical biopsy (most common diagnosis is squamous cell carcinoma).

The next best step in evaluation is metastatic workup: pelvic exam, cystoscopy, and proctoscopy.

Treatment is simple hysterectomy or modified radical hysterectomy if less than stage II. Adjuvant therapy (radiation therapy and chemotherapy) is given when any of the following conditions is present:

- Metastasis to lymph nodes
- Tumor size >4 cm
- Poorly differentiated lesions
- Positive margins
- Local recurrence

Cervical Neoplasia

A 25-year-old woman with a 15-week pregnancy by dates is found to have HGSIL (high-grade squamous intraepithelial lesion) on a recent Pap smear. On pelvic examination there is a gravid uterus consistent with 15 weeks' size, and the cervix is grossly normal to visual inspection. What is the next step in management?

a. Colposcopy and biopsy
b. Cone biopsy
c. Endocervical curettage
d. Hysterectomy
e. Repeat Pap after pregnancy

Answer: **A.** A pregnant woman with abnormal Pap smear is managed in the same way as a nonpregnant woman, with the exception of endocervical curettage which is never performed in pregnancy. An abnormal Pap is evaluated with colposcopy and biopsy. Pregnancy does not predispose to abnormal cytology and does not accelerate precancerous lesion progression into invasive carcinoma.

To prevent cervical dysplasia with vaccination, give quadrivalent HPV recombinant vaccine (Gardasil) to all males and females age 9–45. It protects against the HPV types (6, 11, 16, 18) that cause 70% of cervical cancer and 90% of genital warts. It is not necessary to test for HPV before administering the vaccine.

- The vaccine is especially recommended in immunocompromised populations, as they are at particularly high risk of developing cervical cancer.
- Sexually active women can receive the vaccine, but pregnant women should not.
- Women with previous abnormal cervical cytology, genital warts, or CIN can receive the vaccine, but benefits are limited.

Management of Abnormal Histology During Pregnancy	
Stage	**Management**
CIN/dysplasia	• Repeat Pap and colposcopy 6–8 weeks postpartum; persistent lesions are treated definitively postpartum
Microinvasive cervical cancer	• Cone biopsy to ensure no frank invasion (only performed during pregnancy if finding of invasive cancer will alter timing of delivery) • Deliver vaginally, reevaluate and treat 2 months postpartum
Invasive cancer	**Diagnosed before 24 weeks:** • Definitive treatment (radical hysterectomy or radiation therapy) **Diagnosed after 24 weeks:** • Conservative management up to 32–33 weeks • Cesarean delivery and begin definite treatment

Vaginitis

Women with vaginitis will complain of abnormal vaginal discharge, pruritus, burning, and irritation. It is typically caused by *Candida albicans*, *Gardnerella vaginalis, or Trichomonas vaginalis.*

Diagnosis and Treatment of Vaginitis			
Causative organism	**Clinical symptoms**	**Diagnosis**	**Treatment**
Candidiasis	Clumpy white vaginal discharge	Wet mount shows pseudohyphae	Fluconazole
Bacterial vaginosis	Fishy odor	Wet mount shows "clue cells" (epithelial cells studded with adherent coccobacilli)	Metronidazole
Trichomoniasis	• Strawberry cervix, gray discharge • Sexually transmitted	Wet mount shows motile trichomonads	Metronidazole for patient and partner

Pelvic Pain

The main differentials for a woman with pelvic pain are cervicitis, acute salpingo-oophoritis, chronic PID, and tuboovarian abscess.

The initial workup for pelvic pain:

1. Pelvic exam
2. Cervical culture
3. Laboratory: ESR (sedimentation rate), WBC (include blood culture if fever is present)
4. Sonogram

Dysmenorrhea

- **Primary dysmenorrhea** is the diagnosis when the case describes recurrent, crampy lower abdominal pain along with nausea, vomiting, and diarrhea during menstruation. Symptoms begin 2–5 days after onset of menstruation (ovulatory cycles). There is no pelvic abnormality.
    - Symptoms are related to excessive endometrial prostaglandin F2, which causes uterine contractions and acts on GI smooth muscle.
    - Treatment is NSAIDs or combination OCPs.
- **Secondary dysmenorrhea** has similar symptoms but is caused by another disorder. Most commonly, the cause is endometriosis but another pathology (adenomyosis, leiomyoma) could be responsible.

Cervicitis

This is the diagnosis when cervical discharge is found on routine exam, usually without other symptoms. Get cervical cultures (for chlamydia and gonorrhea).

Treatment is as follows:

- Those with gonorrhea should be treated for both gonorrhea and chlamydia (oral azithromycin and IM ceftriaxone).
- Those with chlamydia should be treated with azithromycin or doxycycline alone.

> - Antibiotics that treat gonorrhea:
>   - Ceftriaxone IM
> - Antibiotics that treat chlamydia:
>   - Azithromycin PO
>   - Doxycycline PO

Acute Salpingo-oophoritis

This is suspected when there is cervical motion tenderness on exam and the patient complains of lower pelvic pain unrelated to menstruation.

Diagnostic testing:

- Cervical cultures
- WBC and ESR (elevated)
- Sonogram to rule out pelvic abscess

Treatment is one dose of IM ceftriaxone + azithromycin for outpatients, and IV cefotetan or cefoxitin + doxycycline for inpatients.

Chronic Pelvic Inflammatory Disease (PID)

Chronic PID classically presents with infertility or dyspareunia. The patient may also have a history of ectopic pregnancy or abnormal vaginal bleeding.

- Cervical culture and lab tests will be negative.
- Sonogram may show bilateral cystic pelvic masses (hydrosalpinges).

Treatment is lysis of tubal adhesions, which may be helpful for infertility. For severe, unremitting pelvic pain, a pelvic clean-out (TAH, BSO) may be needed.

> PID is a risk for ectopic pregnancy because the cilia within the fallopian tubes that normally help move the egg from ovary to uterus become damaged secondary to infection.

Tubo-ovarian abscess is an advanced form of PID, diagnosed when the case describes an ill-appearing woman with severe, lower abdominal/pelvic pain, back pain, and rectal pain, with systemic signs and symptoms (nausea, vomiting, fever, tachycardia).

- WBC and ESR are markedly elevated.
- There is pus on culdocentesis.
- Sonogram shows a unilateral pelvic mass that appears as a multilocular, cystic, complex adnexal mass.
- Blood cultures will grow anaerobic organisms.

Treatment is cefoxitin and doxycycline, with hospital admission. If no response within 72 hours or there is abscess rupture, perform an exploratory laparotomy ± salpingooophorectomy or percutaneous drainage.

When are outpatient antibiotics the answer?

- All cases of cervicitis
- Acute salpingo-oophoritis when there is no systemic infection or pelvic abscess

When are inpatient antibiotics the answer?

- Previous outpatient treatment failure, presence of fever, or pelvic abscess
- All cases of tubo-ovarian abscess

Endometriosis

Endometriosis involves endometrial glands outside the uterus. It classically presents in women age >30 with dysmenorrhea, dyspareunia, dyschezia (painful bowel movements), and infertility.

- The ovary is the most common site, causing adnexal enlargements (endometriomas), also known as a chocolate cyst.
- The cul-de-sac is the second most common site, causing uterosacral ligament nodularity and tenderness on rectovaginal examination. This location is associated with bowel adhesions and a fixed, retroverted uterus.
- Investigations: CA-125 may be elevated. Sonogram may show endometriomas. Definitive diagnosis is made with laparoscopic visualization.

> Don't be fooled! Not all elevations of CA-125 are due to ovarian cancer. It is also elevated in:
> - Cirrhosis
> - Endometriosis
> - Peritonitis
> - Pancreatitis

Treatment is as follows:

- Continuous oral progesterone or OCPs (first-line); progesterone inhibits endometrial growth
- Second-line: testosterone derivatives (danazol) or GnRH analogs (leuprolide)
- Laparoscopic lysis adhesions: laser vaporization of lesions can improve fertility
- TAH and BSO for severe symptoms when fertility is not desired

Vaginal Bleeding and Its Absence

Primary Amenorrhea

Primary amenorrhea is diagnosed with absence of menses at age 14 without secondary sexual development or at age 16 with secondary sexual development.

Diagnostic testing includes:

- Physical exam and ultrasound
  - Are breasts present or absent? Breasts indicate adequate estrogen production.
  - Is a uterus present or absent on ultrasound?
- Karyotype, testosterone, FSH

	Uterus Present	Uterus Absent

Breasts Present	**Work up as secondary amenorrhea**
	• Imperforate hymen
	• Vaginal septum
	• Anorexia nervosa
	• Excessive exercise
	• Pregnancy before the first menses
		Order testosterone levels and karyotype
		• Müllerian agenesis
		  - *XX karyotype, normal testosterone for female*
		• Complete androgen insensitivity (testicular feminization)
		  - *XY karyotype, normal testosterone for male*

Breasts Absent	**Order FSH level and karyotype**
	• Gonadal dysgenesis (Turner syndrome)
	  - *X0 karyotype, FSH elevated*
	• Hypothalamic–pituitary failure
	  - *XX karyotype, FSH low*
		Rare
		Not clinically relevant

A 17-year-old girl is brought to the clinic by her concerned mother because she has never had a menstrual period. The mother reports that her daughter has good grades and studies hard, but seems stressed most of the time which is why she believes her period was delayed. On examination the girl seems to be well-nourished, with adult breast development and pubic hair present. Pelvic examination reveals a foreshortened vagina. No uterus is seen on ultrasound. What is the most appropriate next step?

a. CT scan of the brain to evaluate a pituitary tumor

b. Estrogen and progesterone supplementation

c. Consider in vitro fertilization for future fertility

d. Surgical removal of intra-abdominal testes

e. Vaginal reconstruction

Answer: **E.** This patient has Müllerian agenesis resulting in an absence of uterus, cervix, and upper vagina. Ovaries are intact and estrogen levels are normal. Vaginal reconstruction may be performed to elongate the vagina for satisfactory sexual intercourse.

- Müllerian agenesis: karyotype reveals normal female secondary sexual characteristics and normal estrogen and testosterone levels (ovaries are intact)
    - Only abnormality is absence of all Müllerian duct derivatives (fallopian tubes, uterus, cervix, and upper vagina)
    - Treatment is surgical elongation of the vagina for satisfactory sexual intercourse and counseling about infertility
- Androgen insensitivity: there is no pubic or axillary hair, a karyotype reveals male genotype, and ultrasound reveals testes.
    - The testes produce both normal levels of estrogen for a female and normal levels of testosterone for a male.
    - Treatment is removal of testes before age 20 because of increased risk of testicular cancer; estrogen replacement will then be needed
- Gonadal dysgenesis (Turner Syndrome, XO): karyotyping reveals absence of one X chromosome (45, X), absence of secondary sexual characteristics, and elevated FSH.
    - Because the second X chromosome is essential to the development of normal ovarian follicles, streak gonads develop
    - Treatment is estrogen and progesterone replacement for development of secondary sexual characteristics
- Hypothalamic-pituitary failure: there are no sexual characteristics but uterus is normal on ultrasound and FSH level is low.
    - May be caused by stress, excessive exercise, or anorexia nervosa.
    - Kallmann syndrome is likely diagnosis when anosmia is also described (i.e., hypothalamus doesn't produce GnRH)
    - CNS imaging (CT head) will rule out a brain tumor
    - Treatment is estrogen and progesterone replacement for development of secondary sexual characteristics

> Turner syndrome classically presents with widely spaced nipples, absent breast development, and webbed neck.

Secondary Amenorrhea

This is diagnosed when one of the following conditions presents:

- Regular menses are replaced by an **absence of menses for 3 months.**
- Irregular menses are replaced by an **absence of menses for 6 months.**

Workup of Secondary Amenorrhea	
Steps in the Workup	**Next Step in Management**
1. Pregnancy Test (β-hCG)	
2. Thyrotropin (TSH) (rule out hypothyroidism)	An elevated TRH in primary hypothyroidism → ↑ prolactin. Treat hypothyroidism with thyroid replacement for rapid restoration of menstruation.

3. Prolactin (rule out elevation)	If elevated:
	• Review medications: antipsychotics and antidepressants have antidopamine side effect → ↑ prolactin.
	• CT or MRI of head to rule out pituitary tumor
	  - Tumor <1 cm: bromocriptine or cabergoline (dopamine agonist)
	  - Tumor >1 cm: surgery
	• If the cause of elevated prolactin is idiopathic, treat with bromocriptine.

4. Progesterone Challenge Test (PCT)	• Positive PCT: any withdrawal bleeding is diagnostic of **anovulation** - Treatment: cyclic progesterone to prevent endometrial hyperplasia; clomiphene ovulation induction if pregnancy is desired • Negative PCT: inadequate estrogen or outflow tract obstruction

5. Estrogen–Progesterone Challenge Test (EPCT)	• 3 weeks of oral estrogen followed by 1 week of progesterone
	• Positive EPCT: any withdrawal bleeding is diagnostic of **inadequate estrogen**; next step is to get FSH level
	  - ↑ FSH is ovarian failure. Y chromosome mosaicism may be the cause if patient age <25. Order a **karyotype** for confirmation.
	  - ↓ FSH is hypothalamic–pituitary insufficiency. Order **brain CT/MRI** to rule out a tumor. Give estrogen-replacement therapy to prevent osteoporosis and cyclic progestins to prevent endometrial hyperplasia.
	• Negative EPCT: diagnostic of an outflow tract obstruction or endometrial scarring (e.g., Asherman). Order a **hysterosalpingogram** to identify the lesion. Management: Adhesion lysis followed by estrogen stimulation of the endometrium. An inflatable stent prevents re-adhesion of the uterine walls.

Premenstrual Syndrome

Premenstrual tension is distressing physical, psychological, and behavioral symptoms recurring at the same phase of the menstrual cycle and disappearing during the remainder of the cycle.

Premenstrual dysphoric disorder (PMDD) is more severe, involving major disruption to daily functioning and relationships.

Treatment is SSRIs, which increase extracellular serotonin by blocking the presynaptic receptor. Blocking this receptor leaves more serotonin in the synaptic cleft for the postsynaptic cell to pick up.

Second-line therapy is OCPs. Low doses of vitamin B6 (pyridoxine) may also improve symptoms.

Endocrine Disorders

Polycystic Ovarian Syndrome (PCOS)

Diagnose PCOS when there are 2–3 of the following:

• Gradual-onset hirsutism
• Irregular bleeding
• Polycystic ovaries

- Chronic anovulatory cycles and infertility
- Obesity
- Acne

Diagnosis is mostly clinical, but an elevated LH/FSH ratio is used for confirmation. Bilaterally enlarged ovaries may be found on exam and ultrasound.

- Anovulation → no corpus luteum production of progesterone → unopposed estrogen → hyperplastic endometrium and irregular bleeding → predisposition to endometrial cancer.
- Increased testosterone: ↑ LH levels → ↑ theca cell production of androgens → hepatic production of SHBG is suppressed → ↑ total testosterone and ↑ free testosterone
- Ovarian enlargement: Ultrasound shows a necklacelike pattern of multiple peripheral cysts (20–100 cystic follicles in each ovary). ↑ androgens → multiple follicles in various stages of development, stromal hyperplasia, and a thickened ovarian capsule → bilaterally enlarged ovaries

Diagnostic testing is as follows:

- LH:FSH ratio = 3:1 (normal is 1.5:1)
- Testosterone mildly elevated
- Pelvic ultrasound: shows bilaterally enlarged ovaries with multiple subcapsular small follicles and increased stromal echogenicity

Treatment is as follows:

- OCPs to treat irregular bleeding and hirsutism; the progestin component prevents endometrial hyperplasia
- Spironolactone to suppress hair follicles
- Anastrozole (aromatase inhibitor) for infertility (treatment of choice); clomiphene citrate may also be used
- Metformin to enhance ovulation and manage insulin-resistance

Congenital Adrenal Hyperplasia (21-Hydroxylase Deficiency)

This is the diagnosis when the question describes gradual-onset hirsutism *without* virilization in the second or third decade that is associated with menstrual irregularities and anovulation. Serum 17-hydroxyprogesterone level is markedly elevated. Precocious puberty with short stature is common. Family history may be positive.

Management is corticosteroid replacement, which will arrest the signs of androgenicity and restore ovulatory cycles.

Hirsutism

Hirsutism is excessive male-pattern hair growth in a woman. If there are other masculinizing signs as well (e.g., clitoromegaly, baldness, lowering of voice, increasing muscle mass, and loss of female body contours), that is called virilization.

Anovulation classically presents with a history of amenorrhea followed by unpredictable bleeding (prolonged unopposed estrogen stimulates the endometrium). Consider the following diagnoses:

- Polycystic ovary syndrome (PCOS)
- Hypothyroidism
- Pituitary adenoma
- Elevated prolactin
- Medications (e.g., antipsychotics, antidepressants)

Almost all cases of hirsutism are idiopathic or PCOS. More serious causes of hirsutism (androgen-secreting tumors) need to be excluded in the workup.

Initial diagnostic tests include:

- Testosterone
- DHEAS
- LH/FSH
- 17-hydroxyprogesterone

Idiopathic hirsutism (most common cause) is the diagnosis when all lab tests are normal and there is no virilization.

Treatment is spironolactone. Eflornithine is the first-line topical drug for unwanted facial/chin hair.

Diagnosis	Testosterone	DHEAS	LH/FSH	17-OHP	Next Step in Management
	Produced by ovary & adrenal gland	Produced by adrenal glands	Produced by the anterior pituitary gland	Precursor in cortisol synthesis & converted peripherally to androgens	
Polycystic ovary syndrome	↑	NL /↑	↑ LH ↓ **FSH**	NL	**Ultrasound** to rule out other disorders/tumors Screen lipids and fasting blood glucose
Congenital adrenal hyperplasia	NL/↑	NL /↑	NL/NL	↑↑	**ACTH stimulation** confirms the diagnosis

Menopause

Menopause is defined as 12 months of amenorrhea. The mean age is age 51 years (smokers experience menopause up to 2 years earlier).

FSH will be elevated; however, lab testing is unnecessary for diagnosis.

- Early menopause: menopause occurs age 40–50; most often idiopathic but can also occur after radiation therapy or surgical oophorectomy
- Premature ovarian failure: menopause occurs age <40; may be associated with autoimmune disease or Y chromosome mosaicism

The following menopausal symptoms are related to a lack of estrogen:

- Amenorrhea: menses become anovulatory and decrease in the 3-5 year period known as perimenopause
- Hot flashes (75% of women): unpredictable, profuse sweating and heat; obese women are less likely to experience hot flashes (due to peripheral conversion of androgens to estrone)

- Reproductive tract: decreased vaginal lubrication, increased vaginal pH, and increased vaginal infections
- Urinary tract: increased urgency, frequency, nocturia, and urge incontinence
- Psychic: depressed mood, emotional lability, and sleep disorders
- Cardiovascular disease: most common cause of mortality (50%) in post-menopausal women
- Osteoporosis

Treatment is as follows:

- Topical estrogen cream for vaginal atrophy and dyspareunia
- Prasterone—a dehydroepiandrosterone (DHEA) analogue with weak androgenic and weak estrogenic activity—for dyspareunia in those requiring weaker estrogen exposure

Hormone Replacement Therapy

Hormone replacement therapy (HRT) should be started only for vasomotor symptoms. Never give it to prevent cardiovascular disease.

- Use the lowest dose of HRT to treat symptoms.
- Use the shortest duration of HRT to treat symptoms; reevaluate annually.
- Do not exceed 5 years of therapy (increased risk of breast cancer after 5 years).
  - Women without a uterus can be given continuous estrogen.
  - Women with a uterus must also receive progestin therapy to prevent endometrial hyperplasia.

When is HRT the answer?	When is HRT not the answer?
Treatment of: • Menopausal vasomotor symptoms (hot flashes) • Genitourinary atrophy • Dyspareunia • When topical options fail	• Treatment of osteoporosis • When there is a history of estrogen-sensitive cancer (breast or endometrial); liver disease; active thrombosis; or unexplained vaginal bleeding

Benefits of HRT	Risks of HRT
• Reduced rate of osteoporotic fractures • Reduced rate of colorectal cancer	• Increased risk of DVT • Increased risk of heart attacks and breast cancer in combination therapy • Risk of breast cancer only associated with therapy >4 yrs

Contraception

Low-dose OCPs do not increase the risk of cancer, heart disease, or thromboembolic events in women with no associated risk factors (hypertension, diabetes, or smoking).

	Examples	Absolute Contraindication	Relative Contraindication	Benefits
Barrier methods	• Condoms • Vaginal diaphragm ± spermicides	N/A	N/A	Condoms protective against STDs
Steroid contraception	• Combination (estrogen + progesterone) • Progestin only (OCP called "mini-pill," injectable, implant, morning after pill)	• Pregnancy • Acute liver disease • Vascular disease (e.g., thromboembolism, DVT, CVA, SLE) • Hormone dependent cancer (e.g., breast CA) • Smoker age >35 • Uncontrolled hypertension • Migraines with aura • DM with vascular disease • Thrombophilia	• Migraines • Depression • DM • Chronic HTN • Hyperlipidemia	• ↓ ovarian and endometrial CA • ↓ dysmenorrhea • ↓ abnormal uterine bleeding • ↓ ectopic pregnancy
Intrauterine device	• Levonorgestrel-impregnated • Copper-banded	• Pregnancy • Pelvic malignancy • Salpingitis	• Abnormal uterine size or shape • Immune suppression (including steroid therapy) • Nulligravidity • Abnormal Pap smears • History of ectopic pregnancy	Effective and avoids side effects of hormonal therapy

Emergency contraception can be used when unprotected intercourse occurred and the patient desires pregnancy prevention.

Method	Mechanism	Timing
Copper IUD (**most effective option**)	Prevents fertilization via effect of copper ions on sperm function; prevents endometrial receptivity	Up to 5 days
Ulipristal or mifepristone	Progesterone receptor modulator; delays/inhibits ovulation	Up to 5 days
Levonorgestrel	Progesterone receptor agonist; delays/inhibits ovulation	Up to 3 days
Estrogen + progesterone	Delays/inhibits ovulation (more side effects)	Up to 5 days

Infertility

Infertility is defined as inability to achieve pregnancy after 12 months of unprotected and well-timed intercourse.

> A 35-year-old woman comes to the gynecologist's office complaining of infertility for 1 year. She and her husband have unsuccessfully been trying to achieve pregnancy for more than 1 year. There is no previous history of pelvic inflammatory disease, and she previously used oral contraceptive pills for 6 years. Pelvic examination is normal. Semen analysis is low volume and shows decreased sperm density and low motility. What is the next step in management?
>
> a. Administer testosterone
> b. Measure serum testosterone
> c. Measure thyroid hormone
> d. Repeat semen analysis
> e. Refer for intrauterine insemination
>
> Answer: **D.** Because semen samples are variable, an abnormal semen analysis is repeated in 4–6 weeks to confirm findings.

Steps in workup for infertility are as follows:

- Semen analysis (first step)
- If normal, work up for anovulation
- If semen analysis is normal and ovulation is confirmed, work up for fallopian tube abnormalities.

See the specific expanded steps below:

Step	Diagnosis	Management
1. Semen analysis	Normal values: • Volume >2 mL; pH 7.2–7.8; sperm density >20 million/mL; sperm motility >50%; and sperm morphology >50% normal	• If values abnormal, repeat semen analysis in 4–6 weeks. • **Abnormal semen analysis**: intrauterine insemination, intracytoplasmic sperm injection, and IVF are fertility options. • **No viable sperm**: artificial insemination by donor may be used.
2. Anovulation	• Basal body temperature (BBT) chart: NO midcycle temperature elevation • Progesterone: Low • Endometrial biopsy: Proliferative histology	• Hypothyroidism or hyperprolactinemia are causes of anovulation that can be treated. • Ovulation induction: clomiphene citrate (agent of choice); if that fails, use hMG; ovarian hyperstimulation is the **most common side effect**; monitor ovarian size during induction.
3. Tube abnormalities: hysterosalpingogram and laparoscopy	• Chlamydia antibody: negative IgG antibody test for chlamydia rules out infection-induced tubal adhesions.	• Hysterosalpingogram (HSG): No further testing is performed if the HSG shows normal anatomy. • Laparoscopy: Performed with an abnormal HSG to visualize the oviducts and attempt reconstruction (tuboplasty). If tubal damage is severe, IVF should be planned.

With **unexplained infertility**, the semen analysis is normal, ovulation is confirmed, and patent oviducts are noted. No treatment is indicated. About 60% of patients will go onto achieve a spontaneous pregnancy within the next 3 years.

With **in vitro fertilization**:

1. Eggs are aspirated from the ovarian follicles using an ultrasound-guided transvaginal approach.
2. They are fertilized with sperm in the laboratory, resulting in the formation of embryos.
3. Single embryo is transferred into the uterine cavity with a cumulative pregnancy rate of 55% after 4 IVF cycles.

Gestational Trophoblastic Disease

Gestational trophoblastic disease (GTD) is an abnormal proliferation of placental tissue involving both the cytotrophoblast and/or syncytiotrophoblast. It can be benign or malignant.

- Most common in Taiwan and the Philippines; other risk factors are maternal age extremes (age <20 or age >35) and folate deficiency
- Signs and symptoms often similar to preeclampsia in a woman <20 weeks pregnant
  - Fundus larger than dates, absence of fetal heart tones, bilateral cystic enlargements of ovary (theca-lutein cysts) (most common signs)
  - Bleeding <16 weeks gestation and passage of vesicles from the vagina (most common symptoms); other symptoms of a molar pregnancy include hypertension, hyperthyroidism, and hyperemesis gravidarum and no fetal heart tones appreciated
- The **most common site of distant metastasis** is the lungs.

Benign: H. Mole	
Complete	**Incomplete**
Empty egg	Normal egg
46,XX (dizygotic ploidy)	69,XXY (*triploidy*)
Fetus absent	Fetal parts present
20% → malignancy	10% → malignancy
No chemotherapy; serial β-hCG titers until (–); f/up for 1 year on OCP	

A 32-year-old Filipino woman is 15 weeks' pregnant by dates. She presents with painless vaginal bleeding associated with severe nausea and vomiting. Her uterus extends to her umbilicus but no fetal heart tones can be heard. Her blood pressure is 162/98 mm Hg. A dipstick urine shows 2+ proteinuria. Which of the following is the most likely diagnosis?

a. Chronic hypertension
b. Chronic hypertension with superimposed preeclampsia
c. Eclampsia
d. Molar pregnancy
e. Preeclampsia

Answer: **D.** This presentation is typical of a molar pregnancy. Absence of fetal heart tones eliminates the other options.

Diagnostic testing is sonogram, which reveals homogenous intrauterine echoes without a gestational sac or fetal parts ("snowstorm" ultrasound).

Treatment is as follows:

- Baseline quantitative β-hCG titer; follow serial β-hCG titers monthly until at least 6 consecutive values of zero
- Chest x-ray (rule out lung metastasis)
- Suction dilation and curettage (D&C) (to evacuate the uterine contents)
- Place patient on effective contraception (oral contraceptive pills) to ensure no confusion between rising β-hCG titers from recurrent disease and normal pregnancy

PART 9

Radiology

Choosing an Imaging Study

When is **CT** the best test?

- Noncontrast head CT is best initial test to rule out hemorrhage when trauma or acute neurological change are described
- Contrast head CT to evaluate AV malformation or primary or metastatic tumor
- Abdominal pelvic CT is best test to evaluate retroperitoneal structures: pancreatitis or pancreatic masses or nodal metastasis from colon, prostate, testicular, or renal malignancies
- High-resolution chest CT to evaluate parenchymal lung disease (interstitial fibrosis) and bony structures

When is **MRI** the best test?

- To evaluate demyelinating diseases (e.g., multiple sclerosis and some dementias)
- To evaluate the posterior fossa, base of the skull, and the orbit
- To evaluate acoustic neuromas, pituitary tumors, and small intraparenchymal brain tumors
- Test of choice for bone tumor, bone and soft tissue infection (e.g., osteomyelitis), joint space, and aseptic necrosis of femoral head
- Test of choice to evaluate disease of the spinal cord and spinal column (e.g., herniated discs, degenerative disc disease, and spinal tumors)

When is **nuclear scan** the best test?

- HIDA (hepatobiliary) scan to evaluate biliary obstruction versus acute cholecystitis, biliary leaks postoperatively, and congenital abnormalities of the biliary tract including biliary atresia (not used to evaluate gallbladder stones)

> Regarding CT scan:
> - Do not order CT with contrast for patients with renal disease (creatinine ≥1.5).
> - Similarly, do not order MRI with contrast for patients with renal disease due to the risk of nephrogenic systemic fibrosis.
> - Do not give IV contrast to patients with multiple myeloma.
> - Discontinue metformin before doing a CT scan with IV contrast and resume a full 48 hours after the scan, when renal failure has been ruled out.

- Bone scan to evaluate metastatic bone lesions (prostate, breast, kidney, thyroid, lung), delayed fractures, and osteomyelitis and avascular necrosis of the femoral head
- Adrenal scan is test of choice to localize pheochromocytoma when an MRI/CT scan is nondiagnostic
- V/Q scan is initial test of choice to evaluate for pulmonary embolism (PE)
  - A normal study rules out PE.
  - An indeterminate scan requires further workup with CT angiogram.
  - A perfusion defect with normal ventilation quite probably indicates PE.
  - Do not order a V/Q scan in a patient with COPD or extensive lung disease.
- Gallium scan is test of choice to localize abscess and stage lymphoma/melanoma

When is **ultrasound** the best test?

- To evaluate the gallbladder for stones in the presence of right upper-quadrant pain
- To assess the uterus, adnexa, and ovaries (with the *exception* of cervical carcinoma)
- To evaluate the prostate; it also aids in obtaining biopsy
- To evaluate for deep venous thrombosis (DVT)

Bone scan is not useful in purely lytic metastatic lesions. It is **never the correct answer** in a patient with multiple myeloma.

Recognizing Images

Several conditions are likely to be on the exam in the form of an image. Familiarize yourself with these.

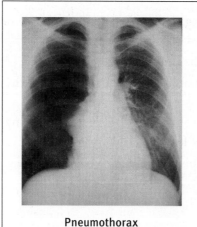

| Pneumothorax | Pneumomediastinum |

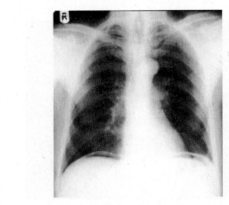

Pneumoperitoneum

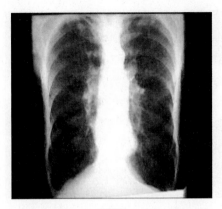

COPD

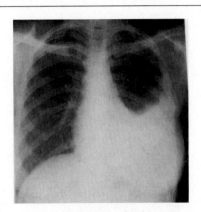

Pleural Effusions

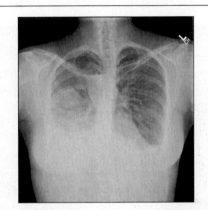

Bilateral Pleural Effusions

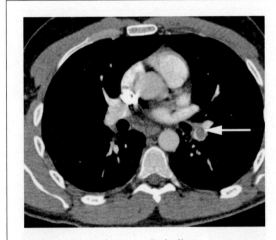

Pulmonary Embolism

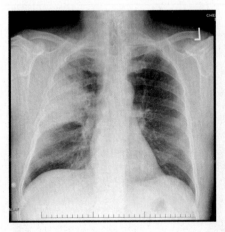

Lobar Pneumonia

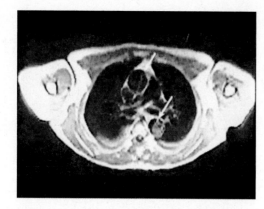

Aortic Dissection

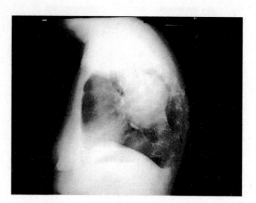

Aortic Aneurysm

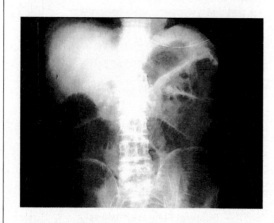

Small Bowel Obstruction

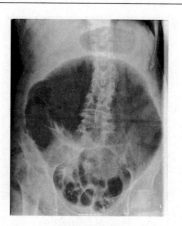

Cecal Volvulus

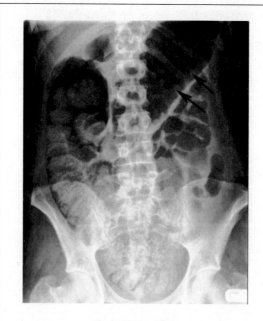

Toxic Megacolon

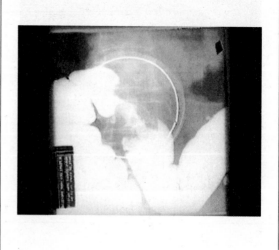

Carcinoma of the Colon

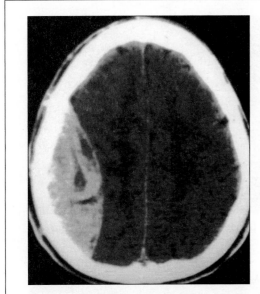

Epidural Hemorrhage

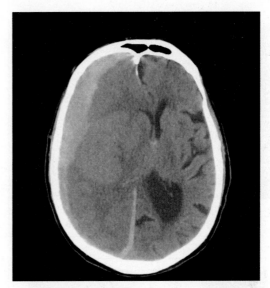

Subdural Hemorrhage

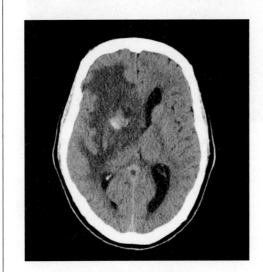

Thalamic Hemorrhage

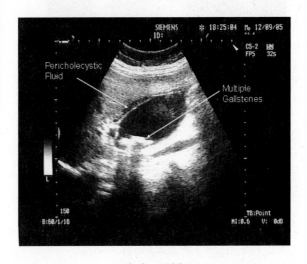

Cholecystitis

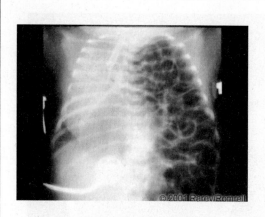

Congenital Diaphragmatic Hernia

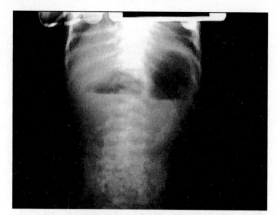

Duodenal Atresia: "Double Bubble" Sign

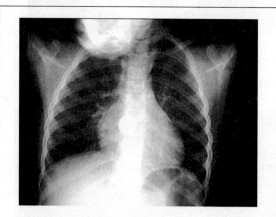

Foreign Body

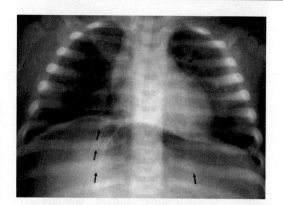

Child Abuse: gastric perforation and intraperitoneal
air and bilateral healing rib fractures
(diagnostic of abuse)

Connecting Images to a Disorder

When you see...	Think of...
Bones	
Lytic bone lesions on x-ray films	Multiple myeloma Primary bone tumor Metastasis (most common: lung, renal or thyroid, breast)
Blastic bone lesions on x-ray films	Metastasis (most common: breast, prostate, lymphoma) Paget disease Medulloblastoma in pediatrics
Chest	
Large mediastinum	Aortic aneurysm Lymphadenopathy
When you see...	**Think of...**
Abdomen/Pelvis	
Small bowel obstruction	Adhesions Hernia Intussusception (pediatrics) Gallstone ileus Carcinoma
Large bowel obstruction	Carcinoma Hernia Diverticulitis Intussusceptions (pediatrics)
Gas in biliary system	Gallstone ileus Gas forming infection Instrumentation
Small kidney(s)	Renal artery disease Chronic hydronephrosis Chronic glomerulonephritis Chronic pyelonephritis
Large kidney(s)	Acute pyelonephritis Acute glomerulonephritis Renal vein thrombosis Carcinoma (unilateral) Wilms tumor (pediatrics)

(continued next page)

Brain/Neurology	
Ring-enhancing lesion in brain	Immunocompetent patients: • Metastatic tumors • Demyelinating disease • Pyogenic abscess Immunocompromised patients: • Toxoplasma encephalitis *(T. gondii)* • Primary CNS lymphoma (Epstein-Barr virus) • Tuberculosis (in endemic areas)
Hemorrhage into basal ganglia, cerebellum, or pons	Hypertensive brain hemorrhage
Hemorrhage into the cerebral hemispheres	Arteriovenous malformation Aneurysm Trauma Metastatic lesions Other causes: vasculitis, cocaine, coagulation abnormalities

PART 10

Psychiatry

Contributing author Niket Sonpal, MD

Psychotic Disorders

Schizophrenia/Schizoaffective Disorder

A 25-year-old woman with hypertension comes to your office, accompanied by her husband, saying she has seen the devil and he is instructing her to commit suicide. She has been having these symptoms for 6 months and has also had several episodes when she believed she was being chased by demons. The patient has a history of 3 suicidal attempts while depressed. On examination she is preoccupied and appears to respond to internal stimuli. Her husband states she has not been formally diagnosed with any illnesses in the past. What is the most likely diagnosis?

a. Schizophrenia
b. Schizophreniform disorder
c. Antisocial personality disorder
d. Temporal lobe epilepsy
e. Schizoaffective disorder

Answer: E. Schizoaffective disorder is a combination of symptoms of schizophrenia and a mood disorder such as depression or bipolar disorder. Symptoms can include delusions, hallucinations, depressed episodes, and manic periods of high energy, and they may occur simultaneously or at different times. Cycles of severe symptoms are often followed by periods of improvement. People with schizoaffective disorder generally respond best to a combination of medication and counseling.

Schizophrenia diagnosis requires persistent symptoms for >6 months, while schizophreniform requires symptoms for >1 month but <6 months. In antisocial personality disorder, the patient shows no regard for rules and/or the feelings of others. Temporal lobe epilepsy would present with seizures, not features of psychosis.

Psychotic disorders present with a combination of positive and/or negative symptoms. The key differentiating feature is the **duration** of symptoms.

- **Positive** symptoms are characteristics that schizophrenics have but that normal individuals would not have.

- **Negative** symptoms are characteristics that schizophrenics lack but that normal individuals would have.

Diagnosing these conditions is as follows:

- Schizophrenia
  - Symptoms must be present ≥1 month, with a significant impact on social or occupational functioning for ≥6 months
  - In addition to having negative symptoms, patient must also have at least one of the following: delusions, hallucinations, or disorganized speech
  - Presents at a younger age in males (age 15–24) than in females (age 25–34)
  - Not diagnosed if symptoms of pervasive developmental disorder are present, unless accompanied by prominent delusions or hallucinations
- Schizoaffective disorder
  - Symptoms of schizophrenia accompany symptoms of a mood disorder such as depression or bipolar disorder
  - Symptoms can occur simultaneously or at different times
  - Cycles of severe symptoms are often followed by periods of improvement
- Schizophreniform disorder, symptoms are present ≥1 month but <6 months
- Brief psychotic disorder
  - Symptoms are present <1 month
  - There is a return to baseline (look for a stressful life event which precipitates the disorder)
- Delusional disorder or personality disorder, when there is a history of symptoms for many years with no impairment of baseline functioning (the key is few if any hallucinations and no bizarre behavior). Treatment for these patients is psychotherapy, as antipsychotics are not effective)
  - There is a history of symptoms for many years with no impairment of baseline functioning
  - The key is few—if any—hallucinations and no bizarre behavior
  - Treatment is psychotherapy, as antipsychotics are not effective

Watch for **suicidal ideation** in patients with schizophrenia or schizophreniform. According to DSM-5:

- About 20% of them attempt suicide at least once, and 5-6% die by suicide.
- They are also at greater risk of depression and suicide after the episode of psychosis resolves.

"Phrenia" >6 months

"Phreniform" >1 month but <6 months

Catatonia is no longer so strongly associated with schizophrenia.

Positive Symptoms	Negative Symptoms
Associated with dopamine receptors	Associated with muscarinic receptors
• Delusions (mostly bizarre) • Disorganized speech/behavior • Hallucinations	• Flattened affect • Social withdrawal • Anhedonia • Apathy • Poverty of thought **Atypical antipsychotics are the most effective treatment for negative symptoms.**

Basic Science Correlate

L-Phenylalanine → L-Tyrosine → L-DOPA → Dopamine

Diagnostic testing starts by ruling out medical illness and other forms of psychosis that are not schizophrenia:

- Drug screen (**best initial test in a patient with psychosis**)
- TSH for hypo- or hyperthyroidism
- Basic electrolytes and calcium to rule out metabolic disorders
- Serology to rule out HIV
- VDRL to rule out syphilis
- Rule out temporal lobe epilepsy, which can present with hallucinations (auditory and olfactory distortions), feeling of *déjà vu,* or dissociation from surroundings

Management is, first, to determine if the patient needs hospitalization. Hospitalize if the patient is suicidal/homicidal (even if against his will) or has bizarre/paranoid symptoms.

Then, give benzodiazepines for agitation and start antipsychotics.

- Antipsychotics (**most effective treatment** to prevent further episodes) are given for 6 months; give for >6 months only with a history of repeat episodes
- Antipsychotics have an immediate quieting effect in acute psychotic attacks of any cause (e.g., schizophrenia, depression with psychotic features, mania in bipolar disorder)
- Antipsychotics delay relapses
- Antipsychotics help to sedate when benzodiazepines are contraindicated or as an adjunct during anesthesia
- Antipsychotics help to suppress tics and vocalization in movement disorders (Huntington disease and Tourette)
- Antipsychotics are chosen based on side effect profile, not efficacy:
  - Low-potency antipsychotics have the highest risk of causing orthostatic hypotension (alpha blockade), acute urinary retention, dry mouth, blurry vision, and delirium (anticholinergic effect). Change to an atypical antipsychotic if these symptoms are present.
  - Thioridazine is associated with prolonged QT and arrhythmias. Always get an EKG if there is chest pain, shortness of breath, or palpitations in a patient taking thioridazine. Thioridazine is also associated with abnormal retinal pigmentation after years of use, so monitor with eye exams.
  - Impotence and inhibition of ejaculation (α-blocker effect) are common reasons for noncompliance in males.
  - Weight gain (due to hyperprolactinemia) is a common reason for noncompliance in females. Also ask about galactorrhea and amenorrhea.

Atypical antipsychotics are used over typical antipsychotics because they have better efficacy and in some cases fewer side effects. They include:

- Quetiapine (causes most sedation of all the atypical antipsychotics)
- Olanzapine (causes most weight gain of all the antipsychotics)
- Clozapine (associated with agranulocytosis in 1% so check CBC with differential before initiating therapy and after starting therapy 1×/week)

The last step in treatment is to initiate long-term psychotherapy.

Long term, the following features indicate a poor prognosis. In general, females respond better to treatment than males, and have a better prognosis.

- Early age of onset
- Negative symptoms
- Poor premorbid functioning
- Family history of schizophrenia

What is the greatest risk factor for progression to schizophrenia?

Answer: **Schizophreniform disorder**, and 70% of cases will eventually progress to schizophrenia.

Basic Science Correlate

Huntington disease is a trinucleotide repeat disorder = CAG repeat = Glutamine.

A 27-year-old woman with a history of refractory psychosis presents to your office for follow-up. She reports coughing productive of green sputum and states that it hurts to take a deep breath. On examination egophony is present on the left lower lung base. Labs reveal an absolute neutrophil count (ANC) of 1,300 cell/mm³. What is the most likely cause of these findings?

a. Olanzapine
b. Quetiapine
c. Risperidone
d. Clozapine
e. Thioridazine

Answer: **D.** The most serious adverse reactions to clozapine include agranulocytosis, seizure, cardiovascular effects, and fever. This patient presents with signs and symptoms consistent with pneumonia, likely due to decreased ANC. Olanzapine causes weight gain, while quetiapine is the most sedating of all the atypical antipsychotics. Thioridazine prolongs the QTc interval in a dose-dependent manner. Risperidone is not associated with changes in white cell count or function.

	Conventional Antipsychotics		Atypical Antipsychotics
	High Potency	**Low Potency**	
Examples	Fluphenazine, haloperidol	Thioridazine, chlorpromazine	Risperidone, olanzapine, quetiapine, clozapine
Advantages	Fewer anticholinergic effects Less hypotension Useful as depot injections (e.g., haloperidol decanoate) for noncompliant patients Give IM route for acute psychosis when patient is unable or unwilling to take PO	Less likely to cause EPS	Drug of choice for initial therapy Greater effect on negative symptoms Little or no risk of EPS
Disadvantages	Greatest association with extrapyramidal systems (EPS)	Greater anticholinergic effects More sedation More postural hypotension	Clozapine is reserved for treatment-resistant patients because of risk of agranulocytosis.

a. A newly diagnosed schizophrenic patient complains of insomnia. What is the most appropriate antipsychotic to initiate therapy?

b. A schizophrenic patient has been maintained on olanzapine for the past 6 months. He complains of daytime sedation, and he has lost 2 jobs in the past month because of impaired performance. What is the next step in management?

Answers:

a. Olanzapine and quetiapine are first-choice medications when insomnia is a problem.

b. Prescribe risperidone, a first-choice medication for the treatment of schizophrenia when sedation is a problem.

Basic Science Correlate

Risperidone affects 6 receptors: 5HT; D1; D2; α1; α2; H1

Movement Disorders

A 35-year-old man presents with poor adherence to chlorpromazine and haloperidol. He complains of tics and other uncontrolled movements. His wife reports that even when he takes his medications, they don't appear to help his paranoia. What is the next step in management?

a. Add risperidone

b. Add diphenhydramine

c. Change to clozapine

d. Increase dose of chlorpromazine

e. Increase dose of haloperidol

Answer: **C.** The case describes 2 main problems in management, poor response to therapy prescribed and movement disorder as a side effect from the regimen. Clozapine is the most effective antipsychotic for schizophrenia and also has no incidence of movement disorders. It is a second-line therapy because of the risk of seizures and agranulocytosis. Remember to monitor CBC to watch for bone marrow suppression.

A 78-year-old man with a slow-growing stomach tumor in palliative care is brought in by the family, who have noticed increased sedation and difficulty eating. They are concerned because he continues to lose more weight. On examination he has repetitive movements of his lips and tongue. He has limited facial expression. His medications include morphine, metoclopramide, and hydrochlorothiazide. Which of the following is the most appropriate management?

a. Decrease morphine
b. Discontinue metoclopramide
c. Start omeprazole
d. Start prochlorperazine
e. Place NG tube for supplemental feedings

Answer: B. Chronic use of dopamine antagonists, including antiemetics (metoclopramide, prochlorperazine), can result in tardive dyskinesia. Management includes discontinuing the offending drug and, if indicated, beginning a newer antipsychotic.

Valbenazine is used to treat tardive dyskinesia in adults. It causes reversible reduction of dopamine release by selectively inhibiting presynaptic human vesicular monoamine transporter type 2 (VMAT2). By selectively inhibiting the ability of VMAT2 to load dopamine into synaptic vesicles, the drug reduces overall levels of available dopamine in the synaptic cleft and, consequently, the symptoms of tardive dyskinesia.

Extrapyramidal symptoms (EPS) are the most common reason for failure to comply with therapy. Be able to identify a patient with a medication-related movement disorder and know how to minimize the symptoms.

> Tardive dyskinesia can be treated with benztropine.

The table shows common medication-related movement disorders and their management.

Acute Dystonia	Bradykinesia (Parkinsonism)	Akathisia	Tardive Dyskinesia	Neuroleptic Malignant Syndrome
Occurs in the first week	Within weeks	Weeks to chronic use	Months to years	Anytime
Muscle spasms (e.g., torticollis), difficulty swallowing **TIP:** Young men are at higher risk.	Bradykinesia, tremors, rigidity, and other signs of parkinsonism **TIP:** Elderly are at higher risk.	Motor restlessness Do not mistake for anxiety for agitation **TIP:** Always review medication list.	Choreoathetosis and other involuntary movements after chronic use; often irreversible	Muscle rigidity, hyperthermia, volatile vital signs, altered LOC, ↑ WBC & CK

• Reduce the dose
• Rx: Anticholinergics
  - benztropine
  - diphenhydramine
  - trihexyphenidyl
	• Reduce the dose
	• Rx: Anticholinergics
	  - benztropine
	  - diphenhydramine
	  - trihexyphenidyl
		• Reduce the dose
		• Add benzodiazepines or beta-blockers
		• Switch to newer antipsychotics
			• Stop older antipsychotics
			• Switch to newer antipsychotics (e.g., clozapine)
			• Add valbenazine or deutetrabenazine (vesicular monoamine transporter 2 [VMAT2] inhibitors)
			
			TIP: *Symptoms commonly worsen after medication discontinuation.*
				• Stop antipsychotic
				
				TIP: *Transfer to ICU for monitoring, mortality rate is 20%.*

> **Basic Science Correlate**
>
> High-potency D2 receptor antagonists produce a dystonic reaction by nigrostriatal dopamine D2 receptor blockade, which leads striatal cholinergic output. Thus, anticholinergics are the first-line treatment.

Anxiety Disorders

Anxiety disorders cause anxiety that cannot be better explained by medical conditions or by the effects of medications/drugs. Other conditions that may present as an anxiety disorder include the following:

- Medical causes: hyperthyroidism, pheochromocytoma, excess cortisol, heart failure, arrhythmias, asthma, and COPD
- Drugs: corticosteroids, cocaine, amphetamines, and caffeine, as well as withdrawal from alcohol and sedatives

A 29-year-old psychiatry resident presents with palpitations, chest pain, and diaphoresis. She is unable to complete her inpatient tasks and is referred to her program director. Her attending states she is agitated and easily distracted, and she reports nausea throughout the day and feeling constantly on the run. She consumes 5 energy drinks, 3 cups of coffee, and 1 pack of cigarettes daily. Urine toxicology is clean on a recent drug screen. What is the most likely diagnosis?

a. Generalized anxiety disorder
b. Manic episode without psychotic features
c. Substance-induced anxiety disorder
d. Agoraphobia
e. Malingering

Answer: **C.** The symptoms are clearly linked to the patient's massive daily caffeine use. With cessation, her substance-induced cardiac and mood symptoms will dissipate. Generalized anxiety disorder cannot be diagnosed in the presence of a confounding factor such as caffeine abuse. You must always rule out substance use before making a psychiatric diagnosis; thus malingering (a diagnosis of exclusion) and mania do not fit at this time. Agoraphobia is a fear of public settings; this vignette makes no mention of symptoms related to public or outdoor settings.

Adjustment Disorder

This is a psychological reaction (anxiety, depression, irritability) that occurs soon after profound changes in a person's life, such as divorce, migration, or birth of a handicapped child. Symptoms are usually experienced within 3 months of the stressful event and are not severe enough to be classified in another category. Adjustment disorder is *not* a true anxiety disorder.

> Do not treat adjustment disorder patients with medications; instead provide counseling to help the patient adjust to the life stressor.

Panic Disorder

Panic disorder is the diagnosis when there are brief attacks of intense anxiety with autonomic symptoms (e.g., tachycardia, hyperventilation, dizziness, and sweating). Episodes occur regularly, without an obvious precipitant and in the absence of other psychiatric illness.

Treatment is cognitive-behavioral therapy and/or relaxation training and desensitization. Relaxation and desensitization may be more useful when agoraphobic symptoms are present. Medications include SSRIs (e.g., fluoxetine) and benzodiazepines (e.g., alprazolam, clonazepam).

Phobic Disorder

Phobic disorder is the diagnosis when the patient has a persistent, unreasonable, intense fear of situations or things. Unlike posttraumatic stress disorder (PTSD) and acute stress disorder (ASD), there is no history of traumatic events (threat to life or limb).

- Social anxiety disorder (most common phobia) is intense anxiety/fear of being judged or rejected in a social situation or performance setting. Patients may worry about appearing visibly anxious. Treatment is a combination of SSRI and CBT.
- Agoraphobia is fear or avoidance of places due to anxiety about not being able to escape (public places, being outside alone, or crowds). Women > men.

Basic Science Correlate

Benzodiazepines work by potentiating the effects of GABA through increased frequency of chloride ions across neuronal cell membranes, resulting in decreased excitability of neurons.

Barbiturates work by potentiating the effects of GABA through increased duration of chloride ions across the neuronal cell membranes, resulting in decreased excitability of neurons.

Generalized Anxiety Disorder

Generalized anxiety disorder (GAD) is excessive, poorly controlled anxiety that occurs daily for >6 months. No single event or focus is related to the anxiety. It often coexists with major depression, specific phobia, social phobia, and panic disorder.

- Distinguish GAD from panic attack or social phobia by what is causing the anxiety.
- If the question describes persistent worry of a panic attack or social encounter, then it is not GAD; in GAD, multiple life circumstances are causing the anxiety, not just one.

Treatment for GAD is supportive psychotherapy, including relaxation training and biofeedback. Medications include SSRIs, venlafaxine, benzodiazepines, and buspirone.

With benzodiazepines, use the following guidelines.

- Do not change dosage abruptly.
- Use the lowest dose in the elderly.
- Advise against using machinery or driving.
- Half-life: alprazolam (shortest); lorazepam (middle); diazepam (longest)

Buspirone is the best option for those whose occupations involve driving or machinery, as there is no sedation or cognitive impairment.

- Therapeutic effect can take up to 1 week
- Can be used safely with other sedative-hypnotics (no additive effect)
- No withdrawal syndrome but lowers seizure threshold

Basic Science Correlate

Buspirone is a serotonin 5-HT1A receptor partial agonist.

Anxiolytic Medications

Anxiolytics Prescribed for Anxiety Disorders		
Anxiety Disorder	Anxiolytic	Benefits
Adjustment disorder with anxious mood	Benzodiazepines with brief psychotherapy	Rapid onset to therapy
Panic disorder	SSRIs, alprazolam, and clonazepam	Decrease frequency and intensity of panic attacks
Generalized anxiety disorder (GAD)	SSRI and buspirone	Decrease overall anxiety
Social phobia	SSRIs and buspirone	Decrease fear associated with social situations

Obsessive-Compulsive Disorder

Obsessive-compulsive disorder (OCD) involves recurrent obsessions or compulsions.

- Obsessions are anxiety-provoking; thoughts are intrusive and are commonly related to contamination, doubt, guilt, aggression, and sex.
- Compulsions are peculiar behaviors which reduce the anxiety and are most commonly habitual hand washing, organizing, checking, counting, and praying.

Obsessive symptoms in psychotic disorders may be misdiagnosed as OCD (but in OCD there are no hallucinations and disorganization, as there are in psychosis).

Those who have OCD also often have depression and substance abuse.

Those who have Tourette syndrome often also have OCD.

Treatment for OCD is behavioral psychotherapy and pharmacotherapy (SSRIs and clomipramine).

Hoarding Disorder

Hoarding disorder is a persistent difficulty discarding or parting with possessions because of a perceived need to save them. Patients experience distress at the thought of getting rid of the items to which they have an excessive attachment.

A lack of functional living space is common among hoarders, whose living conditions may also be unhealthy or dangerous.

Treatment is cognitive behavioral therapy combined with clomipramine or SSRIs.

Trauma- and Stress-Related Disorders

Acute Stress Disorder (ASD) and Posttraumatic Stress Disorder (PTSD)

These disorders involve severe anxiety symptoms that follow a life-threatening event.

- ASD: symptoms last <1 month and occur within 1 month of stressor
- PTSD: symptoms last >1 month

Symptoms fall into 3 key groups:

- Re-experiencing of the traumatic event: dreams, flashbacks, or intrusive recollections
- Avoidance of stimuli associated with the trauma or numbing of general responsiveness
- Increased arousal: anxiety, sleep disturbances, hypervigilance, emotional lability, or impulsiveness

Treatment is benzodiazepines for acute anxiety, and SSRIs and other antidepressants for chronic illness.

A school bus is involved in a major collision. Two children are killed, and 7 others are injured. What is the most important therapy to prevent PTSD?

a. Diazepam
b. Fluoxetine
c. Cognitive behavioral therapy
d. Haloperidol
e. Individual psychotherapy

Answer: **C.** Cognitive behavioral therapy (CBT) seeks to change the way a trauma victim feels and acts by changing the patterns of thinking or behavior, or both, responsible for negative emotions.

Mood Disorders

Major Depressive Disorder

This disorder is characterized by depressed mood or anhedonia and depressive symptoms lasting at least 2 weeks.

Look for other causes of depression where the first step in management is different, such as the following:

- Hypothyroidism
  - Check TSH
  - Treat with thyroxine
- Parkinson disease
  - Treat with anti-Parkinson medications
- Medications
  - Corticosteroids, β-blockers, antipsychotics (especially in the elderly), and reserpine
  - Treat by discontinuing medication and switching to an alternative
- Substance disorders
  - Alcohol (ask CAGE questionnaire), amphetamines, cocaine
  - Treat with detoxification

Treatment is as follows:

- Hospitalization if there is suicidal/homicidal ideation
- Antidepressant medications (SSRI is drug of choice)
- Benzodiazepines for agitation
- Electroconvulsive therapy (ECT) if patient is acutely suicidal (works faster than antidepressants) or if patient worried about side effects from medications; also consider ECT in pregnant patients who are suicidal. If ECT is not available or has failed, consider esketamine.

Persistent Depressive Disorder (Dysthymia)

This disorder is characterized by low-level depression symptoms that are present on most days for at least 2 years. However, the question may describe superimposed acute major depression, which is common in these patients. Do not hospitalize these patients unless there's suicidal ideation.

Treatment is long-term individual, insight-oriented psychotherapy. If that fails, try SSRIs.

Seasonal Affective Disorder

The diagnosis is seasonal affective disorder when the case describes depressive symptoms in the winter months (shorter daylight hours) and absence of depressive symptoms during summer months (longer daylight hours). Treatment is phototherapy or sleep deprivation.

> **SIGECAPS:** Major depressive disorder = Depressed mood +
>
> **S:** changes in sleep
>
> **I:** loss of interests/pleasure
>
> **G:** thoughts of worthlessness or guilt
>
> **E:** loss of energy
>
> **C:** trouble concentrating
>
> **A:** changes in appetite or weight
>
> **P:** changes in psychomotor activity
>
> **S:** thoughts about death or suicide

> In patients with unipolar psychotic depression, the combination of an antidepressant and an antipsychotic is more effective than monotherapy with either drug.

Bipolar Disorder

Bipolar disorder is the diagnosis when there are episodes of depression, mania, or both, that cause distress or impaired functioning for at least 1 week.

Bipolar disorder is the **most commonly missed** diagnosis in the USMLE, because it can easily be mistaken for depression or mania alone. The history will include both manic symptoms and depressive symptoms, as well as periods of normal mood. Rapid cycling bipolar is indicated by >4 episodes of mania per year.

Mania symptoms include grandiosity, less need for sleep, excessive talking or pressured speech, racing thoughts or flight of ideas, distractibility, goal-focused activity at home or at work, or sexual promiscuity. Major depressive symptoms include depressed mood or loss of pleasure or interest.

CCS Tip: If the history suggests drug use, first get a drug screen to rule out amphetamine use as a cause of mania. If the history gives elevated blood pressure or low TSH, consider medical conditions, such as pheochromocytoma and hyperthyroidism.

Treatment is as follows:

- Monotherapy with lithium, lamotrigine, or risperidone (first-line)
- Aripiprazole, divalproex, quetiapine, and olanzapine (second-line)
- Combination therapy for those with multiple recurrences; lurasidone is often added as adjunctive therapy to lithium (**most common side effect** of lurasidone is weight gain and sedation)
- Psychotherapy and cognitive behavioral therapy
- Avoid teratogenic drugs such as lithium, valproate, and carbamazepine in pregnancy

For acute mania:

- Hospitalization and then mood stabilizers to induce remission (lithium is drug of choice); takes 1 week for effect
- Antipsychotics to control the mania; IM depot phenothiazine in noncompliant, severely manic patients
- Antidepressants only for those who have recurrent episodes of depression; administer with mood stabilizers to prevent inducing manic episode

---

Symptoms of mania = **DIG FAST**

D: Distractibility and easy frustration

I: Irresponsibility and erratic, uninhibited behavior

G: Grandiosity

F: Flight of ideas

A: Activity increased with weight loss and increased libido

S: Sleep is decreased

T: Talkativeness

a. What is the most common cause of progression to rapid cycling bipolar?

b. How should you manage rapid cycling bipolar?

c. What other medical conditions predispose a patient to rapid cycling bipolar?

d. What drug has been shown to prevent suicidal ideation in bipolar disorder?

e. A 32-year-old known bipolar patient who is undergoing maintenance therapy with lithium presents with a positive pregnancy test. How will you manage this patient's bipolar disorder?

Answers:

a. **Use of antidepressants:** Do not give antidepressants prophylactically unless the question describes previous severe depressive episodes. In that case, antidepressants are only given for a few weeks.

b. **Gradually stop** all antidepressants, stimulants, caffeine, benzodiazepines, and alcohol.

c. **Hypothyroidism:** Check TSH in any patient with rapid cycling bipolar and replace thyroid hormones if needed.

d. **Lithium**

e. **Discontinue lithium (to avoid heart abnormalities):** Choose ECT therapy for first-trimester patients with manic episodes. Use lamotrigine in 2nd or 3rd trimester.

> Lithium can lead to Ebstein anomaly and diabetes insipidus.

Cyclothymic Disorder

Cyclothymic disorder is a milder form of bipolar disorder, but the mood shifts are less extreme. When a patient presents with a history of episodes of depressed mood and hypomanic mood for at least 2 years, the diagnosis is cyclothymia.

Treatment is psychotherapy. Many people function without medication and learn to manage their hypomanic dispositions (especially artists). Start divalproex when functioning is impaired. Divalproex is more effective in cyclothymia than lithium.

Grief and Depression

Grief	Depression
Sadness, tearfulness, decreased sleep, decreased appetite, decreased interest in the world	
Symptoms wax and wane	Symptoms are pervasive and unremitting
Shame and guilt are less common	Shame and guilt are common
Suicidal ideation is less common	Suicidal ideation is more common
Symptoms can last up to 1–2 years	Symptoms continue for more than 1 year
Patient usually returns to baseline level of functioning within 2 months	Patient does not return to baseline functioning
Treatment includes supportive therapy	Treatment includes antidepressant medications

A 32-year-old woman who gave birth 4 months ago is brought in by her husband because of depressed mood. The husband reports that she has been depressed since the birth of her child, refuses to eat, has trouble sleeping, and is unable to concentrate. The woman reports that she has lost interest in everything and sometimes can't even get out of bed. She has recently had visions of seeing her deceased mother talking to her and criticizing her skills as a new mother. She also admits that she hears her voice talking to her constantly. She denies homicidal or suicidal ideation. Which of the following is the best initial treatment?

a. Psychotherapy
b. Behavioral therapy
c. Sertraline
d. Risperidone
e. Phenelzine

Answer: **D.** Patients with both mood and psychotic symptoms respond to both antidepressants and antipsychotic medication. However, you must treat the worst symptom first. In this case, the antipsychotic would be most indicated to reduce her psychotic symptoms.

A 45-year-old woman presents 2 months after the sudden loss of her son in a car accident. She reports "not coping well with the loss." She is constantly teary, has lost her appetite, and has dropped 2 dress sizes. She finds herself laying out a dinner plate every night for him. Recently, she believes she has heard his voice and every night she has nightmares about the car accident. She denies suicidal ideation. Which of the following is the most appropriate next step in management?

a. Group therapy
b. Amitriptyline
c. Fluoxetine
d. Zolpidem
e. Supportive therapy

Answer: **E.** This patient is undergoing normal grief reaction. Auditory hallucinations without other psychotic symptoms are normal in grief reaction.

Postpartum Depression

	Postpartum Blues or "Baby Blues"	Postpartum Unipolar Depression	Postpartum Psychosis
Onset	After any birth	Usually after second birth	Usually after first birth
Mother's emotions toward baby	Cares about baby	Many have thoughts about hurting the baby	Many have thoughts about hurting the baby
Symptoms	Mild depressive	Severe depressive	Look for psychotic symptoms along with severe depressive symptoms
Treatment	Self-limited; no treatment necessary	Combination of psychotherapy (CBT) and antidepressants if severe	Mood stabilizers or antipsychotics and antidepressants If patient is breastfeeding, choose ECT over medications

Suicide and Suicidal Ideation

Management of the Suicidal Patient	
Ask about risk factors:	**Emergency Assessment**
• **History of suicide threats and attempts is the most important predictor of suicide.** • Family history of suicide • Perceived hopelessness (demoralization) • Schizophrenia/borderline or antisocial PD • Drug use, especially alcohol • Males/age >65 • Socially isolated/recently divorced or widowed • Chronic physical illness • Low job satisfaction or unemployment	• Take all suicide threats seriously • Detain and hospitalize (usually a couple of weeks) • Do not leave patient unsupervised (i.e., always transport patient to ED accompanied by medically trained personnel) • Do not identify with patient • Do not leave patient unsupervised • Treatment of choice = psychotherapy + antidepressant medications (SSRIs are first choice) • For acute, severe risk of self-harm, treatment of choice is ECT

Medical Treatment Options for Mood Disorder

Electroconvulsive Therapy (ECT)

Indications for ECT include:

- Major depressive episodes that are unresponsive to medications
- High risk for immediate suicide
- Contraindications to using antidepressant medications
- Good response to ECT in the past

The biggest complication of ECT is transient memory loss, which worsens with prolonged therapy and resolves after several weeks.

Use of ECT is cautioned in patients with space-occupying intracranial lesions (e.g., brain metastasis), as ECT induces transient intracranial pressure.

It is safe in pregnancy.

Antidepressants and Mood Stabilizers

Choose an antidepressant based on side effect profile. If the patient cannot tolerate the side effects or does not respond after 8 weeks, switch to another antidepressant.

Treat patients for 6 months and attempt to discontinue after tapering. Consider long-term therapy for multiple episodes of depression.

- SSRIs (first-line)
- TCAs are avoided because of risk of toxicity (think: **TCA** may be **T**oxic)
- MAOIs (more helpful in atypical depressive disorders)
- Mirtazapine for a poor appetite, weight loss, or insomnia (mirtazapine is associated with weight gain)
- Bupropion for patients concerned about weight gain or sexual side effects (causes modest weight loss) (bupropion is associated with seizures)
- Amitriptyline or duloxetine for neuropathic pain (duloxetine is safer)

> In TCA overdose, the most urgent next step is to check an EKG for life-threatening arrhythmias.

- Imipramine for enuresis
- Trazodone for depressed patients who have severe insomnia (trazodone is strongly sedating)
- SSRIs and TCAs (except paroxetine) are safe in pregnancy.

Basic Science Correlate

SSRIs inhibit the reuptake of serotonin in the synaptic cleft, resulting in more signaling across the synapses.

> SSRIs are first-line therapy for many conditions because of their therapeutic effect and low side effect profile. Always think of SSRIs first in patients with the following disorders:
>
> - Major depressive disorder
> - Bipolar disorder
> - Anxiety disorders: Panic disorder, OCD, social phobia, generalized anxiety disorder
> - Bulimia nervosa

A young man recently started on antidepressants develops prolonged erection. What is the antidepressant he was most likely taking?

Answer: **Trazodone**

An elderly patient presents with depression and agitation. What is the most appropriate medication?

Answer: Give an **antidepressant with sedative effects** (e.g., doxepin, trazodone). Amitriptyline is also sedating but has anticholinergic effects, which may be problematic in elderly.

A 25-year-old man with history of seizures is diagnosed with depression. Which medications should be avoided?

Answer: Seizures are common with **TCAs and bupropion**, and these medications should be avoided in patients with seizure disorders. The best first-line therapy in patients with seizures is SSRIs.

A middle-aged woman is brought into the ER with confusion and disorientation. An overdose of prescription medications is suspected. Blood pressure is 90/53 mm Hg, HR 111/min. Pupils are dilated, mucous membranes are dry, and she has facial flushing.

1. What is the most likely cause of acute intoxication?
2. What is the most important test to determine severity and prognosis in this patient?

a. EKG
b. EEG
c. Serum sodium
d. Serum tricyclic level
e. Urinalysis

3. EKG is performed and shows PR and QRS prolongation and sinus tachycardia. What is the most appropriate next step in management?

   a. Calcium carbonate
   b. Diazepam
   c. Gastric lavage
   d. Insulin and glucose
   e. Sodium bicarbonate

Answers:

1. **Tricyclic antidepressants (TCAs).** TCAs have anticholinergic effects and are an alpha blocker, causing peripheral vasodilatation and hypotension and also affecting sodium channels in cardiac tissue.

2. **A.** EKG is the single most important test to guide therapy and prognosis. Watch out for prolonged QRS, QT, and PR intervals. Most serious complication is ventricular tachycardia and fibrillation.

3. **E.** Sodium bicarbonate attenuates TCA cardiotoxicity by alkalinization of blood, which uncouples TCA from myocardial sodium channels and increases extracellular sodium concentration, thereby improving the gradient across the channel.

A 42-year-old woman with a history of hypertension, diabetes, and depression presents to the clinic with dry eyes and dry mouth. Her medications include hydrochlorothiazide, metformin, and amitriptyline. Which of the following is the next step in management?

a. Discontinue amitriptyline and change to sertraline
b. Order antinuclear antibodies
c. Order SS-Ro and SS-La
d. Prescribe eye drops
e. Refer to ophthalmologist

Answer: **A.** Discontinue amitriptyline and switch to another antidepressant medication with little/no anticholinergic effects. Anticholinergic effects are most severe with amitriptyline, but there are almost none with most SSRIs.

Lithium

Lithium is the first-line medication for bipolar and schizoaffective disorders and treatment and prophylaxis of mood episodes. Side effects are a major reason for noncompliance. These include the following:

- Acne and weight gain are the most common problems.
- Dose-related tremors, GI distress, and headaches (decrease the dose)
- Hypothyroidism (5%)
- Polyuria secondary to medication-induced diabetes insipidus
- Do not use in first trimester of pregnancy, as it causes cardiac defects. Long-term lithium use also causes nephrotoxicity, and kidney dysfunction is a clear contraindication to lithium therapy.

Divalproex

Divalproex is the first-line choice for rapid-cycling bipolar disorder or when lithium is ineffective, impractical, or contraindicated.

Carbamazepine

Carbamazepine is the second-line choice for bipolar disorder when lithium and divalproex are ineffective or contraindicated. It is not commonly used because of serious agranulocytosis and significant sedation.

> **Basic Science Correlate**
>
> Carbamazepine affects the inactivated state of voltage-gated Na^+ channels, making fewer channels available to open. Carbamazepine is a CYP450 inducer, and it increases the clearance of warfarin, phenytoin, theophylline, and valproic acid.

Somatic Symptom and Related Disorders

A somatic symptom disorder is the diagnosis when there are physical symptoms without medical explanation. The symptoms are severe enough to interfere with the patient's ability to function in social or occupational activities.

> A 47-year-old woman presents to the clinic with shortness of breath, chest pain, abdominal pain, back pain, double vision, and difficulty walking due to weakness in her legs. She remembers being sick all of the time for the past 10 years. According to her husband, she constantly takes medications for all of her ailments. She has visited numerous physicians and none has been able to diagnose her condition correctly. What is the next step in management?
>
> a. ANA
> b. CT of the abdomen
> c. CT of the head
> d. Hospitalize
> e. Schedule regular monthly visits
>
> Answer: **E.** Scheduling regular monthly visits to establish a single physician as the primary caregiver is the most important first step in management. It builds rapport, validates her concerns, and prevents polypharmacy.

Management is as follows:

1. Maintain a single physician as the primary caretaker.
2. Schedule brief monthly visits.
3. *Avoid* diagnostic testing or therapies.
4. Schedule individual psychotherapy.
5. Do *not* hospitalize the patient.

Illness Anxiety Disorder (IAD)

In this disorder, formerly known as hypochondriasis, the patient is preoccupied with having or developing a serious illness despite having only mild symptoms or no symptoms. These patients become easily alarmed about their health.

To be diagnosed with IAD, the patient must have experienced anxiety about illness for at least 6 months. Patient history may include multiple physician and hospital visits.

> A 33-year-old male GI fellow has the persistent belief that he acquired hepatitis C through a needle injury he received while working at an inner-city clinic. Multiple antibody and PCR tests over a period of 1 year have been negative. Despite reassurance to the contrary and a weight gain of 20 pounds, he often thinks he is jaundiced and cachectic. What is the best therapy for this patient?
>
> a. Supportive therapy
> b. Dialectical-based therapy
> c. Cognitive behavioral therapy
> d. Insight-oriented therapy
> e. Psychoanalysis
>
> Answer: **C.** Cognitive behavioral therapy is the best approach for a patient with illness anxiety disorder. Supportive therapy (providing reassurance without challenging the patient to provide further understanding) is not appropriate. Dialectical-based therapy is indicated for patients with borderline personality disorder and not appropriate here. Insight-oriented therapy allows patients express their motivations and fears while gaining understanding of their symptoms; however, changing an aberrant behavior is more important than understanding it. Psychoanalysis is the Freudian approach to uncovering motivations of behavior, taking 5–10 years to complete. While psychoanalysis might eventually lead to understanding of the behavior, it may not change it; it is rarely the correct answer.

Treatment for IAD is primarily therapy-based and aimed at improving patients' ability to understand their health fears rather than eliminating them. It involves establishing a consistent, supportive physician-patient relationship. Cognitive behavioral therapy may help. Medical therapy is reserved for patients who have concomitant GAD or depression.

Conversion Disorder

Conversion disorder is the diagnosis when there are one or more neurologic symptoms that cannot be explained by any medical or neurologic disorder. Most common symptoms are mutism, blindness, paralysis, and anesthesia/paresthesias. Look for psychologic factors associated with the onset or exacerbation of symptoms. A clue to diagnosis is that patients often are unconcerned about their impairment (*la belle indifference*). You must first rule out other medical conditions.

Treatment is a supportive physician-patient relationship and psychotherapy.

Factitious and Malingering Disorders

A 23-year-old nursing student presents to the ED with fever and chills at home. She has had multiple admissions in other hospitals because of pneumonia and chronic pain problems. She was found to be tampering with the blood culture bottles and dipping her temperature thermometer in hot water. Which of the following is the most likely diagnosis?

a. Conversion disorder

b. Factitious disorder

c. Factitious disorder by proxy

d. Malingering

e. Obsessive-compulsive disorder

Answer: **B.**

A 46-year-old homeless man presents to the hospital reporting that he had a seizure this morning. He is adamant that he be admitted; however, he refuses all blood work and imaging studies. He cannot answer questions about the seizure and cannot describe his symptoms at the time of the seizure. Instead he demands to be admitted and is wondering why you're taking so long. When you ask about his social history, he admits that he is homeless at the moment as he was "kicked out of the shelter" because of drug-taking and alcohol abuse. Which of the following is the most likely diagnosis?

a. Conversion disorder

b. Factitious disorder

c. Factitious disorder by proxy

d. Malingering

e. Borderline personality disorder

Answer: **D.**

In both factitious disorder and malingering, the case will suggest that a patient has intentionally feigned symptoms.

- The diagnosis is factitious disorder **imposed on self** if the patient has seen many doctors and visited many hospitals, has large amount of medical knowledge (e.g., health care worker), and demands treatment. The patient is agitated and threatens litigation if tests return negative.

- The diagnosis is factitious disorder **imposed on others** if the signs and symptoms are faked by another person, as in a mother making up symptoms in her child. The motivation is to assume the caretaker role.

- DSM-5 describes malingering as the intentional generation of feigned symptoms. Malingering patients are more preoccupied with rewards or gain (shelter, medications, disability insurance) than with alleviation of presenting symptoms.

Treatment is supportive psychotherapy. Do not confront or accuse the patient, who is likely to become angry and more guarded. Provide only the minimal treatment and workup needed. Aggressive management of the patient's symptoms only reinforces the behavior.

Eating Disorders and Other Impulse Control Disorders

Eating Disorders

Anorexia Nervosa

Anorexia nervosa is seen in young women who are underweight because of food restriction and excessive exercise. They may have a history of purging (50% of patients), but the diagnosis will still be anorexia nervosa.

Bulimia Nervosa

Bulimia nervosa is seen in young women who have normal weight but who have episodes of binge eating followed by guilt, anxiety, and self-induced vomiting, laxative, diuretics, or enema use.

- Episodes must occur at least 1×/week for diagnosis
- Food restriction not a feature
- Look for painless parotid gland enlargement and dental enamel erosions
- Electrolyte disturbances are common (metabolic alkalosis, hypochloremia, and hypokalemia caused by emesis; metabolic acidosis caused by laxative abuse)

Treatment of any eating disorder is first, to hospitalize for IV hydration if electrolyte disturbances are present.

- Olanzapine in anorexia nervosa to help with weight gain
- SSRI antidepressants (especially fluoxetine) to prevent relapses
- Behavioral psychotherapy

Binge Eating Disorder

Binge eating disorder is characterized by recurrent episodes of eating large quantities of food over a short period of time, accompanied by a feeling of loss of control during the binge.

- Binges are followed by feelings of shame, distress, or guilt
- Purging not a feature

Treatment is cognitive behavioral therapy and pharmacotherapy.

Body Dysmorphic Disorder

Body dysmorphic disorder is characterized by young patients (male or female) who are preoccupied with an imagined or slight defect in appearance.

- Preoccupation causes distress and impaired ability to function in a social/occupational setting
- Distress most commonly related to facial features, but not always
- Patients often isolated and housebound

Treatment is high doses of SSRIs.

Impulse Control and Conduct Disorders

These occur in people who are unable to resist impulses. Anxiety prior to the impulse is relieved after the patient acts on the impulse.

- Intermittent explosive disorder: episodes of aggression are out of proportion to the stressor
  - Possible history of head trauma
  - Requirements for diagnosis: age >6 and 2×/week for 3 months or more destructive episodes (assault) 3× in 12 months
  - After an outburst, there is a return to normal mood
  - Treatment is SSRIs and mood stabilizers
- Disruptive mood dysregulation disorder: children with a pervasively angry or irritable mood involving frequent aggressive outbursts that are out of proportion to the stressor
  - Requirements for diagnosis: age <10 and present for 12 months
  - After an outburst, there is not a return normal mood
- Kleptomania: individuals repeatedly steal items to relieve anxiety; the motivation to steal is not *need* of the item. Oftentimes, the patient will later replace the object.
- Pyromania: individuals who repeatedly lights fires; the motivation to set the fire is not personal gain (i.e., insurance money) or anger
  - Children who perform similar acts would be diagnosed with conduct disorder, in which there is a persistent pattern of behavior violating basic rights or societal rules; their motivation is to show anger.
- Pathologic gambling: individuals who are obsessed with gambling despite the consequences. Treatment is group psychotherapy (e.g., Gamblers Anonymous).

> If there is a history of drug intake, intermittent explosive disorder is not the diagnosis.

Psychosocial Problems

Types of Abuse

Class	Child Abuse/Nonaccidental Trauma	Adult Maltreatment/ Elder Abuse	Spousal Abuse
Definition of abuse	• **Physical is most common** (look for bruises, burns, lacerations, broken bones, shaken baby syndrome—do eye exam) • Neglect • Sexual exploitation (STDs) • Mental cruelty	• **Neglect is most common** (50% of all reported cases) • Physical • Psychological • Financial	• **Physical is most common** (#1 cause of injury to American women) • Psychological • Financial
Physician's role in care	1. Mandatory reporting up to age 18; all suspected cases must be reported 2. Protect the child (separate from parents) and consider admission to hospital	1. All suspected cases must be reported 2. Protect patient from abuser and consider admission to hospital	1. Reporting is not indicated 2. Provide information about local shelters and counseling

(continued next page)

Class	Child Abuse/Nonaccidental Trauma	Adult Maltreatment/ Elder Abuse	Spousal Abuse
Those at risk	• Age <1 year • Stepchildren • Premature children • Very active children • "Defective" children	• Caretaker is the most likely source of abuse; spouses are often caretakers	• More frequent in families with drug abuse, especially alcoholism • Victim often grew up in a violent home (50%) • Married at a young age • Dependent personalities • Pregnant, last trimester (highest risk)
Exam points	• Treat female circumcision as abuse • Do not mistake benign cultural practices ("coining," "moxibustion") for child abuse	• Mandatory reporting to Adult Protective Services	

Personality Disorders

Personality disorders (PDs) are pervasive, inflexible, and maladaptive thoughts or behaviors.

- **Males > females**: antisocial and narcissistic PDs
- **Females > males**: borderline and histrionic PDs

Treatment is psychotherapy. Mood stabilizers and antidepressants can be useful for cluster B type PDs.

Features	Examples
Cluster A: Peculiar thought processes, inappropriate affect	
Paranoid PD: • **Distrust and suspiciousness** - Individuals are mistrustful and suspicious of the motivations and actions of others and are often secretive and isolated. - They are emotionally cold and odd. - They often take legal action against other people. • Often confused with schizophrenia. • Main defense mechanism is projection.	A 62-year-old man lives in an apartment and constantly accuses his neighbors of stealing his mail and prying into his apartment. He believes that all his neighbors are conspiring to have him removed from the building.
Schizoid PD: • **Detachment and restricted emotionality** - Individuals are emotionally distant and fear intimacy with others. - They are absorbed in their own thoughts and feelings and disinterested.	A 68-year-old man lives and works in a lighthouse near a remote village. He is seen in town 2–3 times a year to purchase supplies. He has no known friends or family.

(continued next page)

Features	Examples
Schizotypal PD: • **Discomfort with social relationships, thought distortion, eccentricity** - Like schizoid PD except they also have magical thinking, clairvoyance, ideas of reference, or paranoid ideation. • Symptoms aren't severe enough for classification of schizophrenia	A 28-year-old man lives in a small coastal town attempting to start his own internet herbal business. He believes that the herbs have magical powers and he sells their magical properties of healing for a living. He believes that spirits are guiding him to wealth.
Cluster B: Mood lability, dissociative symptoms, preoccupation with rejection	

Histrionic PD:
 	
   - Colorful, exaggerated behavior and excitable, shallow expression of emotions
   - Use of physical appearance to draw attention to self
   - Sexually seductive
   - Discomfort in situations where not the center of attention.
	A 30-year-old woman presents to the doctor's office dressed in a sexually seductive manner and insists that the doctor comment on her appearance. When the doctor refuses to do so, she becomes upset.

Borderline PD: • Unstable affect, mood swings, marked impulsivity, unstable relationships, recurrent suicidal behaviors, chronic feelings of emptiness, identity disturbance, and inappropriate anger. Become intensely angered if they feel abandoned. • **Main defense mechanism is splitting.**	A 30-year-old woman presents to the clinic. She reports that she has been to many doctors, she said they were all wonderful until they started ignoring her or cutting her visits short, then she realized what terrible doctors they were. She starts the visit saying that the assistant at the front desk is the "worst she's ever seen" because she didn't smile at her. The other assistant was just wonderful according to her.
Antisocial PD: • Usually characterized by continuous antisocial or criminal acts, inability to conform to social rules, impulsivity, disregard for the rights of others, aggressiveness, lack of remorse, and deceitfulness.	A 26-year-old man is caught lighting forest fires. He reports that his mother is to blame, and he denies feeling regret. He is found to have had a history of legal problems since childhood. He has no friends and is hostile to everyone at the police station.
Narcissistic PD: • Usually characterized by a sense of self-importance, grandiosity, and preoccupation with fantasies of success. This person believes he is special, requires excessive admiration, reacts with rage when criticized, lacks empathy, is envious of others, and is interpersonally exploitative.	A patient is in the hospital for chest pain and becomes very agitated because he feels he is not getting enough attention. He reports that he is an important CEO and demands a special VIP room and more consideration and a dedicated nurse to attend his needs.
Cluster C: Anxiety, preoccupation with criticism, or rigidity	
Avoidant PD: • Individuals have social inhibition, feelings of inadequacy, and hypersensitivity to criticism. They shy away from starting anything new or attending social gatherings for fear of failure or rejection. They desire affection and acceptance and are open about their isolation and inability to interact with others.	A 45-year-old single man fears an upcoming social party being hosted by his parents. He dreads having to meet other people and doesn't feel comfortable speaking with others. He is planning on staying at home to avoid speaking to others.

(continued next page)

Features	Examples
Dependent PD: • **Submissive and clinging behavior related to a need to be taken care of.** Individuals are consumed with the need to be taken care of. They are clingy and worry about abandonment. They feel inadequate and helpless and avoid disagreements with others. They usually focus dependency on a family member or spouse.	A 28-year-old woman seeks counseling because of a recent relationship breakup. They were dating for 6 months. She continues to call her ex 15–20x/day even though he does not pick up. She says she can't understand why they broke up because she never disagreed with him. She never left the house without him, and she always asked for his opinion, even for little decisions. She cannot imagine a life without him.
Obsessive-Compulsive PD: • Individuals are preoccupied with orderliness, perfectionism, and control. They are often consumed by the details of everything and lose their sense of overall goals. They are strict and perfectionistic, overconscientious, and inflexible. Associated with difficult interpersonal relationships. • **Differentiated from obsessive-compulsive disorder**	A 38-year-old man presents with his wife for marital counseling. The wife reports that he is inflexible and has unrealistic demands of orderliness and an inflexible schedule. Both partners agree that his demands are causing marital problems.

Substance Use Disorders

Step 3 will test your ability to recognize substance abuse and know the best management for acute substance use and acute withdrawal.

Substance	Signs and Symptoms of Intoxication	Treatment of Intoxication	Signs and Symptoms of Withdrawal	Treatment of Withdrawal
Alcohol	Talkative, sullen, gregarious, moody	Mechanical ventilation if severe	Tremors, hallucinations, seizures, delirium	Long-acting benzos No seizure prophylaxis Disulfiram, naltrexone, or acamprosate (all FDA-approved)
Amphetamines, cocaine	Euphoria, hypervigilance, autonomic hyperactivity, weight loss, pupil dilatation, disturbed perception, stroke, myocardial infarction	Short-term use of antipsychotics, benzodiazepines, propranolol, vitamin C to promote excretion	Anxiety, tremors, headache, increased appetite, depression, risk of suicide	Antidepressants
Cannabis	Impaired motor coordination, impaired time perception, social withdrawal, increased appetite, dry mouth, tachycardia, conjunctival redness	None	Depression, irritability, decreased appetite (in chronic, daily users), Cannabinoid hyperemesis Syndrome (think: hot showers)	Supportive care and IV fluids if vomiting
Hallucinogens (e.g., LSD)	Ideas of reference, hallucinations, impaired judgment, dissociative symptoms, pupil dilatation, panic, tremors, incoordination	Supportive counseling (talking down), antipsychotics, benzodiazepines	None	None

(continued next page)

Substance	Signs and Symptoms of Intoxication	Treatment of Intoxication	Signs and Symptoms of Withdrawal	Treatment of Withdrawal
Inhalants	Belligerence, apathy, assaultiveness, impaired judgment, blurred vision, stupor, coma	Antipsychotics if delirious or agitated	None	None
Opiates	Apathy, dysphoria, constricted pupils, drowsiness, slurred speech, impaired memory, coma, death	Naloxone	Fever, chills, lacrimation, runny node, abdominal cramps, muscle spasms, insomnia, yawning	Clonidine, methadone, buprenorphine
PCP	Panic reactions, assaultiveness, agitation, nystagmus (vertical), HTN, seizures, coma, hyperacusis	Talking down, benzodiazepines, antipsychotics, support respiratory function	None	None
Barbiturates and benzodiazepines	Inappropriate sexual or aggressive behavior, impaired memory or concentration	Flumazenil (only in acute overdose, never in chronic) **(always the wrong answer on the exam)**	Autonomic hyperactivity, tremors, insomnia, seizures, anxiety	Substitute short-acting with long-acting (e.g., chlordiazepoxide) and then taper; use lorazepam or oxazepam in comorbid liver disease

> **Basic Science Correlate**
>
> Cocaine blocks the reuptake of norepinephrine serotonin and dopamine, while amphetamines induce the release of dopamine.

> **Basic Science Correlate**
>
> Opiates bind to mu, kappa, and/or delta receptors.

Alcohol Use Disorder

The presence of ≥**2** of these symptoms indicates an alcohol use disorder (AUD):

- Alcohol often taken in larger amounts or over a longer period than was intended
- Persistent desire or unsuccessful efforts to cut down or control alcohol use
- Investment of significant time in obtaining, using, or recovering from the effects of alcohol
- Craving for alcohol (i.e., strong desire or urge to use)

- Failure to fulfill major role obligations at work, school, or home as a consequence of recurrent alcohol use
- Continued alcohol use despite ongoing social/interpersonal problems caused or exacerbated by its effects
- Reduction or cessation of important social, occupational, or recreational activities because of alcohol use
- Recurrent alcohol use in situations in which it is physically hazardous
- Continued use despite knowledge of a physical or psychological problem arising from alcohol
- Tolerance, as defined by a need for markedly increased amounts of alcohol to achieve intoxication or desired effect *or* a markedly diminished effect with continued use of the same amount of alcohol
- Withdrawal, as manifested by characteristic alcohol withdrawal syndrome *or* use of alcohol/related substance e.g., benzodiazepine to relieve or avoid withdrawal symptoms

The severity of AUD is assessed based on how many symptoms are present:

- Mild: 2–3 symptoms
- Moderate: 4–5 symptoms
- Severe: 6 or more symptoms

Basic Science Correlate

Ethanol is converted to acetaldehyde by alcohol dehydrogenase.

Basic Science Correlate

Alcohol follows zero-order elimination kinetics, in which a constant quantity per time unit of the drug is eliminated.

The CAGE questionnaire is a widely used screening tool to identify problems with alcohol. It does not diagnose AUD; rather, a positive screen (≥ 2 "yes" answers) indicates the need for a more formal review of the diagnostic criteria to determine whether a diagnosis is warranted.

CAGE: "yes" to any 2 of the following questions is suggestive of AUD:

- Have you ever felt that you should **C**ut down your drinking?
- Have you ever felt **A**nnoyed by others who have criticized your drinking?
- Have you ever felt **G**uilty about your drinking?
- Have you ever had an **E**ye-opener to steady your nerves or alleviate a hangover?

On the Step 3 exam, when the question describes a patient with alcohol use, do the following:

- Order toxicology to look for use of other drugs: breath, blood, and urine drug screens.
- Look for secondary effects of alcohol use (but *not* for diagnosis): elevated GGTP, AST, ALT, and LDH.
- If there's suggestion of IV drug use (e.g., track marks), order HIV, hepatitis B, hepatitis C, and PPD (for tuberculosis).
- Alcoholics Anonymous (AA) is the **most effective treatment** for alcohol use disorder or prevention of relapse.

Other treatment measures include:

- Naltrexone implant for long-term treatment of opioid- and alcohol use disorders
- Acamprosate and disulfiram for alcohol use disorder
- Antidepressants only for alcohol use disorder when there is a comorbid psychiatric disorder

---

Basic Science Correlate

Disulfiram inhibits the enzyme acetaldehyde dehydrogenase, leading to a rise in acetaldehyde when alcohol is consumed. Acetaldehyde is responsible for the vomiting, headache, tachycardia, and sweating.

Acute Outpatient Management of Alcohol Use Disorder	Acute Inpatient Management Pearls	Chronic Maintenance Management
- Prevent further ETOH intake - Prevent individual from driving a car, operating machinery - Sedate patient if she becomes agitated - Transfer to inpatient	- Look for withdrawal symptoms - Prevent Wernicke-Korsakoff (ataxia, nystagmus, ophthalmoplegia, amnesia): Give IV or IM thiamine and magnesium ASAP; also give B12 and folate. - Benzodiazepine of choice is **chlordiazepoxide** or **diazepam** - Choose short-acting benzodiazepine *only* if the question describes patient with severe liver disease (prevent toxic metabolites)—**lorazepam** or **oxazepam** - Do *not* give seizure prophylaxis; repeated seizures should be treated with diazepam - Haloperidol is *never* the answer (reduces seizure threshold)	- Refer to inpatient rehabilitation or outpatient group therapy (e.g., AA) - Never give drug therapy without group psychotherapy - Naloxone and acamprosate decrease relapse rate only when given with psychotherapy - Disulfiram has poor compliance and hasn't been shown to be effective

Withdrawal Syndrome	Minor Withdrawal Symptoms	Alcoholic Hallucinosis	Withdrawal Seizure	Delirium Tremens
Onset after last drink	6 hours	12–24 hours	48 hours	48–96 hours
Symptoms	Insomnia, tremulousness, mild anxiety, headache, diaphoresis, palpitations	Visual hallucinations There may also be auditory and tactile hallucinations.	Tonic-clonic seizures	Hallucinations, disorientation, tachycardia, hypertension, low-grade fever, agitation, and diaphoresis
Exam tips	Give thiamine, folate, multivitamin, and glucose.	If there are hallucinations with disorientation, altered mental status, alcoholic hallucinosis is *not* the answer.	Get CT scan if repeated seizures to rule out structural or infectious cause.	Time of onset is important. This is the diagnosis if the case describes symptoms 2 days after last drink.

A 38-year-old man presents to the ED with acute-onset, right lower quadrant abdominal pain. He undergoes an appendectomy. Two days later he is found in his room disorientated and agitated, and is claiming to see snakes around him. Physical exam reveals tachycardia and temperature of 101.2°F. Which of the following is the most likely diagnosis?

a. Alcoholic hallucinosis

b. Delirium tremens

c. Korsakoff psychosis

d. Fentanyl withdrawal

e. Pulmonary embolism

Answer: **B.** Delirium tremens should always be suspected. The clue is that symptoms occur more than 2 days after the last drink. The question doesn't need to give you a history of alcohol use.

Cannabis Withdrawal

Longtime heavy users of marijuana experience psychological and physiological symptoms upon stopping use. A typical Step 3 patient case will describe a patient who uses cannabis daily for several months to years and then abruptly stops.

Symptoms typically manifest within 24–72 hours and commonly include irritability, difficulty sleeping, depression, fevers, and nausea and vomiting. It is unknown what amount, duration, and frequency of cannabis use are required to produce an associated withdrawal disorder during a quit attempt.

Treatment is supportive care.

A 27-year-old woman is brought to the ED by EMS in response to a bystander's report that she was yelling, singing, and dancing in the street. A bag of "K2" was found in her possession. The patient is agitated and slamming her chair against the walls. On examination her eyes are not injected. Urine toxicology is negative for all usual substances. What is the most likely diagnosis?

a. Cocaine intoxication
b. Synthetic cannabinoid use
c. Alcohol intoxication
d. LSD use
e. PCP use

Answer: **B.** The lack of a positive toxicology screen in this patient and the findings of euphoria, aggression, and altered mental status help make the diagnosis. Synthetic cannabinoids such as K2 are a commonly abused street drug that, like LSD or PCP, present with aggression, but the symptoms wear off more quickly. Synthetic cannabinoids fit into the same receptors in the brain as THC and thus can induce similar euphoric effects.

Caffeine Withdrawal

Any withdrawal syndrome that occurs after abrupt cessation of caffeine intake is regarded as caffeine withdrawal. Headache is the most common symptom, but depression, anxiety, difficulty concentrating, and fatigue may also be seen.

If caffeine abstinence is unintentional, the patient can simply consume caffeine to relieve withdrawal symptoms. If abstinence is intentional, however, symptoms typically resolve within days.

Human Sexuality

Homosexuality

Homosexuality is *not* a mental illness but instead is classified as a variant of human sexuality.

Sexual Dysfunction

Pharmacological Agents That Cause Sexual Dysfunction	
Drug	**Effect**
α1-blockers	Impaired ejaculation
SSRIs	Inhibited orgasm
β-blockers	Erectile dysfunction
Trazodone	Priapism
Dopamine agonists	↑ erection and libido
Neuroleptics	Erectile dysfunction

Paraphilic Disorder

Paraphilias involve recurrent, sexually arousing preoccupations, which are usually focused on humiliation and/or suffering and the use of nonliving objects and nonconsenting partners. Occurs for more than 6 months and causes impairment in patient's level of functioning.

Treatment is individual psychotherapy and aversive conditioning. For severe impairment, antiandrogens or SSRIs can help to reduce patient's sexual drive.

- Voyeurism (earliest paraphilia to develop): recurrent urges to observe an unsuspecting person who is engaging in sexual activity or disrobing
- Pedophilia (most common paraphilia): recurrent urges or arousal toward prepubescent children
- Exhibitionism: recurrent urge to expose oneself to strangers
- Fetishism: involves the use of nonliving objects usually associated with the human body
- Frotteurism: recurrent urge or behavior involving touching or rubbing against a nonconsenting partner
- Masochism: recurrent urge or behavior involving the act of humiliation
- Sadism: recurrent urge or behavior involving acts in which physical or psychological suffering of a victim is exciting to the patient

Premenstrual Dysphoric Disorder

Premenstrual dysphoric disorder is a severe form of premenstrual syndrome that includes physical and behavioral symptoms. The underlying etiology is unknown.

- Extreme mood shifts that can disrupt work and damage relationships, including extreme sadness, hopelessness, irritability, and anger
- Physical symptoms include breast tenderness and bloating

Diagnosis is made with ≥ 5 of the following symptoms:

- Marked lability
- Marked irritability or anger
- Markedly depressed mood
- Marked anxiety and tension
- Decreased interest in usual activities
- Difficulty concentrating
- Lethargy and marked lack of energy
- Marked change in appetite
- Hypersomnia or insomnia
- Feeling overwhelmed or out of control
- Physical symptoms

Symptoms usually resolve with the onset of menstruation. For severe cases, treat with cognitive behavioral therapy and SSRIs.

Gender Dysphoria Disorder

Patients with gender dysphoria disorder experience significant distress in response to the sex they were assigned at birth. Symptoms in children include anxiety with regard to their own genitalia, social isolation from their peers, anxiety, loneliness, and depression. Patients have a strong desire to be acknowledged and treated as the other gender or to alter their current sex characteristics surgically.

Diagnosis is made in adolescent or adult patients who have experienced symptoms ≥6 months.

Treatment may include psychotherapy or may support the individual's preferred gender through hormone therapy, gender expression and role, and/or surgery.

PART 11

Emergency Medicine/ Toxicology

Overdose

Acetaminophen

The clinical course of acetaminophen overdose is as follows:

- First 24 hours: nausea and vomiting, which resolve
- 48–72 hours later: hepatic failure

It is safe to give charcoal and N-acetylcysteine (NAC) at the same time. Know the following about treating an acetaminophen overdose:

- Give NAC to anyone with possible overdose of a toxic amount; it is benign
- NAC is useful to prevent liver toxicity for up to 24 hours after the ingestion. After 24 hours, there is no specific therapy to prevent or reverse the liver toxicity of acetaminophen.
- Vomiting patients can get NAC through the IV route.

If the amount of ingestion is equivocal, then get an acetaminophen level to determine if there will be toxicity but do not wait for the results to give NAC if the overdose is large.

- 10 g → toxic
- 15 g → fatal

The amounts needed for toxicity and fatality are lower if there is underlying liver disease or alcohol abuse.

Extra NAC never hurt anyone. Untreated acetaminophen overdose will kill the patient.

A man is brought to the ED a few hours after ingesting a bottle of extra-strength acetaminophen. What is the next best step in management?

a. Urine toxicology screen
b. N-acetylcysteine
c. Acetaminophen level
d. Transfer to the ICU
e. Liver function tests
f. Gastric emptying

Answer: **B.** The specific antidote is more important than waiting for a level with acetaminophen overdose. On a CCS case, do both. Do not transfer patient to the ICU without doing something for him first.

Aspirin/Salicylates

Aspirin acts as a direct stimulant to the brainstem, causing hyperventilation. A patient with an aspirin overdose will always be hyperventilating.

In addition, aspirin is a toxin to the lungs, causing acute respiratory distress syndrome (ARDS).

Other findings with aspirin overdose include:

- Metabolic acidosis, from the loss of Krebs cycle in mitochondria; the result is lactic acidosis from hypoxic metabolism and anion gap is elevated
- Respiratory alkalosis, which always precedes the metabolic acidosis
- Renal insufficiency: salicylates, like other NSAIDs, are directly toxic to the kidney tubule
- Elevated PT: aspirin interferes with the production of vitamin K-dependent clotting factors
- CNS: confusion; severe cases can lead to seizures and coma
- Fever

> The easiest way to identify the aspirin overdose patient is tinnitus.

On CCS, order a CBC, chemistry panel, ABG, PT/INR/PTT, and salicylate (ASA) level.

Treatment is alkalinization of the urine to increase excretion and charcoal to block absorption. Use dialysis for severe cases.

CCS Tip: Alkalinize the urine with D^5W with 3 amps of bicarbonate. Alkalinization of the urine facilitates excretion of the following:

- Salicylates (ASA)
- Tricyclic antidepressants (will show up on the urine tox you ordered)
- Phenobarbital
- Chlorpropamide

Benzodiazepines

Benzodiazepine overdose by itself is not fatal. Let the patient sleep! Move the clock forward on CCS, and the overdose will pass.

Do not administer flumazenil for benzodiazepine overdose to patients in the ED. You do not know who has chronic dependency, and flumazenil can induce benzodiazepine withdrawal and seizures.

Burns and Carbon Monoxide

When a patient has been in a fire, the most important step is to give 100% oxygen. The most common cause of death in fires is carbon monoxide (CO) poisoning, i.e., it causes 60% of deaths in the first 24 hours. (Later on, the most common cause of death is infection.)

After that, determine who needs to be intubated and who can be managed with just fluids.

- Intubate if hoarseness, wheezing, stridor, or burns inside the nose or mouth is present
- If respiratory injury is not present, manage with fluids in high volume.
  - Calculate the replacement fluid on the percentage of skin with second and third degree burns.
  - Give 4 mL of Ringer's or normal saline for each kilogram x the percentage of body surface burned.

Carbon Monoxide Poisoning

Carboxyhemoglobin (COHg) does not release oxygen to tissues, so CO poisoning is the same as anemia and asphyxiation.

Presentation includes:

- Shortness of breath
- Lightheadedness and headaches
- Disorientation
- Metabolic acidosis due to tissue hypoxia (in severe disease)

CO poisoning commonly presents in families that are "snowed in" and can't leave their house with a wood-burning stove. Everyone is fatigued and has a headache. Look for the phrase "He feels better when he is shoveling snow."

If CO poisoning is suspected, call an ambulance. Treat all survivors of a fire with 100% oxygen until you have their CO level.

> On CCS, order aspirin, acetaminophen, and alcohol (ETOH) level on all overdose patients. There is a very high frequency of co-ingestion.

Digoxin

Digoxin overdose presents with GI disturbance (most common), e.g., nausea, vomiting, diarrhea, and pain, as well as the following:

- Blurred vision and seeing yellow "halos" around objects
- Arrhythmia: anything is possible (you may see PR prolongation and you may see "paroxysmal atrial tachycardia with block")
- Encephalopathy

*Hypo*kalemia may lead to digoxin toxicity, but digoxin toxicity leads to *hyper*-kalemia from poisoning of the sodium/potassium ATPase.

Treatment is digoxin-binding antibodies (Digibind) for severe disease (i.e., CNS and cardiac abnormalities)

Ethylene Glycol and Methanol

Overdose from ethylene glycol and methanol presents with intoxication and metabolic acidosis with increased anion gap.

Ethylene glycol presents with:

- Renal insufficiency from direct toxicity
- Hypocalcemia from precipitation of the oxalic acid with the calcium
- Kidney stones

Methanol presents with:

- Visual disturbance
- Retinal hyperemia from the toxicity of the formic acid

Treatment is ethanol or fomepizole. Dialysis will remove them from the body before they are metabolized into the toxic metabolite.

Methemoglobinemia

Methemoglobinemia involves hemoglobin locked in an oxidized state that will not allow it to pick up oxygen. Symptoms include:

- Cyanosis
- Shortness of breath
- Dizziness, headache, confusion
- Seizures

Look for a history of use of nitrate, anesthetics, dapsone, or other oxidants, as well as any of the drugs ending in *-caine.* (lidocaine, benzocaine).

Methemoglobinemia can caused by something as small as the anesthetic sprayed into the throat of someone who is to undergo intubation. It can also be caused by nitroglycerin.

Diagnostic testing is as follows:

- Normal pO_2 on ABG with chocolate-brownish blood (oxidized blood)
- Methemoglobin level

Treatment is 100% oxygen. Methylene blue restores the hemoglobin to its normal state.

> If cyanotic + normal pO_2, think of methemoglobinemia.

Neuroleptic Malignant Syndrome/Malignant Hyperthermia

This syndrome is unrelated to dosage or previous drug exposure. Patients are often those who recently started taking antipsychotics (particularly haloperidol) or Parkinson patients who have recently stopped levodopa.

Look for high fever, tachycardia, muscle rigidity, altered consciousness, elevated CPK, and autonomic dysfunction. Mortality rate is 20%.

Treatment starts with transferring to the ICU and giving IV fluids.

- Discontinue antipsychotic
- Give bromocriptine to overcome dopamine receptor blockade (bromocriptine is a potent dopamine D2 receptor agonist)
- Give muscle relaxant dantrolene or diazepam to reduce muscle rigidity

A 46-year-old woman is brought to the ED by her husband after a suicide attempt. She is confused, lethargic, and disoriented. Her respiratory rate is 8/min and blood pressure 120/80 mm Hg. What is the most important next step?

a. Oxygen
b. Bolus of normal saline
c. Naloxone, thiamine, dextrose
d. Endotracheal intubation
e. Gastric emptying
f. Urine toxicology screen

Answer: **C.** With an acute change in mental status of unclear etiology, administer antidotes such as naloxone, dextrose, and thiamine. Oxygen does nothing specific. Gastric emptying is less useful than a specific antidote, and should be used only if the overdose clearly occurred during the last hour. With an acute change in mental status, hypoglycemia is a very common cause, as is an opiate overdose.

In a CCS case, give naloxone, dextrose, and thiamine, and give oxygen and saline while checking the toxicology screen—all at the same time.

Lithium

Suspect lithium toxicity when the question describes an elderly patient who takes lithium with renal failure or hyponatremia (may be caused by diuretics, vomiting, dehydration). The question will describe nausea, vomiting, acute disorientation, tremors, increased DTRs, and even seizures.

Treatment is dialysis.

For the exam, know the different features of lithium toxicity, MAOI-induced hypertension, serotonin syndrome, and neuroleptic malignant syndrome.

Basic Science Correlate

Lithium can also result in nephrogenic diabetes insipidus. Lithium accumulates in the collecting duct through epithelial sodium channels. This leads to resistance to ADH by increasing urinary prostaglandin E2, which induces lysosomal degradation of aquaporin 2 water channels.

Basic Science Correlate

Antipsychotics cause NMS through D2 receptor blockade in the hypothalamus, nigrostriatal pathways, and spinal cord. This leads to muscle rigidity, tremor, and elevated temperature. In the periphery, antipsychotics lead to increased calcium release from the sarcoplasmic reticulum, which leads to rigidity and muscle cell breakdown.

Serotonin Syndrome

Serotonin syndrome is the diagnosis when the case describes a history of SSRI use and the use of migraine medication (triptans) or an MAOI. Symptoms include agitation, hyperreflexia, hyperthermia, and muscle rigidity with volume contraction secondary to sweating and insensible fluid loss.

Treatment is as follows:

- IV fluids
- Cyproheptadine (a histamine-1 receptor antagonist with nonspecific 5-HT1A and 5-HT2A antagonistic properties) to decrease serotonin production
- Benzodiazepine to reduce muscle rigidity

MAOI-Induced Hypertensive Crisis

Consider this diagnosis if the history describes a patient with acute hypertension and a history of MAOI use and either antihistamines, nasal decongestants, or consumption of tyramine-rich foods (cheeses, pickled foods). May also be seen in patients who take an MAOI and a TCA concurrently.

Basic Science Correlate

MAOIs inhibit the breakdown of dietary amines. This raises levels of tyramine, which in turn displaces norepinephrine from the storage vesicles, leading to hypertensive crisis.

Treat as hypertensive crisis. There is no specific antihypertensive indicated.

A 40-year-old woman with a history of bipolar disorder presents with confusion, ataxia, and tremors. She was recently treated for acne with clindamycin and has had diarrhea for 2 weeks. She began to have nausea and vomiting yesterday. On examination her deep tendon reflexes are 4+ and brisk, but no other focal neurologic deficits are discerned. What is the most likely diagnosis?

a. Lithium toxicity
b. Sepsis
c. Serotonin syndrome
d. Parkinson disease
e. Stroke

Answer: **A.** Lithium toxicity presents with disorientation, tremors, nausea, vomiting, and increased deep tendon reflexes. The most common cause of lithium toxicity is dehydration, which this patient is likely suffering from due to her antibiotic exposure (which, incidentally, was for acne that is also a side effect of lithium!).

Basic Science Correlate

Lithium can also result in nephrogenic diabetes insipidus. Lithium accumulates in the collecting duct through epithelial sodium channels. This leads to resistance to ADH by increasing urinary prostaglandin E2, which induces lysosomal degradation of aquaporin 2 water channels.

Basic Science Correlate

Antipsychotics cause NMS through D2 receptor blockade in the hypothalamus, nigrostriatal pathways, and spinal cord. This leads to muscle rigidity, tremor, and elevated temperature. In the periphery, antipsychotics lead to increased calcium release from the sarcoplasmic reticulum, which leads to rigidity and muscle cell breakdown.

Opiates

Opiate toxicity leads to death from respiratory depression. One cannot die from opiate withdrawal.

Treatment is naloxone for acute overdose.

Use buprenorphine, a partial opioid receptor moderator, to treat opioid addiction. Like methadone, it can be used to detoxify a patient from opioid addiction or to maintain a patient with chronic use.

Serotonin Syndrome

Serotonin syndrome is the diagnosis when the case describes a history of SSRI use and the use of migraine medication (triptans) or an MAOI. The patient will present with agitation, hyperreflexia, hyperthermia, and muscle rigidity with volume contraction secondary to sweating and insensible fluid loss.

Treatment is as follows:

- IV fluids
- Cyproheptadine to decrease serotonin production. Cyproheptadine is a histamine-1 receptor antagonist with nonspecific 5-HT1A and 5-HT2A antagonistic properties.
- Benzodiazepine to reduce muscle rigidity

Treat as hypertensive crisis. There is no specific antihypertensive indicated.

> **What is the first assessment prior to prescribing antidepressants?**
>
> a. CBC
> b. Family history of depression
> c. Previous use of antidepressants
> d. Suicidal ideation
> e. Thyroid function tests
>
> Answer: **D.** Always assess for suicidal ideation prior to starting antidepressants, as there is an increased risk in suicidal ideation in some patients within the first 2 weeks. If the patient is acutely suicidal, you must hospitalize and consider electroconvulsive therapy.

Heat

All heat disorders present with rhabdomyolysis. When severe, possible confusion or seizures may result, as well as a potentially life-threatening rhythm disturbance from the hyperkalemia.

All the heat conditions have similar symptoms (confusion, seizures, hyperkalemia, arrhythmias), but their treatments are entirely different.

- Neuroleptic malignant syndrome (NMS)
  - Look for ingestion of neuroleptic medication, e.g., phenothiazines
  - No specific diagnostic test
  - CPK and potassium can be elevated; muscle rigidity is common
  - Treatment is a dopamine-agonist (cabergoline or bromocriptine) or dantrolene
- Malignant hyperthermia (no clinical distinction from NMS, just different risks of medications)
  - Look for a history of anesthetic use
  - Treatment is dantrolene

- Heat stroke (heat disorder from exertion and high outside temperatures)
  - Look for outside activity with high temperature, along with exertion and dehydration
  - Treatment is physical removal of heat from the body; spray patient with water and fan with air-conditioning or ice baths/packs, but do not infuse iced saline into the body since that could stop the heart

	Heat Exhaustion	Heat Stroke
Presenting symptoms	Excessive sweating Nausea/vomiting	Dry skin Altered mental status
Body temperature	Elevated	Elevated
Treatment	Normal saline IV (room temp) and remove patient from hot environment	Spray patient with water and apply ice baths/packs

The table compares heat stroke, neuroleptic malignant syndrome, and malignant hyperthermia.

	NMS	Malignant Hyperthermia	Heat Stroke
Risk	Antipsychotic medications	Anesthetics	Exertion on hot days
Presentation	• High temperature • Confusion • Arrhythmia • Hyperkalemia	Same	Same
Lab testing	CPK and potassium elevated	Same	Same
Treatment	Bromocriptine Dantrolene	Dantrolene	Hydration and external cooling (ice baths/packs, spraying with water and evaporation)

When is **gastric emptying** the answer?

- Almost never. Gastric emptying is useful only in the first hour after an overdose.
  - 1 hour: 50% of pills can be removed
  - 1–2 hours: 15% of pills can be removed
  - 2 hours: it is useless
- Furthermore, gastric emptying can never be performed when caustics (acids and alkalis) have been ingested.
- Intubation and lavage can rarely be performed if the patient has ingested the substance within the last 1–2 hours and there is no response to naloxone, dextrose, and thiamine.

When is **naloxone, thiamine,** and **dextrose** the answer?

- When there is an acute mental status change of unclear etiology

When is **charcoal** the answer?

- Most overdose cases. If you have a toxicology case and don't know what to do, give charcoal. It won't harm anyone.

Ipecac syrup can never be used in a patient with altered mental status because the patient will aspirate (and you will fail). Ipecac is never used in children.

CCS Tip: In overdose cases, do multiple things simultaneously. If there is a change in mental status, give naloxone, thiamine, and dextrose at the same time you check a toxicology screen, give oxygen, and do routine labs.

Following is the overdose case "menu":

- Specific antidote if the etiology is clear
- Toxicology screen
- Charcoal
- CBC, chemistry, urinalysis
- Psychiatry consultation if overdose is the result of a suicide attempt
- Oxygen for carbon monoxide poisoning or any dyspneic patient

The table lists antidotes for overdose.

Substance	Antidote
Acetaminophen	N-acetylcysteine
Aspirin	Bicarbonate to alkalinize the urine
Benzodiazepines	Do *not* give flumazenil; it may precipitate a seizure
Carbon monoxide	100% oxygen, hyperbaric in some cases
Digoxin	Digoxin-binding antibodies
Ethylene glycol	Fomepizole or ethanol
Methanol	Fomepizole or ethanol
Methemoglobinemia	Methylene blue
Neuroleptic malignant syndrome	Bromocriptine, dantrolene
Opiates	Naloxone
Organophosphates	Atropine, pralidoxime
Tricyclic antidepressants	Bicarbonate protects the heart

Neuroleptics/Anesthetics/Heat

All heat disorders present with rhabdomyolysis. When severe, possible confusion or seizures may result, as well as a potentially life-threatening rhythm disturbance from the hyperkalemia.

Neuroleptic Malignant Syndrome (NMS)

Look for the ingestion of neuroleptic medication, such as phenothiazines. NMS has no specific diagnostic test. CPK and potassium levels can be elevated. Muscle rigidity is common.

Treat with the dopamine agonists cabergoline or bromocriptine. Dantrolene is also effective.

Malignant Hyperthermia

Look for a history of anesthetic use. There is *no* clinical distinction between NMS and malignant hyperthermia, just different risks of medications. Treat with dantrolene.

Heat Stroke

Heat stroke is a heat disorder from exertion and high outside temperatures. You can only get heat stroke when the outside temperature is high and you are dehydrated or exerting yourself.

Although the symptoms of confusion, seizures, hyperkalemia, and arrhythmias are the same as those seen in NMS and malignant hyperthermia, the treatment is entirely different.

Treatment is physical removal of heat from the body. Spray the patient with water and fan the patient with air-conditioning or ice baths/packs.

Do not infuse iced saline into the body, since that could stop the heart.

	Heat Exhaustion	Heat Stroke
Presenting symptoms	Excessive sweating Nausea/vomiting	Dry skin Altered mental status
Body temperature	Elevated	Elevated
Treatment	Normal saline IV (room temp) and remove patient from hot environment	Spray patient with water and apply ice baths/packs

The table compares heat stroke, neuroleptic malignant syndrome, and malignant hyperthermia.

	NMS	Malignant Hyperthermia	Heat Stroke
Risk	Antipsychotic medications	Anesthetics	Exertion on hot days
Presentation	• High temperature • Confusion • Arrhythmia • Hyperkalemia	Same	Same
Lab testing	CPK and potassium elevated	Same	Same
Treatment	Bromocriptine Dantrolene	Dantrolene	Hydration and external cooling (ice baths/packs, spraying with water and evaporation)

Tricyclic Antidepressants

Death from overdose on tricyclic antidepressants tends to occur from seizures or arrhythmia.

A patient with a history of depression comes in with an overdose resulting from a suicide attempt. There was a bottle of amitriptyline nearby. What is the most urgent step?

a. Charcoal
b. Gastric lavage
c. Transfer to ICU
d. EKG
e. EEG
f. Head CT
g. Administer bicarbonate

Answer: **D.** In tricyclic overdose, the most urgent step is to perform an EKG to see if there is widening of the QRS. Those with a wide QRS are most likely to develop ventricular tachycardia or torsade de pointes. If there is a wide QRS or an arrhythmia, give bicarbonate and transfer to the ICU. Gastric lavage is not as important as protecting the heart. Alkalinizing the patient with bicarbonate carries its own risks. Therefore, you would want to find out first whether the patient really needs the bicarbonate.

Other effects of tricyclics are related to their anticholinergic effects:

- Dilated pupils
- Dry mouth
- Constipation
- Urinary retention

Organophosphate Poisoning

Organophosphates inhibit acetylcholinesterase, blocking the metabolism of acetylcholine and, therefore, enormously increasing the effect of acetylcholine.

Presentation includes:

- Salivation
- Lacrimation
- Urination
- Diarrhea
- Wheezing from bronchospasm

In the presentation, look for a crop duster exposed to insecticides or a survivor of nerve-gas attack.

Treatment is first with atropine and then pralidoxime (**most effective treatment**). Remove the clothes and wash the rest off the patient.

> Make sure not to spread the contaminant. When caring for victims of a nerve-gas attack, be certain you are protected. The toxin is absorbed through the skin.

Bites

Arachnid Bites

- Black widow spider
  - Presents with abdominal pain, rigidity, and hypocalcemia
  - Presents as if there were a perforated abdominal organ but there is pain without tenderness
  - Treatment is antivenin
- Brown recluse spider
  - Presents with local necrosis, bullae, and dark lesions
  - Treatment is debridement of the wound; steroids and dapsone may help
- Centruroides scorpion (inhabits the U.S. Southwest and Mexico, warm/dry environments)
  - Presents with local pain and paresthesia as a result of the neurotoxin that scorpion injects
  - Severe CN nerve defects (vision, eye movement, slurred speech)
  - Neuromuscular skeletal muscle dysfunction (**most severe effect**)
  - Cholinergic excess causes bradycardia, secretions, and vomiting.
  - Diagnosis made by history of sting, pain on tapping site, and abnormal eye movements with normal mental status; there is no diagnostic test
  - Treatment is management of secretions, pain, and airway; use antivenin and atropine for very severe cases

Rabies

Bats are the most common rabies vector; raccoons, skunks, and dogs are less common.

After any bat bite or other suspicious animal bite, give postexposure prophylaxis (PEP) immediately with **rabies immune globulin and vaccine.** Also give PEP if patient wakes to find a bat flying in the room.

Symptoms are encephalopathy, hydrophobia (fear of water), and aerophobia (fear of air). Once rabies has become symptomatic, however, there is no treatment.

Hypothermia

Look for an alcoholic falling asleep outside in winter. Hypothermia kills with rhythm disturbance.

The most urgent step is to perform an **EKG: "J-waves of Osborn,"** which look like ST segment elevation, are the most specific finding.

Acute Altitude Sickness

Ascending to an altitude above 8,000 feet (2,500 meters) leads to:

- Headache (like an alcohol hangover)
- Malaise, slurred speech, abnormal coordination
- Sleep disturbance
- Acute pulmonary edema

The only way to stop the symptoms is rapid descent from altitude.

Prevent altitude sickness by **acclimating to 6,000 feet** before ascending higher and using **acetazolamide**. Other preventive medications are dexamethasone, nifedipine, and tadalafil.

Climbing with inhaled oxygen markedly reduces the likelihood of developing altitude sickness.

PART **12**

Ethics

Autonomy

Autonomy is the most frequently tested subject on Step 3. The most fundamental ethical concept is that an adult with the capacity to understand his medical problems can refuse any therapy or test.

- It does not matter if the treatment or test is simple, safe, and risk-free.
- It does not matter if the person will die without the treatment or test.
- As long as the patient can understand the situation, he has the right to refuse the treatment or test.

Respecting autonomy is more important than trying to do the right thing for a patient. Trying to do the right thing for a patient is called beneficence.

An adult who is alert and not mentally handicapped is deemed to have capacity to understand his own medical procedures and treatments. Capacity is determined by physicians.

"Competence" (a legal term) is determined by courts and judges.

A 35-year-old mentally intact patient is refusing radiation for a stage I lymphoma. The treatment has a 95% chance of cure and virtually no adverse effects. What do you do?

a. Try to discuss it with him
b. Honor his wishes
c. Order a psychiatric consultation
d. Arrange an ethics committee consultation
e. Get a court order

Answer: **A.** Even though an adult patient with capacity can refuse anything, the USMLE wants you to discuss things first. Even though you may eventually honor his wishes, if an answer says "meet," "confer," or "discuss," then do that first.

When a patient's capacity to understand is not clear, the answer should be "psychiatry consultation."

In other words, psychiatry consultation is not needed when the patient is clearly competent. Nor is it needed when the patient is in a coma and clearly doesn't have the capacity to understand.

Minors

Minors, by definition, are not determined to have the capacity to understand their medical problems until age 18. However, the Step 3 exam does like to test your understanding of the emancipated minor.

- **Emancipation** means that, although the patient is age <18, he can make his own decisions. Emancipated minors are living independently and self-supporting, married, or in the military.
- **Partial emancipation** is considered to be present for the following issues: sex; reproductive health; and substance abuse
  - If the patient is a minor and seeks treatment for contraception, STDs, HIV, or prenatal care, she is partially emancipated.
  - In other words, she can make these decisions on her own, and her privacy is to be respected like that of an adult.
  - **An exception is abortion**: 36 states have parental notification laws for abortion.

How does the USMLE exam get around issues that are not universal across the United States?

- The answer is a safe and universally correct answer, e.g., "Recommend that the patient inform the parents."

Another topic of concern with respect to minors is that parents cannot refuse life-saving therapy for minors. If a blood transfusion would save the life of their child, the parents cannot refuse. Doing so would be considered child abuse.

Jehovah's Witnesses may refuse therapy for themselves but not for a child.

Informed Consent

Informed consent is based on autonomy. Only a fully informed patient with the capacity to understand the issues can grant "informed consent."

For the consent to be informed, the patient must be informed of the following:

- Benefits of the procedure (how will it help)
- Risks of the procedure
- Alternatives to the procedure
- Information is in a language patient can understand
- The informed consent must be given for each procedure (specificity)

Emergencies

Consent is implied in an emergency when there is not sufficient time to determine capacity or prior wishes. If prior wishes are fully known, then this information takes precedence.

Consent obtained via telephone is considered valid. If the patient's proxy is not present at the time of the procedure, consent obtained via the telephone counts.

Pregnancy

- Treatment: Pregnant women can refuse treatment, even if the life of the fetus is at risk. Until the fetus comes out, it is considered part of the woman's body. So a woman could refuse a blood transfusion during pregnancy, even if the life of the fetus is at risk. Once the baby is born, however, she cannot refuse treatment for the baby.
- Abortion: A woman's right to an abortion varies by trimester of pregnancy. Consent of the father is not required for the abortion.
  - First trimester: woman has an unrestricted right to an abortion
  - Second trimester: woman has access but her rights are less clear
  - Third trimester: there is no clear access to abortion in the third trimester; in third trimester, the fetus is potentially viable
- Donation of gametes: Patients have an unrestricted right to donate sperm and eggs. There is no ethical problem with being a paid donor for sperm and eggs (note, however, that one cannot be a paid donor for organs, e.g., the kidney or corneas).

Confidentiality

The patient has an absolute right to privacy concerning his own medical information. The following persons do not have a right to any of the medical information of the patient:

- Relatives, employers, friends, and spouses
- Other physicians: If a physician seeks medical information about a patient, you cannot release it without the express consent of the patient.
- Members of law enforcement: You cannot release medical information to courts or police without a court order or subpoena.

Hence, only a patient can obtain or ask for her medical information to be released. A current physician cannot obtain a patient's previous medical records without her direct consent.

Breaking Confidentiality to Prevent Harm to Others

An exception to the privacy rule is in the circumstance of protecting other people.

- If a patient has a transmissible disease, such as tuberculosis or HIV, the physician can violate the patient's confidentiality to protect innocent third parties. If you have tuberculosis, for example, your doctor can contact your close associates without your consent if they are at risk. If you have syphilis, HIV, or gonorrhea, your doctor can safely inform others without your consent that they may be at risk.

- The classic example is of a patient with a psychiatric illness who may be planning to harm others. The physician has the right to break your confidentiality to alert the person at risk to prevent harm.

This issue comes down entirely to whether another person may be harmed by the patient's illness or actions. If you have a dangerous disease and your doctor does *not* inform the innocent third party at risk, then that physician is liable for harm that befalls the innocent person.

End-of-Life Issues

Autonomy as applied to end-of-life issues is the most important subject for the test and for patient autonomy.

Withholding and Withdrawing of Care

Withholding of care and withdrawing of care are considered indistinguishable from the point of view of the test and of proper ethical behavior. An adult with capacity can withhold or withdraw any form of therapy. If the patient begins therapy, he has the right to withdraw that care. The reasons for the withdrawal or withholding of care are *not* important.

Advance Directives

An advance directive is a set of instructions from an adult patient with capacity directing the care of himself or herself prior to losing capacity.

Health Care Proxy

The strongest advance directive is a health care proxy. The proxy is both a document describing the care the person desires as well as the appointment of an agent to be the decision maker. The agent as a decision maker does not take hold until the patient loses the capacity to make a decision. If I appoint a proxy but I am still here, alert, and communicative, you cannot ask the agent for consent for my procedures.

Living Will

A living will is a written document outlining the care desired by the patient. If a patient does not have a health care proxy, the living will can be very useful to outline the care she wants. If the patient writes out, "I never want to be intubated," this is valid. If she writes, "No heroic measures," this is not valid. To be useful, a living will must be clear and precise.

Do Not Resuscitate (DNR) Orders

The DNR order means the refusal of endotracheal intubation and cardiopulmonary resuscitation in the event of the loss of the ability to breathe or the heart stopping. A DNR order does not mean the elimination of testing or medical therapy.

Patient with No Capacity and No Advance Directive (Proxy or Living Will)

This is the most complex and the most common circumstance. In this case, the care is based on the best understanding of the patient's wishes for herself. Family and friends attempt to outline what they heard the patient say she wanted. This is *not* the same as saying "This is what is best for the patient." Decisions are based on the best possible understanding of clearly expressed wishes. If there is no clear expression of wishes, then the weakest basis on which to act is the "best interests of the patient."

Ethics Committee

The ethics committee is used for cases in which the following are true:

- The patient is not an adult with capacity.
- There are no clearly stated wishes on the part of the patient.

Also, the ethics committee is the answer if:

- The caregivers, such as the family, are split or in disagreement about the nature of the care. If some family members say, "He never wanted to be on a ventilator, ever," and some family members say, "He might have wanted a ventilator sometime," then this is a case for an ethics committee.

Court Order

This option comes into play only when all the other options have not given clarity. If there is disagreement after all the other steps, including an ethics committee, which cannot reach a clear determination of care, then a court order is the answer. You do *not* need a court order if the proxy clearly states wishes or the family is in agreement.

Fluid and Nutrition Issues

An adult patient with capacity may refuse all forms of nutrition. There is no ethical basis for forcing fluids or nutrition upon a patient. If the patient is not an adult with the capacity to understand, the proxy or living will can direct the removal of fluid and nutrition, provided the patient's clearly expressed wishes while competent stated that no artificial nutrition be started. In the absence of clearly stated wishes on the issue of fluids and nutrition, they should be given.

Physician-Assisted Suicide and Euthanasia

- **Physician-assisted suicide** means providing the patient with the means to end her own life. **This is always wrong.**
- **Euthanasia** means the physician directly administers the means of ending the patient's life. **This is always wrong.**

These are *not* the same as providing pain medications that may end the patient's life. It is ethical to give pain medication, even if the only way to relieve pain may result in the inadvertent shortening of life. The primary difference is intent:

- In physician-assisted suicide, the primary intent is to end life.
- With a life shortened by pain medication, the primary intent is to relieve suffering.

Futile Care

There is *no* obligation on the part of the physician to provide care that will not work. There is no obligation to provide treatments without possible benefit.

> A patient with widely metastatic cervical cancer develops renal failure. The family insists that dialysis be started. What do you tell them?
>
> Answer: You do not have to provide dialysis to a person who will certainly die and not benefit from the treatment.

Brain Death

You are not obliged to provide care for a brain-dead patient.

Brain death = dead.

HIV Issues

A **patient has a right to confidentiality** of his HIV status. However, this confidentiality can be broken to protect the uninfected, such as sexual and needle-sharing partners.

There is **no obligation for HIV-positive health care workers to disclose their HIV status.** This includes surgeons. A surgeon does *not* have to disclose her HIV status to patient.

Physicians have the legal right to refuse to treat any patient. It is *not* illegal to refuse to take care of HIV-positive persons—it is **unethical** to refuse care to HIV-positive patients simply because they are HIV-positive, but it is **legal** to do so.

Doctor-Patient Relationship

A physician has no obligation to accept a patient. If there is only one neurosurgeon at a hospital and a patient needs neurosurgery, that would not compel the physician to accept the patient.

Once the patient has been accepted, however, **the physician cannot simply abandon him**. Should the physician prefer that the patient find care elsewhere, she has an obligation to inform the patient that he must find another physician, and must render care until a substitute caregiver can be identified.

Gifts

- **Ethically acceptable:** Gifts from patients that are **small** and **not tied to specific treatments and tests**
- **Ethically unacceptable:** Gifts given with the intention of getting **a specific prescription**

Sexual Contact

- Psychiatrists: Sexual contact between a patient and a psychiatrist is never acceptable.
- Other physicians: They must end the doctor-patient relationship first.

Elder Abuse

Elder abuse can be reported even against the will of the patient. Elder abuse does not imply a specific age; it has to do with the **fragility** of the patient. If the patient is frail and vulnerable, the abuse can be reported even against the patient's will.

Impaired Drivers

Impaired drivers, such as patients suffering from a seizure disorder, cannot have their license taken away by a physician. Only the department of motor vehicles can remove or restrict a license. These laws are not clear from state to state.

Torture

Physician participation in torture, on any level, is always wrong. You cannot even agree to certify the patient dead.

Impaired Physicians

Impaired physicians must be reported to an authority figure:

- For physicians in training, the reporting should be to the program director or department chair.
- For faculty, reporting is to the department chair or the dean of the medical school.
- For those in practice, reporting is to the state medical board of the office of professional medical conduct.

The impairment must involve **potential danger to medical care:**

- If you see a physician stealing a car, his behavior is not reportable to the department chair.
- If you see a physician dancing naked on a table at a bar but her medical performance is not impaired, that is not reportable.

PART 13

Patient Safety

General Patient Safety Goals

Hand Washing

The single most important measure for reducing transmission of infection from one person to another (or from one site to another on the same patient) is hand washing with soap and water. Wearing gloves does not replace the need for hand hygiene.

Isolation Practice

Three isolation categories reflect the major modes of pathogen transmission in nosocomial settings.

- **Contact precautions:** Health care workers should perform hand hygiene and wear gloves and gowns upon room entry (*C. difficile* is most commonly tested infection).
- **Droplet precautions**: Health care workers should wear a mask when standing within 6 feet of patients on droplet precautions. No special air handling systems are required.
- **Airborne precautions**: Patients requiring airborne isolation need a private room with negative air pressure. Health care workers must wear a mask with filtering capacity of 95%.

Falls

Falls in older persons occur commonly, caused by multiple factors.

- Risk of falls increases as the number of medications increases. With every visit, review all medications and discontinue unnecessary drugs.
- Exercise is the most consistently positive intervention to reduce the risk of falls and injurious falls. On CCS, order physical therapy.
- Vitamin D supplementation has no benefit in the prevention of falls.

Fall prevention is highly tested on the USMLE Step 3 exam.

- A cardiac pacemaker can reduce the rate of falls in those with carotid sinus hypersensitivity.
- Nutritional supplementation for 3 months can reduce the rate of falls in those who are older and malnourished.
- Cataract surgery can reduce the rate of falls.

Medical Errors

Medical errors are unintended acts or omissions with the potential to harm patients.

On the exam, the most commonly tested point is that patients should be informed of all medical errors, regardless of whether there was an adverse outcome. This will strengthen informed decision-making, promote trust, and reduce patient stress.

Nosocomial Infections

Catheter-Associated Urinary Tract Infection (CAUTI)

CAUTI is the most common type of health care-associated infection and leading cause of nosocomial bacteremia.

The diagnosis is made when a patient has catheter-related bacteriuria combined with fever, suprapubic tenderness, costovertebral angle tenderness, and evidence of a systemic inflammatory response syndrome. The **most accurate** test is UA with WBCs and urine culture.

Treatment involves prompt removal of the catheter and antibiotics to reduce the risk of CAUTI. For those with long-term indwelling bladder catheterization, do intermittent catheterization.

Central Line-Associated Bloodstream Infection (CLABSI)

All catheters can introduce bacteria into the bloodstream. If a patient with a central line develops signs of infection, blood cultures are taken from a peripheral vein. If the cultures yield the same organisms, remove the central line and give antibiotics.

- Start antibiotics immediately after blood cultures are obtained.
- Change antibiotics based on sensitivities.
- The most common CLABSI bugs are *S. aureus*, coagulase-negative *staphylococci*, and *Candida* species.

Pressure-Induced Skin Injuries

Pressure-induced skin injuries are localized areas of damage to the skin and underlying tissue, usually over a bony prominence. They commonly develop as a result of chronic immobility.

The goal for pressure-induced skin injuries is prevention.

- Chronically immobile patients should be positioned and repositioned at least every 2 hours to relieve tissue pressure.
- Nutritional intake should be optimized to aid in wound healing.
- If necrotic tissue is seen, then wound debridement should be the next step in management.

Staging of Pressure-induced Skin Injuries	
Stage	**Description**
1	Skin intact with non-blanchable redness for >1 hour after relief of pressure
2	Blister or other break in the dermis with partial thickness loss of dermis, with or without infection
3	Full thickness tissue loss. Subcutaneous fat may be visible; destruction extends into muscle with or without infection. Undermining and tunneling may be present.
4	Full thickness skin loss with involvement of bone, tendon, or joint, with or without infection. Often includes undermining and tunneling.
Unstageable	Full thickness tissue loss in which the base of the ulcer is covered by slough and/or eschar in the wound bed

Complementary and Alternative Medicine

The Step 3 exam will want you to know the most commonly taken herbal and nutritional supplements and their adverse reactions.

How does one know if a patient **is taking a specific supplement**?

- On each visit, review the patient's medications (prescription, over-the-counter, and supplements) and document in the medical record.

How does one know if a patient **should take a specific supplement**?

- Encourage the patient to discuss the risks and benefits with you in an office-based setting.

Common Herbs and Nutritional Supplements				
Name	**Intended goal**	**Adverse effects**	**Drug interactions**	**Effectiveness**
St. John's wort	Treatment of depression	Insomnia, anxiety and vivid dreams	• Do not use with antidepressants • Induces CYP3A4	Inconsistent evidence for efficacy
Saw palmetto	Treatment of BPH	Nausea	Bleeding with antiplatelet and anticoagulants	No more effective than placebo
Red yeast rice	Treatment of hyperlipidemia	Abnormal LFTs and myalgias	• Do not take with statins or fibrates • Induces CYP3A4	Does not appear to be effective
Milk thistle	Reduction of liver inflammation	Nausea and dyspepsia	Interacts with medications metabolized by CYP2C9 and CYP3A4	Does not appear to be effective
Ginseng	Immune system enhancement	Hypertension, diarrhea, and pruritus	Interacts with MAOs and warfarin	Inconsistent evidence for efficacy
Ginkgo biloba	Improved cognition	Increased risk of bleeding	INH, NNRTI, and warfarin	Inconsistent evidence for efficacy
Echinacea	Treatment of URI	Unpleasant taste and GERD	None	Does not appear to be effective
Cranberry	Prevention of UTI	None	None	Does not appear to be effective
Black cohosh	Treatment of post-menopausal symptoms	Headache	None	Does not appear to be more effective than placebo

PART 14

Ophthalmology

Retinal Diseases

Diabetic Retinopathy

Non-proliferative retinopathy means there are microaneurysms, retinal hemorrhages, and cotton-wool spots. The seriousness of the condition is based on the degree of macular edema. Treatment is glucose control to a target HgA1C <7%.

Retinopathy is "proliferative" (**proliferative retinopathy**) if there is neovascularization or vitreous hemorrhage. Treatment is laser photocoagulation of the retinal or injection of vascular endothelial growth factor (VEGF) inhibitors.

Treatment is in the form of prevention, i.e., tight glycemic control.

Refer patients to an ophthalmologist for screening (dilated retinal exam or retinal photography) as follows:

- **Type I**: screen after 1 year of having been diagnosed with diabetes
- **Type II**: screen within 5 years of having been diagnosed with diabetes
- Screening is then done annually in everyone.

Retinal Artery and Vein Occlusion

Occlusion of the vasculature of the eye presents with the sudden unilateral loss of vision. Both arterial and venal occlusion can be diagnosed only by direct examination of the arteries and veins of the retina. Arterial occlusion gives a pale retina with markedly diminished blood flow. Venous occlusion shows a backup of blood into the eye.

- Aspirin as primary or secondary prevention of diabetic retinopathy does not work. Fish oil has zero utility.

- There is weak data on lipid management, but overall, controlling hyperlipidemia of BP has not had an effect on microvascular disease in the eyes.

Treatment is as follows:

- Arterial occlusion: no proven treatment
  - Attempt to open the artery with thrombolytics, ocular massage, and arterial dilators such as nitroglycerin.
  - Anterior chamber paracentesis with a knife may suddenly decrease intraocular pressure and dislodge the clot from the artery.
- Central retinal vein occlusion: vascular endothelial growth factor (VEGF) inhibitors (ranibizumab, bevacizumab) to treat the vascular overgrowth of diabetic retinopathy and wet macular degeneration. Central retinal vein occlusion is associated with macular edema, so VEGF inhibitors can relieve the pressure brought on by the clot and release this edema.

Macular Degeneration

Age-related macular degeneration (AMD) is the most common cause of blindness in adults in resource-rich countries. AMD presents with loss of central vision and can only be diagnosed by retinal examination.

- **Dry AMD** (more common)
  - Treatment is antioxidant vitamins, A, C, E and zinc
  - Continued tobacco smoking is especially destructive to vision in AMD
- **Wet AMD** (less common but much more likely to progress toward blindness) means there is a proliferation of abnormal blood vessels.
  - Treatment is antioxidant vitamins and intravitreal injections of a VEGF inhibitor (e.g., bevacizumab, ranibizumab, pegaptanib, or aflibercept), which are very effective
  - Photodynamic therapy is an alternative for those who cannot be treated with an intravitreal VEGF inhibitor

VEGF inhibitors are stunningly effective in wet AMD and can stop over 90% of cases from progressing.

Retinal Detachment

Retinal detachment presents with a sudden loss of vision like "a curtain coming down." Consult ophthalmology and perform a dilated retinal examination.

Treatment is:

- Tilt the head back.
- Reattach the retina with surgery, cryotherapy, or by injecting an expansile gas into the eye.
- If that fails, place a band around the eye to get the retina close to the sclera.

Glaucoma

Acute angle closure glaucoma is an ophthalmologic emergency. It presents with a red eye and fixed midpoint pupil.

Treatment is pilocarpine drops to constrict the pupil. Mannitol can be used as an osmotic diuretic to help open the angle. Other therapies include:

- Acetazolamide to decrease production of aqueous humor
- Prostaglandin analogs (latanoprost, travoprost, bimatoprost) to increase outflow of aqueous humor
- Beta blockers topically: timolol
- Alpha agonists (apraclonidine, brimonidine) to increase outflow and decrease production

If medication cannot control intraocular pressure, do laser or surgical trabeculoplasty.

Optic Neuritis

Optic neuritis is inflammation of the optic nerve, and it is extremely dangerous. It is usually caused by an autoimmune disease such as multiple sclerosis, but it can also exist as an isolated syndrome or as a result of an infection such as meningitis or encephalitis. In 90% of patients, it occurs in only one eye.

- Happens over hours to days, so is much slower than a retinal detachment or artery/vein occlusion.
- An afferent pupillary defect occurs, meaning the pupil in the affected eye will constrict if a light is shown in the normal eye.
- One-third of cases have an inflamed nerve visible on funduscopic exam, while two-thirds are retro-orbital.

The MRI is essential in diagnosing demyelinating disease as a cause of optic neuritis. It detects an inflamed optic nerve and orbits in 95% of cases.

Optic neuritis can blind the patient. Even after treatment with steroids there can be significant residual visual disturbance and atrophy of the optic nerve.

> Color desaturation in optic neuritis means colors appear "washed out." Red looks orange or pink.

> In 90% of optic neuritis cases, pain is present.

Red Eye

Diagnosing and treating "red eye" requires knowing the basic ophthalmology expected on Step 3. The table summarizes the various causes of red eye.

	Glaucoma	Conjunctivitis	Uveitis	Abrasion
Presentation	Midpoint fixed pupil Rock-hard, painful eye Corneal haziness	Viral: Bilateral watery discharge, itchy eyes Bacterial: Unilateral purulent discharge, eyelids stuck together	Photophobia	History of trauma, most commonly from contact lenses
Diagnosis	Tonometry	Clinical presentation	Slit lamp examination	Fluorescein stain picks up on the damaged cornea
Treatment	Pilocarpine drops Acetazolamide Mannitol Topical beta blockers	Bacterial form is treated with topical antibiotics	Steroids	*No* specific therapy Do *not* patch abrasions caused by contact lenses

Herpes Keratitis

With keratitis, the eye is extremely red and painful. There is tearing and blurry vision.

Testing is fluorescein stain, which confirms the damage. PCR or viral culture confirms the lesion as herpes. Serology for herpes is always a wrong answer.

Treatment is topical trifluridine, ganciclovir, or acyclovir.

> Herpes keratitis is the only time that topical acyclovir is effective.

- Disease that is incompletely treated can lead to scarring and blindness that will require replacement of the cornea.
- Topical steroids are extremely dangerous and can lead to blindness.

Cataracts

Cataracts are characterized by painless, progressive loss of vision that is often bilateral. Look for a question stem that describes an older person who is having a hard time driving at night because of increased glare.

Cataracts do not need a diagnostic test. They can be seen on examination with direct ophthalmoscopy.

There is no medical therapy. Cataract removal is the most common surgical procedure in the United States.

Cavernous Sinus Thrombosis (CST)

The cavernous venous sinus travels just outside the nasal sinuses. This is why infectious sinusitis can infarct or thromboses the venous sinus.

Since CN III, IV, and VI travel through the venous sinus, patients present with diplopia and multiple gaze palsies (because the extraocular muscles lose their innervation). Orbital pain and proptosis are common.

Staphylococcus aureus is the causative organism in 70% of cases.

Diagnosis is done with MRI.

Treatment is treatment of the infection and anticoagulation. The best empiric coverage includes vancomycin for MRSA and anaerobic coverage if it is from the sinuses.

PART 15

Ear, Nose, and Throat

Head and Neck Infections

Otitis Externa

Simple Otitis Externa

This is a form of cellulitis of the skin of the external auditory canal. Due to the swelling of the canal, it can be difficult to visualize the tympanic membrane.

Otitis externa is associated with swimming, because swimming washes out the acidic environment normally found in the external auditory canal. Other causes include foreign objects in the ears (e.g., repeated use of cotton swabs, hearing aids, etc.).

Symptoms include:

- Itching and drainage from the external auditory canal
- Pain, especially when the tragus of the ear is manipulated

No specific tests are necessary; diagnosis is based on exam. Do not perform a routine culture of the ear canal.

Treatment is a topical antibiotic (ofloxacin, ciprofloxacin, polymyxin/neomycin). A topical hydrocortisone can decrease swelling and itching, and an acetic acid and water solution to reacidify the ear can help eliminate the infection.

Cerumen impaction can make treating otitis externa impossible. The function of cerumen (earwax) is to make the external auditory canal acidic. Acid wax suppresses bacteria; it is like the lactobacilli in the vagina in this regard. Cerumen blocks water (hydrophobic), and a low-water environment suppresses bacteria. Pseudomonas likes to grow in water.

Treat the impaction by removing the cerumen (which will be visible on otoscopy).

- Direct mechanical removal by curette/spoon (most effective)
- "Blast" it out with saline irrigation via syringe
- Use mineral oil, hydrogen peroxide, or carbamide peroxide to break down the earwax

Malignant Otitis Externa

Extremely different from simple otitis externa, malignant otitis externa is really osteomyelitis of the skull from *Pseudomonas* in a patient with diabetes. It is an extremely serious condition because it can lead to a brain abscess and destruction of the skull.

Diagnose it as you would diagnose osteomyelitis.

CT or MRI is the **best initial test**. Bone biopsy is the **most accurate test**.

Treatment is surgical debridement and antibiotics active against *Pseudomonas* (ciprofloxacin, piperacillin, cefepime, carbapenem, aztreonam).

> **Basic Science Correlate**
>
> Quinolone antibiotics, such as ciprofloxacin, work by inhibiting DNA gyrase (topoisomerase). DNA gyrase unwinds DNA so it can be replicated. By preventing DNA from unwinding, you prevent DNA from copying and reproducing itself.

Otitis Media

Key features include the following:

- Redness
- Bulging
- Decreased hearing
- Loss of light reflex
- Immobility of the tympanic membrane (**most sensitive finding**)

If the tympanic membrane is freely mobile on insufflations of the ear, then otitis media is not present. The physical exam may also describe the absence of the light reflex.

There is no radiologic test to confirm the diagnosis, which is based entirely on physical examination. Patients may complain of decreased or muffled hearing.

Treatment is amoxicillin; usual course is 7–10 days but longer for younger patients and shorter for older patients.

For recurrent cases that fail therapy, perform tympanocentesis (**most accurate test**) and aspirate of the tympanic membrane for culture, but this is rarely needed.

> ### Basic Science Correlate
>
> Otitis media is caused by swelling of the Eustachian tube. When the narrowest portion (or isthmus) becomes inflamed, it blocks the egress of secretions. Pneumococcus, nontypeable *Haemophilus*, and Moraxella are the most common causes. *Haemophilus* vaccine does not prevent the type of infections that cause sinusitis and otitis. Vaccine prevents only invasive group B *Haemophilus*.

CCS Tip: On CCS, advance the clock 3 days. If the infection is not improving, switch the amoxicillin to one of the following:

- Amoxicillin-clavulanate
- Cefdinir
- Ceftibuten
- Cefuroxime
- Cefprozil
- Cefpodoxime

Sinusitis

For acute sinusitis, look for a patient with nasal discharge, fever, headache, facial tenderness, tooth pain, bad taste in the mouth, and decreased transillumination of the sinuses. Most cases are viral, but bacterial causes include the same group that causes otitis media: *Streptococcus pneumoniae*, *Haemophilus influenzae*, and *Moraxella catarrhalis*.

> Sinusitis best initial test: If x-ray and CT are both in the answer options, **choose CT.**

Diagnostic testing includes CT (**best initial test**) and **sinus aspirate for culture** (most accurate)

Treatment is antibiotics (same as for otitis media) with added inhaled steroids. Use amoxicillin/clavulanate if there is fever and pain; persistent symptoms despite 7 days of decongestants; and purulent nasal discharge.

For chronic rhinosinusitis, use nasal saline irrigation and nasal steroid spray.

> ### Basic Science Correlate
>
>
> Clavulanic acid (pictured here) is a beta-lactamase inhibitor that confers a broader spectrum of antimicrobial activity to penicillin. Clavulanic acid is similar in structure to the beta-lactam ring of penicillin. The enzyme beta lactamase destroys the clavulanic acid instead of the penicillin. This is why it is a "suicide inhibitor." The other beta-lactamase inhibitors, tazobactam and sulbactam, work the same way.

Pharyngitis

The diagnosis of streptococcal pharyngitis is certain if the following are present:

- Pain/sore throat
- Exudate
- Adenopathy
- *No* cough/hoarseness

Diagnostic testing includes:

- "Rapid strep test" (**best initial test**)
  - A positive rapid strep test is just as specific as a positive throat culture, but it is performed instantly and can tell if the organism is of the type (group A strep) that might lead to rheumatic fever or glomerulonephritis.
  - In adults, the sensitivity of the rapid strep test is enough; if result is negative, no further testing or treatment with antibiotics is necessary.
- Culture: **most accurate test**

Treatment is penicillin or amoxicillin. With penicillin allergy, use azithromycin or clarithromycin (if allergy is just a rash, use cephalexin).

Influenza

Look for a patient with arthralgia, myalgia, cough, headache, fever, sore throat, and feeling of tiredness.

Diagnostic testing is viral rapid antigen detection testing of a nasopharyngeal swab. This is the best next step if the diagnosis is unclear.

Treatment is oseltamivir, zanamivir, or baloxavir if the patient presents within the first 48 hours after the onset of symptoms. These are neuraminidase inhibitors that work against both influenza A and B.

- Peramivir is an IV neuraminidase inhibitor comparable in efficacy to oseltamivir.
- Amantadine and rimantadine would be wrong answers, as they are effective only against influenza A.

Vaccination Against Influenza

Influenza vaccine is **indicated** in the general population at any age. The strongest indications are:

- COPD, CHF, dialysis patients, steroid use, health care workers, everyone age >50
- Step 3 will expect you to know that there is a **live attenuated vaccine administered by inhalation**.
  - Live vaccine is effective only in those age <50 with none of the medical problems described.
  - Injected inactivated virus is required by anyone with illness and/or those age >50.
  - **Egg allergy is no longer an absolute contraindication to flu vaccine.**

> - Isolate flu patients for 7 days.
> - Being at home is considered "isolation." Stay at home.

> An allergy to eggs is not a contraindication to flu vaccine.

Allergic Rhinitis

Allergic rhinitis presents with recurrent episodes of nasal itching, stuffiness, rhinorrhea, and paroxysms of sneezing. There is also often eye itching, dermatitis, and wheezing.

Allergic rhinitis may be associated with the development of asthma.

Treatment is as follows.

- Avoidance of the allergen (mainstay of all therapy for those with extrinsic allergies)
  - Close windows and stay in air-conditioned rooms to avoid pollen
  - Avoid pets if there is an allergy to animal dander
  - Cover mattresses and pillows with mite- and dust-proof casings
- Drug therapy: intranasal corticosteroids; antihistamines (loratadine, fexofenadine, cetirizine); intranasal antihistamines (azelastine); cromolyn; ipratropium bromide; leukotriene inhibitors (montelukast); nasal saline spray and wash

- Immunotherapy (desensitization) for extrinsic allergens that cannot be avoided
  - Must stop beta blockers first, before desensitization (a favorite question on Step 3)
  - If anaphylaxis occurs during desensitization, then epinephrine is used, but if the person is on a beta blocker then the action of epinephrine will be blocked.

> Intranasal steroids are the single most effective treatment for allergic rhinitis.

Basic Science Correlate

Cromolyn and nedocromil work by stabilizing mast cells. They prevent degranulation of mast cells so that histamine and leukotrienes are not released. This mechanism is entirely preventive in nature: After exposure to the allergen has stimulated the mast cells, cromolyn will not work.

Dizziness/Vertigo

All patients with vertigo will have a subjective sensation of the room spinning around them. This is often associated with nausea and vomiting.

All patients with vertigo will have nystagmus (horizontal). When a patient thinks the room is spinning, the eyes should naturally dart back and forth to give the feeling of looking at a single point.

There are a number of conditions that can cause vertigo.

Disease	Characteristics	Hearing Loss/Tinnitus
Benign positional vertigo	Changes with position	No
Vestibular neuritis	Vertigo occurs without position changes	No
Labyrinthitis	Acute	Yes
Meniere disease	Chronic	Yes
Acoustic neuroma	Ataxia	Yes
Perilymph fistula	History of trauma	Yes

Diagnostic testing is MRI of the internal auditory canal.

Benign Positional Vertigo (BPV)

This presents as vertigo alone with no hearing loss, no tinnitus, and no ataxia. The question may describe a positive Dix-Hallpike maneuver. History may describe onset of symptoms when quickly changing positions.

Manage BPV by repositioning the head to reposition the otoliths of the vestibular system. Use the Epley maneuver to do so. BPV responds modestly to meclizine.

Vestibular Neuritis

This is an idiopathic inflammation of the vestibular portion of the 8th cranial nerve. Because only the vestibular portion is involved, there is no hearing loss and no tinnitus. Presumably, this condition is viral. It is entirely characterized by vertigo and dizziness and is not related to changes in position.

There is no specific diagnostic test. Treat with steroids. Symptomatic relief can be achieved with antihistamines such as meclizine or diphenhydramine, benzodiazepines and antiemetics.

Labyrinthitis

Labyrinthitis is inflammation of the cochlear portion of the inner ear. There is hearing loss as well as tinnitus. This condition is acute and self-limited and may be treated with meclizine and steroids. Acute hearing loss may respond to steroids.

> Steroids can improve acute hearing loss.

Ménière Disease

Same presentation as labyrinthitis (vertigo, hearing loss, tinnitus), but Ménière is chronic with remitting and relapsing episodes. Treat with salt restriction meclizine and diuretics. For severe disease, ablation of 8th cranial nerve on one side may be needed.

Acoustic Neuroma

This is an 8th cranial nerve tumor that can be related to neurofibromatosis or Von Recklinghausen disease. It presents with ataxia in addition to hearing loss, tinnitus, and vertigo.

Diagnostic testing is MRI of the internal auditory canal.

Treatment is surgical resection.

Perilymph Fistula

Head trauma or any form of barotrauma to the ear may rupture the tympanic membrane and lead to a perilymph fistula. Fix the hole surgically.

Wernicke-Korsakoff Syndrome

Wernicke-Korsakoff syndrome presents as follows:

- History of chronic heavy alcohol use
- Confusion with confabulation
- Ataxia
- Memory loss
- Gaze palsy/ophthalmoplegia
- Nystagmus

With memory loss, it is very important to perform the following tests:

- Head CT
- B12 level
- Thyroid function (T4/TSH)
- RPR or VDRL

Treatment is thiamine (if the condition is acute, give IV dose and switch to oral later). Also give glucose with thiamine, but administer thiamine first, then the glucose.

Index

A

Abdomen
  abscess, 322
  aortic aneurysm, 62, 270, 349–350
  hernias, 347–348
  pelvic CT, 477
  sonogram, 407
  trauma, 311–312
Abiraterone, 267
Abortion, 434–436
  minors, 532
  right to an abortion, 533
Abrasion of eye, 546
Abruptio placenta, 413–414, 415–416
  disseminated intravascular
    coagulation, 413, 414, 445
Abscesses
  abdominal, 322
  brain, 19–20
  diverticular, 319
  epidural, 23
  pancreatic, 319–320
  perinephric, 89–90
  pilonidal cyst, 327
  retropharyngeal, 377
  spinal epidural, 24
  tubo-ovarian, 466
Absence seizures, 399
Absolute risk reduction, 288–289
Abuse and neglect
  child abuse, 375, 482, 506–507
  elder abuse, 506–507, 537
  mandatory reporting, 370, 375,
    506–507, 537–538
  refusal of treatment for minor, 532
  spousal abuse, 506–507
Accelerations in fetal heart rate, 440
Accepting a patient, 537
Accuracy, 278
ACE inhibitors
  acute coronary syndrome, 37
  angioedema from, 110
  aortic regurgitation, 53
  ARBs interchangeable, 39, 47–48
  cardiomyopathy, 59–60

chronic angina, 39
congestive heart failure, 47, 48
diabetic nephropathy, 117–118
handgrip *vs.* amyl nitrate, 51–52
hyperkalemia and, 252
hypertension, 261
mitral regurgitation, 57–58
neonate effects, 366
Takotsubo cardiomyopathy, 60
valvular disease, 53, 57–58
Acetaldehyde from alcohol, 511
Acetaminophen overdose, 517–518
Acetazolamide, 140
Acetylcholine, 165, 210
Achalasia, 209
Achilles tendon rupture, 340
Acid reflux, 29
Acne, 307
Acromegaly, 131–132
ACTH levels, 127–128, 129, 130
Actinic keratosis, 304
Actinomyces, 102
Acute abdomen, 315–322
  inflammation, 318–320
  ischemia, 321–322
  obstruction, 317–318
  perforation, 316
  peritonitis, 237
  surgical consultation, 321
Acute fatty liver of pregnancy (AFLP),
  433
Acute respiratory distress syndrome
  (ARDS), 153–154, 332
Acute tubular necrosis (ATN), 242
Acyanotic heart defects, 381, 382–383
Acyclovir, 19, 74
Addison disease, 128–129
  hyponatremia, 256
Adefovir, 75
Adenomyosis, 457
Adhesive capsulitis, 177
Adjustment disorder, 491, 493, 539
Adjuvant hormonal therapy, 453–454
Adrenal disorders, 126–130

congenital adrenal hyperplasia,
  129–130, 470–471
Adrenal scan, 478
Adult maltreatment/abuse, 506–507, 537
Advance directives, 534–535
  none and no capacity, 535
Aganglionic megacolon, 336
Aggressive mood disorders, 506
Agonist drugs, 452
Agoraphobia, 491–492
AIDS/HIV, 90–95
Airway in trauma, 309
Akathisia, 490
Alcohol withdrawal, 509, 512–513
  hypomagnesemia and, 257
  newborn, 366
  seizures, 512–513
Alcohol/alcoholic
  abuse, 509, 510–513
  acute pancreatitis, 232, 319
  CAGE questionnaire, 511
  celiac disease, 222
  chronic pancreatitis, 223
  cirrhosis, 237
  delirium tremens, 513
  depression, 495
  elimination kinetics, 511
  esophageal cancer, 210
  fetal alcohol syndrome, 368
  folate deficiency, 184
  hallucinosis, 513
  hypothermia, 529
  Klebsiella pneumonia, 150
  porphyria cutanea tarda, 292
  use disorder, 510–513
  variceal bleeding, 229
Aldosterone
  Conn syndrome, 253
  hyporeninemic hypoaldosteronism,
    259
  potassium levels and, 252, 256
Alkalinization of urine, 244, 518
Allergic bronchopulmonary
  aspergillosis, 152
  cystic fibrosis, 379–381